TENTH EDITION

LANGE Q&A™

PSYCHIATRY

Sean M. Blitzstein, MD
Director, Psychiatry Clerkship
Clinical Associate Professor of Psychiatry
University of Illinois at Chicago
Chicago, Illinois

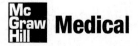 **Medical**

New York Chicago San Francisco Lisbon London Madrid Mexico City Milan
New Delhi San Juan Seoul Singapore Sydney Toronto

The McGraw·Hill Companies

Lange Q&A Psychiatry, Tenth Edition

Copyright © 2011 by The McGraw-Hill Companies, Inc. All rights reserved. Printed in the United States of America. Except as permitted under the United States Copyright Act of 1976, no part of this publication may be reproduced or distributed in any form or by any means, or stored in a data base or retrieval system, without the prior written permission of the publisher.

1 2 3 4 5 6 7 8 9 0   QDB/QDB   15 14 13 12 11

ISBN 978-0-07-170345-1
MHID 0-07-170345-4

This book was set in Palatino by Glyph international.
The editors were Kirsten Funk and Brian Kearns.
The production supervisor was Sherri Souffrance.
Project management was provided by Manisha Singh, Glyph International.
The cover design was by The Gazillion Group.
Quad/Graphics was printer and binder.

This book is printed on acid-free paper.

Library of Congress Cataloging-in-Publication Data

Lange Q & A. Psychiatry / [edited by] Sean M. Blitzstein.—10th ed.
    p. ; cm.
  Q & A
  Psychiatry
  Includes bibliographical references and index.
  ISBN-13: 978-0-07-170345-1 (pbk. : alk. paper)
  ISBN-10: 0-07-170345-4 (pbk. : alk. paper)
  1. Psychiatry—Examinations, questions, etc.   I. Blitzstein, Sean.
II. Title: Q & A. III. Title: Psychiatry.
  [DNLM: 1. Mental Disorders—therapy—Examination Questions.   2. Mental Disorders
diagnosis—Examination Questions.   3. Psychiatry—Examination Questions.   WM 18.2]   RC457.E18 2011
616.890076—dc22
                                                                          2011000441

McGraw-Hill books are available at special quantity discounts to use as premiums and sales promotions, or for use in corporate training programs. To contact a representative please e-mail us at bulksales@mcgraw-hill.com.

Contents

Contributors

Shetal M. Amin, MD
Department of Psychiatry
University of Illinois at Chicago
Chicago, Illinois
Legal and Ethical Issues in Psychiatry and Medicine

Martina R. Gunaratnam, MD
Department of Psychiatry
University of Chicago at Illinois
Chicago, Illinois
Psychological Treatment and Management

Jacqueline Haimes, MD
Child, Adolescent, and Adult Psychiatrist
Private Practice
Evanston, Illinois
Childhood and Adolescent Psychiatry

Sonya Rasminsky, MD
Assistant Professor
Department of Psychiatry and Behavioral
    Sciences
Northwestern University
Feinberg School of Medicine
Chicago, Illinois
Somatic Treatment and Psychopharmacology

Anoop K. Vermani, MD
Department of Psychiatry
University of Illinois at Chicago
Chicago, Illinois
Differential Diagnosis

Marika I. Wrzosek, MD
Department of Psychiatry
College of Medicine
University of Illinois at Chicago
Chicago, Illinois
Adult Psychopathology

Student Reviewers

Melanie Zupancic, MD
Psychiatry/Medicine Resident (PGY2)
SIU School of Medicine
Division of Psychiatry
Springfield, Illinois

Lindsey Shultz
Medical Student (M4)
Weill Cornell Medical School
New York, New York
Class of 2010

Brandon McKinney
Medical Student (M4)
University of Michigan Medical School
Ann Arbor, Michigan
Class of 2010

Preface

Welcome to *Lange Q&A: Psychiatry*, 10th edition. It is my sincere pleasure to provide you with this edition in support of your ongoing education in psychiatry. Far from being a "soft science," psychiatric research and practice are at the forefront of medicine, incorporating pharmacology, psychology, sociology, and neurosciences; the result being a genuine biopsychosocial approach to patient care. Such a sizeable integration yields a broad field in which to study and test. Because of this, this 10th edition covers the gamut of topics, from adult and child psychiatry, to psychopharmacology and ethics. All major diagnoses are covered, with the emphasis being on differential diagnosis and treatment (whether psychological or somatic). In fact, this edition consists of eight chapters with over 800 questions. Reviewer feedback suggested that psychological testing questions are rarely seen on board exams so rather than eliminate this pertinent information—even if viewed as "low yield"—this subject area has been incorporated into the two practice exams at the end of the book.

As this book is geared toward medical students studying for their psychiatry clerkship exams, as well as for their United States Medical Licensing Examination (USMLE) Step 2 CK examination, each and every question is clinically focused comprising of a patient-centered vignette. Consistent with the USMLE format, the answers are either multiple-choice or extended matching items. In order to promote self-assessment and formative learning, all answers include detailed explanations regarding *why* the incorrect choices are flawed. A list of references is included for those students who wish to further research a particular issue.

All questions, answers, and explanations have been reviewed and updated, and, similar to the 9th edition, the diagnostic criteria are based on the American Psychiatric Association's *Diagnostic and Statistical Manual of Mental Disorders, Fourth Edition, Text Revision (DSM-IV-TR)*. While draft revisions of the *DSM-V* are currently available for review, it is not scheduled for publication until mid-2013. Although some diagnostic criteria will undoubtedly change, the final form of the *DSM-V* remains in development at this time, so a conscious decision was made to use the *DSM-IV-TR* for this edition.

Finally, a few suggestions on how best to use this book. This book should be used as a supplement to your primary learning. It neither replaces reading a basic text on Psychiatry, nor seeing live patients during a rotation. Chapters 1 through 6 can be used to reinforce or complement certain areas. The final two chapters (Chapters 7 and 8) are practice tests of consisting of 116 and 118 randomly ordered questions, respectively, that simulate an actual board examination.

Sean M. Blitzstein, MD

Acknowledgments

This book continues to reflect the hard work and dedication of a large group of contributors to past editions of the predecessor book, *Appleton & Lange Review of Psychiatry*:

Ivan Oransky, MD
R. Andrew Chambers, MD
Joseph R. Check, MD
Vladimir Coric, MD
Frank G. Fortunati, MD, JD
Brian Greenlee, MD
Julie E. Peters, MD
Greer Richardson, MD
William Roman, MD
Louis Sanfilippo, MD
Raziya Sunderji, MD
Blake Taggart, MD
Elizabeth Walter, MD
Chung-Che Charles Wang, MD

Thank you to my endlessly patient, understanding, and supportive editor at McGraw-Hill, Kirsten Funk. I would also like to thank all of my contributors, many of whom were former residents and mentees—you've given me more than I can ever say.

Sean M. Blitzstein, MD

CHAPTER 1

Child and Adolescent Psychiatry
Questions

DIRECTIONS (Questions 1 through 75): For each of the multiple choice questions in this section, select the lettered answer that is the one *best* response in each case.

Questions 1 and 2

A 17-year-old girl with a history of major depressive disorder (MDD) comes to your primary care office for a routine visit. When you walk into the examining room, you notice that she is sitting slumped forward with her head bent down. She does not make eye contact and says nothing. She admits that she uses marijuana approximately twice per week and cuts on her arm when stressed. Her mother reveals that she is particularly worried as the girl's paternal uncle committed suicide 10 years ago. You suspect that she is having a recurrence of depressive symptoms and are concerned about her risk for suicide.

1. Which of the following factors most increases this patient's risk of committing suicide?

    (A) cutting behavior
    (B) diagnosis of depression
    (C) gender
    (D) relative who committed suicide
    (E) substance use

2. Further history is obtained, and the patient reveals that she has, in fact, been feeling more depressed recently, with difficulty sleeping, low appetite, fatigue, and problems concentrating. She denies suicidal ideation, however.

Which of the following would be the most appropriate plan for treatment?

    (A) Admit her to the hospital given her history and potential risk.
    (B) Ask your psychiatric colleague to see her within the next few days.
    (C) Prescribe antidepressant medications and schedule a follow-up appointment in 1 month.
    (D) Refer her to a social worker.
    (E) Tell the mother you'll follow up with her at your next routine visit.

Questions 3 and 4

A mother brings her 7-year-old son to you because she is worried about him. She tells you that he sits up in bed in the middle of the night and screams. She says he is inconsolable but eventually falls back to sleep.

3. Which of the following is the most likely diagnosis?

    (A) intermittent explosive disorder
    (B) narcolepsy
    (C) nightmare disorder
    (D) sleep terror disorder
    (E) sleepwalking disorder

4. During which stage of sleep do these episodes most likely occur?

(A) stage 1
(B) stage 2
(C) stages 3-4
(D) rapid eye movement (REM) stage
(E) any stage

Questions 5 and 6

A 17-year-old girl with a history of asthma presents for a physical examination prior to entering college. You note that she appears angry. Upon further questioning, you learn that she has felt irritable for the past 6 months since breaking up with her boyfriend of 2 years. She says she feels tired all the time and comes home from school every day, lies on the couch, and watches television. Her grades have dropped because she cannot concentrate. Despite her fatigue, she complains of difficulty sleeping. She has lost 12 lb over the last 6 months. She reports that she quit the senior celebration committee, no longer "hangs out" with her friends, cannot imagine things will improve, and is considering not going to college. Her physical and laboratory examination is normal.

5. Which of the following medications would be the most appropriate to treat this patient?

(A) carbamazepine (Tegretol)
(B) imipramine (Tofranil)
(C) lithium
(D) olanzapine (Zyprexa)
(E) sertraline (Zoloft)

6. According to the *DSM-IV-TR*, which of the following symptoms in this patient differentiate her disorder from that in an adult?

(A) anhedonia
(B) decreased concentration
(C) insomnia
(D) irritable mood
(E) weight loss

Questions 7 and 8

A 6-year-old boy is brought to the clinic by his parents at the request of the boy's teachers. The teachers report that he is quiet in class. When he does talk, he frequently makes errors with verb tense. His parents recall that his speech was delayed. On examination, the boy is friendly and cooperative. His speech is clear, but he uses simple sentences with a limited vocabulary. Otherwise, his physical and laboratory examinations are normal.

7. Which of the following is the most likely diagnosis?

(A) developmental coordination disorder
(B) disorder of written expression
(C) expressive language disorder
(D) phonological disorder
(E) stuttering

8. By what age would failure to speak 200 words be most consistent with a speech delay in this patient?

(A) 1
(B) 2
(C) 3
(D) 4
(E) 5

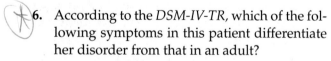

Questions 9 and 10

A 15-year-old boy without prior psychiatric history is on his school concert trip. He is brought to a local emergency room because of the acute onset of increased anger, agitation, and paranoia. On interview, he reports feeling unsafe because a government agency is spying on him.

9. Which of the following tests would be the most important to order first?

(A) electroencephalogram (EEG)
(B) glucose tolerance test
(C) PET (positron emission tomography) scan of his head
(D) thyroid function tests
(E) urine toxicology screen

10. All appropriate laboratory evaluations and studies come back within normal limits. Which of the following disorders would be most likely consistent with this patient's presentation?

(A) anorexia nervosa
(B) bipolar disorder, manic
(C) borderline personality disorder
(D) generalized anxiety disorder
(E) major depressive disorder

Questions 11 and 12

An 8-year-old boy is referred to you by a school nurse because he has been complaining of stomachaches every morning in school. On interviewing the boy's mother, you learn that he does not like to go to school, insists on coming home immediately after school each day, and sleeps in his parents' bed at night. The mother denies other complaints.

11. Which of the following is the most likely diagnosis?

(A) post-traumatic stress disorder (PTSD)
(B) reactive attachment disorder of early childhood
(C) separation anxiety disorder
(D) social phobia
(E) specific phobia

12. Which of the following would you most likely find in this patient's history?

(A) low levels of parental control
(B) parent with an anxiety disorder
(C) parents with a warm and accepting style
(D) secure attachment
(E) temperament characterized by sociability and extroversion

Questions 13 and 14

A 12-year-old boy is brought to the pediatric emergency department by his grandmother who reports he is not acting like himself. He reports that he feels "incredibly great" and doesn't need a doctor because he has powers to heal himself of all sickness. He speaks rapidly and his grandmother reports he has not slept more than 6 hours over the past 3 days. She reports that he appears extremely revved up and hyperactive.

13. Which of the following is the most likely diagnosis?

(A) attention-deficit/hyperactivity disorder (ADHD)
(B) bipolar disorder, manic phase
(C) major depressive disorder with psychotic features
(D) panic disorder
(E) schizophrenia

14. Ingestion of which of the following substances would most likely bring about similar symptoms?

(A) alcohol
(B) cannabis
(C) cocaine
(D) heroin
(E) phencyclidine (PCP)

15. A 9-year-old boy walks into your office accompanied with his mother. They are arguing about his wanting a new portable video gaming system. His mother, exasperated with her son's behavior, tells you that they were late because it took him a long time to finally agree to get into the car to come to the appointment with you. Alone with you in your office, he appears irritated and refuses to answer your questions or look up from his lap. After 10 minutes, he tells you about the "annoying kids" in his class and how they "made me get in trouble." Further history from the mother reveals that, despite the above behavior, he does not have a history of aggression toward peers or property and has not had any legal problems. Which of the following is the most likely diagnosis?

(A) agoraphobia
(B) attention-deficit/hyperactivity disorder (ADHD)
(C) conduct disorder
(D) generalized anxiety disorder (GAD)
(E) oppositional defiant disorder (ODD)

Questions 16 through 18

A 15-year-old girl who is a competitive figure skater presents with concerns about her weight. She believes that she would be a better skater if she could lose weight and feels very upset and frustrated that she has failed in her attempts. You are suspicious she may have bulimia nervosa. The girl reluctantly admits that she sometimes eats "a whole lot" of food at one time such as a quart of ice cream, a large bag of potato chips, and a jar of peanut butter. You then notice abrasions on the back of her right hand.

16. Which of the following opening statements would be the most appropriate?

    (A) "Tell me about the scratches on your hand."
    (B) "I've noticed the cuts on your hand. Are you trying to hurt yourself?"
    (C) "How did the scratches happen?"
    (D) "I see you have scratches on your hand. Do you have a cat?"
    (E) "Sometimes I see girls who make themselves throw up. Have you ever done that?"

17. Which of the following laboratory abnormalities would you most likely find in this patient?

    (A) elevated iron
    (B) elevated protein
    (C) hyperchloremia
    (D) hypokalemia
    (E) hyponatremia

18. Which of the following types of psychotherapy would be the most effective for this particular patient?

    (A) cognitive-behavioral therapy
    (B) family therapy
    (C) group therapy
    (D) psychoanalysis
    (E) psychodynamic psychotherapy

Questions 19 through 21

An 8-year-old boy with a history of major depressive disorder (MDD) treated with fluoxetine (Prozac) is brought to the pediatric emergency department after running into the street in front of a car on the way home from school. He refused to speak to the emergency room doctor. You are asked to consult as you are on your psychiatry rotation. The emergency room doctor is suspicious that the boy's behavior reflected underlying suicidal impulses.

19. Which of the following opening statements would be the most valuable in facilitating the boy's discussion of the situation?

    (A) "You sure were lucky the car swerved at the last minute."
    (B) "You weren't trying to actually get hit by the car, were you?"
    (C) "What *were* you thinking when you ran into the street?"
    (D) "It sounds like quite a day. Can you tell me about what happened after school today?"
    (E) "Children who try to hurt themselves are very confused. Are you confused?"

20. Which of the following symptoms of MDD would be more likely in this patient compared to an adolescent with MDD?

    (A) drug abuse
    (B) hopelessness
    (C) hypersomnia
    (D) psychomotor agitation
    (E) weight change

21. Which of the following would be this child's most likely method of attempting suicide in the future?

    (A) firearms
    (B) hanging
    (C) jumping from buildings
    (D) stabbing
    (E) substance ingestion

22. An 11-year-old boy with enuresis presents to the clinic for routine follow-up. His bed-wetting has not responded to behavioral interventions, so you had previously initiated treatment with intranasal desmopressin (DDAVP)

after completion of a full physical and laboratory examination. Which of the following signs and symptoms would be the most likely adverse effect?

(A) headache

(B) hypotension

(C) liver toxicity

(D) sedation

(E) tremor

Questions 23 and 24

A 9-year-old boy with a history of panic disorder treated with cognitive-behavioral therapy is brought to your office by his mother because he has been irritable and depressed. On physical examination, the boy appears depressed but otherwise normal. Laboratory examination is normal.

23. What would be the likelihood of this patient having comorbid major depressive disorder (MDD)?

(A) 10%

(B) 25%

(C) 33%

(D) 50%

(E) 75%

24. After a thorough history and mental status examination, you diagnose the boy with MDD and decide to initiate treatment with fluoxetine. You inform the boy and his mother of possible adverse effects of fluoxetine. Which of the following would be the most likely adverse effect of fluoxetine?

(A) hypotension

(B) liver toxicity

(C) nausea

(D) sedation

(E) weight gain

Questions 25 and 26

A 24-month-old girl is brought to the clinic by her mother for a routine visit. The mother tells you that the girl has not spoken her first clear word yet, at times seems she does understand what people say to her, and does not play with her 4-year-old brother. The mother also tells you that her daughter seems clumsy and has started to make odd, repetitive movements with her hands. According to the girl's chart, she had a normal head circumference at birth, at 6 months, and at 12 months, and had seemed to be developing normally. On physical examination, you note that her rate of head growth has slowed.

25. Which of the following is the most likely diagnosis?

(A) Asperger disorder

(B) autistic disorder

(C) childhood disintegrative disorder

(D) pervasive developmental disorder, not otherwise specified

(E) Rett disorder

26. The mother informs you that the child has an identical twin sister and is concerned about her risk of developing this disorder. What do you tell her is the most likely risk of the twin developing the same illness?

(A) 10%

(B) 25%

(C) 50%

(D) 75%

(E) 100%

Questions 27 and 28

A 12-year-old boy is referred by the court for evaluation. He skips school, stays out late at night, and verbally abuses his parents. He has run away from home on three separate occasions prompting his parents to call the police. He has been caught shoplifting and has been in numerous physical fights with his peers.

27. Upon further history, which of the following would most likely be found in this patient?

(A) absence of a biological father

(B) absence of a biological mother

(C) mother with an anxiety disorder

(D) patient being an only child

(E) parents who promote pacifism

28. Which of the following personality disorders is this boy most likely to develop?

    (A) antisocial personality disorder
    (B) avoidant personality disorder
    (C) paranoid personality disorder
    (D) schizoid personality disorder
    (E) schizotypal personality disorder

Questions 29 and 30

A 10-year-old girl who has recently been diagnosed with diabetes mellitus Type I is referred to you by her pediatrician for an evaluation. You notice that she seems sad. Her parents are concerned about her being "depressed." Consideration is given for diagnosing adjustment disorder with depressed mood versus major depressive disorder (MDD).

29. Which of the following criteria for the diagnosis of adjustment disorder most distinguishes it from MDD?

    (A) Symptoms cause marked distress or significant impairment in functioning.
    (B) Symptoms develop following an identifiable stressor.
    (C) Symptoms develop within 3 months of the onset of the stressor.
    (D) Symptoms do not persist for more than 6 months following termination of the stressor.
    (E) Symptoms do not represent bereavement.

30. Approximately what percentage of children who are diagnosed with diabetes mellitus Type I develop adjustment disorder following their medical diagnosis?

    (A) 1%
    (B) 5%
    (C) 10%
    (D) 33%
    (E) 75%

Questions 31 and 32

A 9-year-old boy is referred to you for evaluation because of repeated teasing at school related to his inappropriate peer interactions. The teachers report that at any time, without warning, the boy will make a disruptive sound or shout out in class. They describe him as polite and neat but restless and jumpy.

31. Which of the following is the most likely diagnosis?

    (A) conduct disorder
    (B) oppositional defiant disorder
    (C) panic disorder
    (D) separation anxiety disorder
    (E) Tourette disorder

32. Which of the following medications would be the most appropriate to prescribe?

    (A) bupropion (Wellbutrin)
    (B) clonidine (Catapres)
    (C) haloperidol (Haldol)
    (D) paroxetine (Paxil)
    (E) venlafaxine (Effexor)

Questions 33 and 34

A 7-year-old boy with leukemia is referred to you because of concerns about his mood. His parents report that he fluctuates between appearing depressed and acting angry. At times he plays quietly in his room, but at other times he displays anger outbursts, often hitting his 4-year-old brother. His mother admits that she has decreased her expectations of him, and feels that since he is ill he should not receive any punishments.

33. Which of the following methods would be the most effective way to engage his mother in a discussion regarding the role of her actions on the boy's behavior?

    (A) Acknowledge her guilt and anxiety about her son's illness but explain the importance of providing limits and structure for his emotional well-being.
    (B) Empathize with the trauma of having a sick child.
    (C) Refer her to a parent support group.
    (D) Sit quietly and make no comments about her parenting style.
    (E) Tell her that treating her son like a baby is hurting him emotionally.

34. It is determined that the boy is suffering from major depression. You speak to the mother about possible treatment options, both psychopharmacological and psychotherapeutic, but she is concerned about his ongoing leukemia treatment. Which of the following approaches is most appropriate regarding the treatment of both his leukemia and major depression?

(A) Treat the depression prior to the leukemia.

(B) Treat the depression after the leukemia.

(C) Treat the depression concurrent with the leukemia.

(D) Treat the leukemia first and the depression will resolve.

(E) Treat the leukemia only as treatment of the depression will not be effective in the setting of a medical illness.

Questions 35 and 36

An 8-year-old boy presents to your office for a routine visit. One month earlier, you diagnosed him with Tourette disorder and prescribed medication. He and his parents report that the medication has been helpful.

35. Which of the following is the most common comorbid disorder associated with Tourette disorder?

(A) autistic disorder

(B) bipolar disorder

(C) expressive language disorder

(D) obsessive-compulsive disorder

(E) separation anxiety disorder

36. Which of the following is necessary for the diagnosis of Tourette disorder?

(A) at least one motor tic and multiple vocal tics

(B) both multiple motor tics and at least one vocal tic

(C) multiple motor tics and multiple vocal tics

(D) only motor tics

(E) only vocal tics

Questions 37 and 38

An 8-year-old boy with a family history of tic disorders is referred to you for an evaluation of behavioral difficulties in school. His teachers report that he is unable to sit still, constantly fidgets, and is unable to complete class work because he is so easily distracted. The boy's mother reports that he has always had a lot of energy. She says that preparing to leave for school in the morning is extremely difficult because of her son's disorganization and forgetfulness. Otherwise, she has no complaints. She denies that her son produces any repetitive movements or sounds.

37. Which of the following is the most likely diagnosis?

(A) attention-deficit/hyperactivity disorder (ADHD)

(B) bipolar disorder

(C) conduct disorder

(D) disruptive behavior disorder not otherwise specified

(E) oppositional defiant disorder

38. The patient is subsequently treated for the above condition. He returns to an appointment after several weeks, now with repetitive grimacing and blinking movements which has resulted in his getting teased in school. Which of the following classes of medications is most likely to be responsible?

(A) benzodiazepines

(B) D_2 antagonists

(C) monoamine oxidase inhibitors (MAOIs)

(D) selective serotonin reuptake inhibitors (SSRIs)

(E) stimulants

Questions 39 and 40

A 6-year-old boy is referred to you by his school to evaluate his difficulty with keeping up with reading and math despite his above average intelligence. It is suspected that he suffers from a reading and math disorder, so further testing and evaluation is indicated.

39. Which of the following findings would be required for a diagnosis of reading disorder?

 (A) The child has an above average IQ (intelligence quotient) but below average reading achievement.
 (B) The child has an average IQ and below average reading achievement.
 (C) The child's reading achievement is substantially below the child's IQ.
 (D) The child's reading achievement is substantially above the child's IQ.
 (E) The child's reading achievement and IQ are both below average.

40. What would be the approximate risk of this child having a comorbid psychiatric disorder?

 (A) 5%
 (B) 10%
 (C) 25%
 (D) 50%
 (E) 75%

Questions 41 and 42

An 8-year-old child is referred to you for an evaluation of bed-wetting. Several behavioral interventions have been attempted, including eliminating fluid intake in the evening, scheduled awakenings at night to use the bathroom, and a urine alarm (a bell and pad). These techniques have been unsuccessful, and the child continues to urinate in bed every night.

41. What is the likelihood of this patient having a comorbid mental illness?

 (A) 10%
 (B) 20%
 (C) 30%
 (D) 40%
 (E) 50%

42. Which of the following medications should you prescribe to treat this patient?

 (A) benztropine (Cogentin)
 (B) desmopressin (DDAVP)
 (C) methylphenidate (Ritalin)
 (D) paroxetine (Paxil)
 (E) trazodone (Desyrel)

Questions 43 through 45

A 10-year-old boy is referred to you because his pediatrician suspects that he may have attention-deficit/hyperactivity disorder (ADHD). After a thorough history, physical examination, and laboratory investigation you make the diagnosis of ADHD. After discussing the adverse effects of medications, you prescribe methylphenidate to be taken in the morning and at lunch on school days.

43. Which of the following is the most common adverse effect of methylphenidate?

 (A) hypotension
 (B) insomnia
 (C) liver toxicity
 (D) tremor
 (E) weight gain

44. What is the likelihood that this patient will significantly benefit from the methylphenidate?

 (A) 10%
 (B) 25%
 (C) 33%
 (D) 50%
 (E) 70%

45. Despite education and reassurance, the mother is adamantly opposed to stimulant medications but still wishes her son to receive treatment for his ADHD. Which of the following medications would be the most appropriate?

 (A) aripiprazole (Abilify)
 (B) atomoxetine (Strattera)
 (C) citalopram (Celexa)
 (D) mixed amphetamine salts (Adderall)
 (E) valproic acid (Depakote)

Questions 46 and 47

During a routine office visit, the mother of a 37-month-old girl tells you that she is concerned about her daughter's behavior. Since the birth of her son 4 months earlier, the mother states that her daughter has been more irritable and angry. The child has told her mother that she doesn't want the baby anymore and to take him back. The mother is especially concerned because her daughter tried to bite the baby the week before.

46. Which of the following statements is the most appropriate response to this mother?

    (A) "If you simply ignore your daughter's behavior, it will pass."
    (B) "It is understandable that your daughter is angry and experiences jealousy with the new baby joining the family."
    (C) "The next time she tries to bite him, you should bite her back so she knows how it feels."
    (D) "Tell your daughter she is being a very bad girl and you won't love her if she bites the baby."
    (E) "Tell your daughter that she needs to love the baby and be a wonderful big sister."

47. Which of the following tasks would this girl be able to perform at her current age?

    (A) Acknowledge her angry and competitive feelings toward her sibling.
    (B) Be able to state her age and gender.
    (C) Count to 50.
    (D) Recognize that water poured from one glass into another of a different size is the same amount.
    (E) Ride a bicycle.

Questions 48 and 49

A 4-year-old boy is referred to you for evaluation because he has poor social relatedness. Upon interview, he appears healthy and well-kempt. He grabs your office key off your desk. At your office door, he takes the key and locks and unlocks your door repeatedly. Despite attempts to redirect and distract him, he remains preoccupied with this task. After about 10 minutes, you attempt to take the key away from him and he becomes extremely upset, making an insistent, piercing cry.

48. Which of the following areas would you most likely expect additional difficulties in this patient?

    (A) attention
    (B) fine motor skills
    (C) gross motor skills
    (D) language skills
    (E) potty training progress

49. Which of the following qualities would be most associated with a more favorable prognosis in this child?

    (A) easily toilet trained
    (B) interested in mechanical toys
    (C) organized in play
    (D) reciprocal conversation
    (E) reciting songs and poems from memory

Questions 50 and 51

A 17-year-old girl comes to your office for a routine visit. She states that she feels fine and offers no complaints. On physical examination, you find that her weight is 92 lb and her height is 65 in. One year earlier, her weight had been 126 lb, and her height was 65 in. After further discussion, you learn that she is terrified of gaining weight and believes that she is fat and needs to lose more weight. She reports that she has not menstruated in the past 6 months.

50. Which of the following laboratory abnormalities are you most likely to find?

    (A) hypercholesterolemia
    (B) hyperkalemia
    (C) hypocarotenemia
    (D) increased thyroid-stimulating hormone (TSH)
    (E) leukocytosis

51. Which of the following complications would be the best indication for admitting this patient to the hospital?

    (A) anemia
    (B) arrhythmia
    (C) bradycardia
    (D) hypotension
    (E) lanugo

Questions 52 and 53

An 8-month-old boy is brought to the clinic by his mother. She complains that her son has been experiencing screaming and crying fits when she leaves him with a babysitter. She says that in the past he did not object to being left with a babysitter and asks you why he becomes so upset now, and what she can do about it.

52. Which of the following statements would be the most appropriate response?

    (A) "This behavior is characteristic of autistic children."
    (B) "It is possible that your son has separation anxiety disorder."
    (C) "This behavior suggests that you're not spending enough time with your son."
    (D) "It sounds as though your son is overly attached to you."
    (E) "This behavior is normal at your son's age and will pass with time."

53. Which of the following diagnoses would be most appropriate if the boy in the previous question (Question 52) were an 8-year-old boy with similar behavior?

    (A) agoraphobia
    (B) normal behavior
    (C) obsessive-compulsive disorder
    (D) separation anxiety disorder
    (E) social phobia

Questions 54 and 55

A 10-year-old boy is referred to you due to extreme difficulties in school. He has been held back a grade and is still not passing his classes. During the course of your evaluation, you learn that the boy hears voices telling him that he is stupid and to leave the classroom. Afraid to disobey, he goes to the bathroom frequently. He also has difficulty falling asleep at night because the voices keep him awake. In addition, you learn that the boy believes others can read his thoughts. Physical and laboratory examinations are normal. You suspect that the boy may be suffering from schizophrenia.

54. Which of the following items in his history would be most consistent with your provisional diagnosis?

    (A) always social and outgoing
    (B) father with schizotypal personality disorder
    (C) parents getting divorced
    (D) recently transferred schools
    (E) recently used marijuana

55. Which of the following features would indicate a poorer prognosis in this patient?

    (A) acute onset
    (B) affective symptoms
    (C) good premorbid adjustment
    (D) onset before the age of 10
    (E) well-differentiated symptoms

Questions 56 through 58

A 9-year-old girl with a family history of bipolar disorder is referred to you by her school because of disruptive behavior in class that has been worsening over the past 3 months. Her teachers report that her energy level is high. Both attention-deficit/hyperactivity disorder (ADHD) and a manic episode are considered.

56. Which of the following symptoms would be more consistent with ADHD rather than mania?

    (A) distractibility
    (B) impulsivity
    (C) low self-esteem
    (D) motoric overactivity
    (E) pressured speech

57. If this child's school is unable to manage her behavior in her classroom despite outpatient treatment and medication, which of the following long-term options would be the most optimal school placement?

(A) home schooling

(B) parochial school

(C) school for children with learning disabilities

(D) residential treatment

(E) therapeutic day school

58. Further history and evaluation over time result in the diagnosis of bipolar disorder, manic. Which of the following medications would be the most appropriate treatment?

(A) bupropion (Wellbutrin)

(B) duloxetine (Cymbalta)

(C) methylphenidate (Ritalin)

(D) mixed amphetamine salts (Adderall)

(E) valproic acid (Depakote)

Questions 59 and 60

An 8-year-old boy is brought to your office by his mother for evaluation of an upper respiratory infection. The mother mentions that her son has started wetting the bed again. In addition, she mentions that the boy's grandmother died recently and wonders if this is affecting him.

59. At which of the following ages would a child normally be able to appreciate that death is irreversible?

(A) 2 years

(B) 3 years

(C) 5 years

(D) 7 years

(E) 12 years

60. Which of the following defense mechanisms is the boy most likely employing when he is wetting the bed?

(A) acting out

(B) denial

(C) regression

(D) repression

(E) somatization

Questions 61 and 62

A 12-year-old boy with Tourette disorder comes to your office for a routine visit. Two weeks earlier, you had prescribed clonidine for his illness. The boy reports that his tics have subsided slightly since starting the clonidine, but complains about the medicine.

61. Which of the following adverse effects is this boy most likely experiencing?

(A) dry mouth

(B) hypotension

(C) nausea

(D) sedation

(E) tremor

62. The parents bring in the boy's 7-year-old brother for evaluation. After further history is obtained, he is diagnosed with attention-deficit/hyperactivity disorder (ADHD). Which of the following classes of medications would be the most appropriate choice for the brother?

(A) antipsychotic

(B) monoamine oxidase inhibitor (MAOI)

(C) serotonin-specific reuptake inhibitor (SSRI)

(D) stimulant

(E) tricyclic antidepressant (TCA)

63. A 6-year-old boy is brought to the emergency department by his mother, who reports that he was playing on some steps in front of the house when he slipped and fell. She tells you that she is concerned that he might have broken his arm. An x-ray of the boy's arm shows a fracture of the ulna, as well as signs of several old fractures of varying ages. Which of the following is the most appropriate course of action?

    (A) Recommend calcium supplements and a multivitamin daily.
    (B) Refer the boy to an orthopedist for further evaluation.
    (C) Set the current broken bone in a cast and recommend that the boy see his pediatrician for follow-up care.
    (D) Tell the boy that you notice that he has had multiple broken bones and ask him how each of these fractures happened.
    (E) Tell the mother that you notice that the boy has had multiple broken bones and recommend that she limit the boy's sports activities.

64. The mother of a 6-year-old patient calls and asks you for advice. She says that her son still sucks his thumb, and she is concerned about this behavior. Which of the following suggestions is the most appropriate?

    (A) The mother should coat her son's thumb in hot pepper sauce.
    (B) The mother should ask the dentist to construct a mouth appliance that will not allow him to suck.
    (C) The mother should ignore the behavior.
    (D) The mother should give him gum frequently.
    (E) The mother should encourage him to stop sucking by designing a behavioral system to reward stopping.

Questions 65 and 66

A 14-year-old girl presents to her pediatrician complaining that she has been "freaking out." The girl describes episodes of shaking, gasping for air, and feeling like she is going to die. The feelings intensify for a few minutes and resolve spontaneously. These episodes have occurred at various times, in various situations, and the girl is worried that she is going crazy. A complete history and physical does not reveal any further relevant symptoms or signs.

65. Which of the following is the most appropriate treatment?

    (A) aripiprazole
    (B) carbamazepine
    (C) risperidone
    (D) sertraline
    (E) valproic acid

66. Prior to prescribing medications, which of the following should the pediatrician order next?

    (A) electrocardiogram (ECG)
    (B) electroencephalogram (EEG)
    (C) neurology consult
    (D) pulmonary function tests
    (E) routine laboratory studies

67. A 5-year-old girl diagnosed with lupus is seen by her female pediatrician for a routine visit. After returning home from the clinic, the girl asks her friend to "play doctor." Which of the following defense mechanisms best describes this behavior?

    (A) displacement
    (B) dissociation
    (C) identification
    (D) rationalization
    (E) reaction formation

Questions 68 and 69

A 10-year-old girl with a history of asthma is brought to the clinic after a recent increase in her asthma symptoms. During the visit, you learn that she is being beaten by her mother's boyfriend on a regular basis.

68. Under which of the following circumstances does the law require mandatory reporting by a physician of suspected child abuse?

(A) in all cases

(B) only in cases in which the child shows behavioral manifestations of abuse

(C) only when consent of a parent or guardian is obtained

(D) only when the physician believes it is in a child's best interest

(E) only when the physician has examined all children in the family

69. Which of the following manifestations would be the most likely outcome of the abuse?

(A) aggression

(B) dissociative disorder

(C) generalized anxiety disorder

(D) major depressive disorder

(E) post-traumatic stress disorder

70. A 4-year-old boy is referred to you because he will not speak in preschool. Over the course of about 2 months, he gradually stopped talking. His mother reports that he initially objected to going to preschool, but now no longer complains. She states that at times her son is quiet and stays in his room, but that she has not otherwise noticed a significant change in his speech or behavior. Which of the following is the most likely diagnosis?

(A) dysthymic disorder

(B) major depressive disorder (MDD)

(C) selective mutism

(D) separation anxiety disorder

(E) social phobia

71. A 2-year-old boy is referred to you for evaluation due to the suspicion that the child is the victim of physical abuse secondary to factitious disorder by proxy. Which of the following family members is the most likely perpetrator fabricating the illness?

(A) father

(B) brother

(C) mother

(D) sister

(E) uncle

72. A frustrated mother brings her 14-year-old son to a child psychiatrist after he is expelled from three high schools in 1 year. She reports the boy has tried twice to set his school on fire, has slashed school bus tires, and has broken into the principal's office to steal athletic trophies. In addition, he has been suspended numerous times for getting into fights with other students. She shudders and tearfully relates that she recently caught him singeing one of the family cats with a cigarette butt. Which of the following personality disorders is this boy most at risk of developing in the future?

(A) antisocial

(B) borderline

(C) histrionic

(D) obsessive-compulsive

(E) schizotypal

73. An 8-year-old boy is brought in by his mother who complains that she can't get her son to listen to her. She is frustrated because he frequently ignores her requests and instructions. Consideration is given toward the diagnosis of oppositional defiant disorder (ODD). Which of the following features would best support the diagnosis in this child?

(A) aggression to people

(B) depressive symptoms

(C) disobedience toward teachers

(D) lack of participation in tasks requiring attention

(E) violation of rules

74. A 13-year-old girl is seen by her psychiatrist 1 year after an automobile accident. She demonstrates intact language ability and complex motor skills. She has no identifiable abnormalities in the perception of stimuli, but she has lost the ability to read since the accident. Which of the following deficits is she most likely demonstrating?

(A) agnosia

(B) alexia

(C) anomia

(D) aphasia

(E) apraxia

75. A 10-year-old girl without significant medical history is brought by her father to the pediatrician for evaluation. Over the past school year, she has been having increasing difficulties going to sleep. Although she has "always had bedtime rituals," they have extended in complexity and length. Most of her time in the evening is now spent going around the house numerous times, locking and unlocking the doors and windows. While she knows the chances of a burglary are slim, she is extremely anxious about her safety, and she "can't stop" the urges to perform these behaviors. As a result, she only obtains 5 hours of sleep, and she has been falling asleep in class with diminishing grades. Which of the following therapeutic interventions is considered the first-line treatment for this disorder?

(A) cognitive behavioral therapy (CBT)
(B) family therapy
(C) group therapy
(D) short-term psychodynamic therapy
(E) supportive therapy

DIRECTIONS (Questions 76 through 93): The following group of numbered items are preceded by a list of lettered options. For each question, select the one lettered option that is *most* closely associated with it. Each lettered option may be used once, multiple times, or not at all.

Questions 76 through 79: Match the patient IQ with the intelligence level.

(A) normal intelligence 70 - 100
(B) mild mental retardation 55 - 70
(C) moderate mental retardation 40 - 55
(D) severe mental retardation 25 - 40
(E) profound mental retardation

76. A 14-year-old boy with an IQ of 34. D

77. An 8-year-old girl with an IQ of 96. Normal A

78. An 11-year-old boy with an IQ of 68. B

79. A 17-year-old boy with an IQ of 52. C

Questions 80 through 83: Match the disease or disorder with the patient.

(A) anorexia nervosa
(B) Asperger disorder
(C) bulimia nervosa
(D) hypochondriasis
(E) obsessive-compulsive disorder
(F) panic disorder
(G) pica
(H) pyromania
(I) Tourette disorder
(J) trichotillomania

80. A 14-year-old girl with episodes of palpitations, chest pain, shortness of breath, and diaphoresis who has a normal physical and laboratory examinations. F

81. A 10-year-old girl with physical findings that include hypotension, bradycardia, and lanugo hair. A

82. An 8-year-old boy with erythematous, chapped hands, and an otherwise normal physical and laboratory examination. E

83. A 13-year-old girl with a bald patch on the back of her head and an otherwise normal physical and laboratory examination. J

Questions 84 through 87: Match the disease or disorder with the patient.

(A) Asperger disorder
(B) attention-deficit/hyperactivity disorder (ADHD)
(C) autistic disorder
(D) expressive language disorder
(E) Rett disorder
(F) selective mutism

84. A 6-year-old girl whose parents are going through a divorce will not speak while at school. F

85. A 9-year-old boy who frequently blurts out comments in class without waiting his turn to be called on.

86. A 7-year-old boy who performs well in school, but seems to talk as if reciting a monologue rather than interacting in conversation and generally avoids other children.

87. A 6-year-old boy, who is having difficulty in school, avoids interactions with his classmates and others. He is noted making repetitive rocking movements.

Questions 88 through 93: Match the age range with the corresponding developmental milestone.

   (A) infant (0-18 months)
   (B) toddler (18-36 months)
   (C) preschool age (3-6 years)
   (D) school age (7-12 years)
   (E) adolescence (13-17 years)

88. Focus on following the rules.

89. Establishing self as autonomous, separate from caregiver, by practicing leaving and returning to the caregiver.

90. Establishing trust in the world through responsiveness and empathy of a caregiver.

91. Preoccupation with superheroes who represent idealized caregivers as a result of conflicted feelings toward caregivers.

92. The development of the ability to think about and manipulate ideas abstractly.

93. The development of the ability to apply reasoning so that the child is not limited only by perceptions.

DIRECTIONS (Questions 94 and 95): For each of the multiple choice questions in this section, select the lettered answer that is the one *best* response in each case.

94. A 16-year-old girl is brought to you by her mother because of dropping grades, apathy, and poor motivation. You learn that she has recently started smoking marijuana on a regular basis. Which of the following symptoms would most support the diagnosis of cannabis dependence?

   (A) Driven while under the influence of marijuana.
   (B) Grades have dropped substantially.
   (C) Ongoing desire to reduce marijuana use.
   (D) Smoked marijuana alone.
   (E) Smokes marijuana at least 2 days a week.

95. As the school psychologist, you are asked to see a fourth grader who has been consistently acting out in class. He often lies about things he has done in class, such as trying to cheat on tests. You learn that at home he practices shooting his BB gun at squirrels as well as at the family dog. He expresses no concern for these creatures nor remorse at his behavior. Which of the following is the most likely diagnosis?

   (A) autistic disorder
   (B) bipolar disorder
   (C) childhood schizophrenia
   (D) conduct disorder
   (E) oppositional defiant disorder

Answers and Explanations

1. **(B)** Suicide is a considerable risk in depressed adolescents, and should be specifically addressed during an interview with a patient who appears depressed or agitated, or has a history of a suicide attempt. In fact, the adolescent suicide rate has increased substantially during the past few decades. Male gender, a prior suicide attempt, history of psychiatric illness, family history, and substance abuse are all risk factors for a completed suicide. A history of a prior suicide attempt is the largest risk factor for suicide for both males and females in all age groups; the majority of those who complete suicide have attempted suicide in the past. Greater than 90% of youths who commit suicide have a comorbid psychiatric illness, frequently depression. Although cutting behavior is concerning in adolescents, it is not associated with the intent to kill oneself. More girls than boys demonstrate suicidal behavior and attempts, but nearly five times more teenage boys complete suicide than do teenage girls. This is because boys more frequently use guns and other violent methods to attempt suicide.

2. **(B)** Given the adolescent's history of depression and risk factors of substance abuse and family history, it is very important to ensure appropriate treatment for her quickly. It would be optimal for a psychiatrist to evaluate her as soon as possible. She does not necessarily need to be admitted to a hospital, since she does not appear at imminent risk of self-harm. If antidepressants are prescribed, the adolescent initially needs to be followed more closely than in 1 month. Certainly, waiting more than that without any intervention would be inadequate and inappropriate. She would likely benefit from medication management, so a psychiatrist would be preferable to a social worker in this situation.

3. **(D)** Sleep terror disorder (or night terrors) involves repeated episodes of sudden awakening from sleep accompanied by panic symptoms that begin with a scream and is associated with unresponsiveness to comfort or attempts to awaken them. It typically lasts just a few minutes. Intermittent explosive disorder does not occur during sleep and involves outbursts of anger and sometimes violent behavior. Narcolepsy is characterized by the triad of sleep attacks, cataplexy (sudden loss of muscle tone), and hypnopompic/hypnagogic hallucinations or sleep paralysis. Nightmare disorders occur in the latter third of the night and during REM sleep, in contrast to sleep terrors. When awakened, the individual quickly becomes oriented, unlike other parasomnias where the individual is disoriented, confused, and difficult to arouse. Like sleep terror disorder, sleepwalking disorder is also a parasomnia. It involves the child sitting up or leaving their bed but is not accompanied by terror or autonomic arousal.

4. **(C)** Episodes of sleep terror, as well as of sleepwalking, occur during deep sleep (stages 3-4). Nightmare disorder occurs during REM sleep.

5. **(E)** This patient is suffering from a major depressive disorder (MDD), single episode. A selective serotonin reuptake inhibitor (SSRI) such as sertraline is a first-line agent for MDD in children and adolescents. Tricyclic antidepressants (TCAs) such as imipramine cause

more adverse effects than SSRIs typically do, and in overdose is much more likely to be lethal. Mood stabilizers such as carbamazepine and lithium are used for bipolar disorder and as adjuncts to the treatment of MDD refractory to antidepressant medications alone. Antipsychotics such as olanzapine are usually reserved for use as adjuncts when psychosis develops or in bipolar disorder.

6. **(D)** In the *Diagnostic and Statistical Manual of Mental Disorders, Fourth Edition, Text Revision* (DSM-IV-TR), major depressive disorder requires a depressed mood for at least 2 weeks for adults to receive the diagnosis, but in the case of children and adolescents, an irritable mood may substitute for having a depressed mood. The required symptoms that involve sleep, appetite, anhedonia, concentration, and psychomotor functioning are the same for adults and adolescents in diagnosing major depressive disorder.

7. **(C)** This boy most likely suffers from expressive language disorder. Typical symptoms include having a markedly limited vocabulary, making errors in tense, and having difficulty recalling words or producing sentences with developmentally appropriate length or complexity. In addition, the boy's difficulties are interfering with academic functioning. There is no indication that he has difficulty with motor coordination, so a diagnosis of developmental coordination disorder would be inappropriate. There is no indication that this boy has difficulty with written expression. This boy does not suffer from a phonological disorder because his speech is clear and he has not failed to develop expected speech sounds. Similarly, he is not suffering from stuttering (a communications disorder diagnosis) because there is no disturbance in the fluency and time patterning of his speech.

8. **(C)** Speech delay refers to expressive language development and number of words spoken. The average number of words a 2-year-old speaks is 200 words. Therefore, the inability to speak 200 words by age 3 would constitute a speech delay.

9. **(E)** It is most likely that the boy used illicit substances during his trip that caused him to experience the acute psychotic symptoms. While it is important to rule out other medical causes, they are less likely to present acutely with psychotic symptoms in a teenager. Seizure disorder, head injury, diabetes, and thyroid disease are unlikely to present initially with psychotic symptoms.

10. **(B)** Mania in bipolar disorder can often present with psychotic symptoms including hallucinations, delusions, and disorganized thinking. Anorexia nervosa (an eating disorder) and generalized anxiety disorders do not present with psychotic symptoms. Individuals with borderline personality disorder may have psychotic-like symptoms especially when they are regressed, but they are much more likely to present with depression, suicidal thinking, and substance abuse. While major depressive disorder can be accompanied by psychotic features, it does not commonly present this acutely or as often as in bipolar disorder.

11. **(C)** This boy's behavior and symptoms are most consistent with separation anxiety disorder, characterized by developmentally inappropriate and excessive anxiety concerning separation from the home or from those to whom the individual is attached. Consistent with this diagnosis, the boy does not like to go to school, comes home immediately after school, sleeps in his parents' bed at night, and has repeated physical symptoms when at school. The boy is not suffering from PTSD because there is no evidence of a traumatic event that is persistently reexperienced and has caused symptoms of increased arousal and avoidance of associated stimuli. For a diagnosis of reactive attachment disorder of infancy or early childhood, the boy would need to have suffered markedly disturbed social relatedness, in most contexts, beginning before the age of 5. The boy's symptoms are not consistent with social phobia because he does not have a marked and persistent fear of social or performance situations with exposure causing intense anxiety. Finally, a diagnosis of specific phobia would require the display of marked and persistent fear cued by the presence of anticipation of a specific object or situation.

12. **(B)** Children with parents who have a history of an anxiety disorder are at increased risk for developing an anxiety disorder themselves. Other risk factors for developing a childhood anxiety disorder include parents who have an overly controlling and rejecting style, an insecure attachment with ones primary caregiver, and an inhibited and shy temperament.

13. **(B)** These symptoms are consistent with a manic episode of bipolar disorder. Attention-deficit/hyperactivity disorder is associated with hyperactivity and impulsivity but not grandiosity and delusional thinking. Major depression may have psychotic symptoms if severe, but it would not present with an inflated mood or increased energy. Panic disorder would present with recurrent panic attacks and significant anxiety. Although schizophrenia can present with delusional symptoms, they are usually not grandiose delusions; in addition, this patient has significant mood symptoms.

14. **(C)** Cocaine is a stimulant and can produce both manic and psychotic symptoms. Alcohol, cannabis, heroin, and PCP ingestion can induce a psychotic state including hallucinations and paranoia, but it would not classically be accompanied by manic symptoms.

15. **(E)** This boy likely has ODD. ODD is an externalizing behavior disorder that involves a pattern of hostile and defiant behavior. Children with ODD are often angry, argumentative, and easily annoyed by others. In order to confirm the diagnosis, you would need to gather additional information regarding the length of time the behavior has been present (at least 6 months is required), as well as rule out a mood, psychotic, or conduct disorder. Although anxiety disorders can present with tension, irritability, and even noncompliance when a child is placed in a new situation (such as a doctor's office), this child does not appear to have anxiety in places where escape may be difficult if having a panic attack (such as in agoraphobia) or excessive worry about a number of events (such as in GAD). While the patient's presenting symptoms are not primarily involving inattention, distractibility, or hyperactivity consistent

with ADHD, there is considerable comorbidity between ADHD and ODD. His lack of violence or serious violation of rules is not consistent with conduct disorder; however, ODD (especially if untreated) may lead to conduct disorder over time.

16. **(A)** Signs of bulimia nervosa include erosion of tooth enamel caused by acidic vomitus and abrasions on the dorsum of the hand due to scraping by the upper teeth as the individual pushes the hand to the back of the throat to induce vomiting. A direct but open-ended statement, such as "Tell me about the scratches on your hand," is most likely to be helpful in this situation. It is not a secret that the abrasions are there, but the patient has not mentioned them. Usually, a patient appreciates a direct question rather than wondering if you ignored or did not notice something obvious. Questions such as "Do you scratch yourself?" or "Do you have a cat?" are not open-ended; they require "yes" or "no" answers and are unlikely to yield new information. "Are you trying to hurt yourself?" or "How did the scratches happen?" may sound accusatory; patients are more likely to offer information if you seem nonjudgmental. If this girl does not volunteer information that confirms to you that she is not inducing vomiting, you may need to use a more direct but reassuring statement such as "Sometimes I see girls who make themselves throw up. Have you ever done that?"

17. **(D)** Medical complications can arise for bulimic patients who vomit or use laxatives or diuretics. A hypokalemic-hypochloremic alkalosis (due to vomiting) is a possible serious finding that can contribute to a cardiac arrhythmia. Anemia (as opposed to increased iron) can be seen, as well as decreased protein. The reduced chloride can lead to elevated sodium due to sodium resorption. Because of these changes, it is important to monitor bulimic patients for electrolyte or acid-base imbalance.

18. **(A)** Bulimia nervosa is most effectively treated with cognitive-behavioral therapy. Family therapy, group therapy, and longer-term, insight-oriented therapies (such as psychoanalysis and

psychodynamic psychotherapy) may be used as adjuncts to cognitive-behavioral therapy, but they have not been demonstrated to be as effective in changing the behaviors associated with bulimia nervosa.

19. **(D)** When attempting to engage a child in a clinical setting, it is important to choose words carefully in an attempt to establish an open, trusting connection, especially with a troubled and resistant child. It is always preferable to initiate the interview with more open-ended rather than closed-ended questions. The questions should optimally reflect empathy for the child and their situation without appearing too sentimental or judgmental. Also, it is important to avoid assumptions about the patient's feelings without checking with the patient first. The statement, "You sure were lucky the car swerved at the last minute" assumes the boy wanted to avoid being hit by the car, and also is a comment that does not lead to any elaboration from the patient. Statements **(B)** and **(C)** are both judgmental and more likely to shut down conversation than facilitate it. Also, asking a child if they are confused is a close-ended question that comes across as condescending.

20. **(D)** Psychomotor agitation is more commonly seen in children with MDD compared to adolescents with MDD. Children with MDD may appear more anxious and irritable than sad and depressed. Hypersomnia, hopelessness, weight change, and drug abuse are more commonly seen in adolescents with MDD compared to children with MDD.

21. **(E)** Substance ingestion is the most common method children use when attempting suicide. Firearms are used less frequently than substance ingestion, but are more often lethal. Other methods frequently used by children include stabbing, cutting, jumping from buildings, hanging, running in front of vehicles, and gas inhalation. It is important to note that some suicide attempts may be mistaken for accidents, so it is important to directly ask children if they intended to hurt or kill themselves.

22. **(A)** Headaches and nausea are common adverse effects associated with the synthetic antidiuretic hormone, DDAVP. Hypotension, liver toxicity, sedation, and tremor are not associated with desmopressin.

23. **(D)** The approximate comorbidity of childhood anxiety disorders (overanxious disorder, separation anxiety disorder, panic disorder) and MDD is 50%.

24. **(C)** The most common adverse effects of fluoxetine include gastrointestinal symptoms (eg, nausea, lose stools), insomnia, agitation, and headaches. In general, hypotension, liver toxicity, sedation, and weight gain are not side effects associated with fluoxetine.

25. **(E)** This girl's history and presentation are consistent with Rett disorder, which is characterized by normal prenatal and perinatal development, normal head circumference at birth, and normal psychomotor development through the first 5 months of life. Between the ages of 5 and 48 months, there is deceleration of head growth, loss of hand skills with development of stereotyped hand movements such as hand wringing, loss of social interaction (which may improve later), appearance of poorly coordinated gait or trunk movements, and severely impaired expressive and receptive language development with severe psychomotor retardation. Children with Asperger disorder do not show delay in language development (eg, single words are used by the age of 2). Autistic disorder and pervasive developmental disorder, not otherwise specified, are not appropriate diagnoses because this girl's presentation is better accounted for by Rett disorder. Children with childhood disintegrative disorder have at least 2 years of normal development before showing marked regression in multiple areas of functioning.

26. **(E)** Rett disorder is only seen in girls. It is likely that it has a genetic component. Case reports in monozygotic twins demonstrate 100% concordance.

27. **(A)** This patient's presentation is consistent with conduct disorder. There are many factors that are associated with an increased risk of a child developing conduct disorder. These include the child's biological father being absent, having a mother with somatization disorder or alcohol abuse, having a large family, and having aggressive, unsupportive, and conflict-ridden parents.

28. **(A)** Children and adolescents who are diagnosed with conduct disorder are at increased risk for antisocial personality disorder as adults. Antisocial personality disorder is not diagnosed until after the age of 18, and one of the criteria is evidence of conduct disorder prior to the age of 15. Earlier onset of conduct disorder is associated with an increased risk of developing antisocial personality disorder. Conduct disorder is not as closely associated with avoidant personality disorder, paranoid personality disorder, schizoid personality disorder, or schizotypal personality disorder.

29. **(D)** By definition, symptoms of adjustment disorder do not last longer than 6 months after a stressor or the termination of its consequences. If depressive symptoms persist, MDD may be diagnosed. In both adjustment disorder and MDD, symptoms must cause marked distress or significant impairment in functioning, may develop following a stressor, may develop within 3 months of the onset of a stressor, and must not represent bereavement.

30. **(D)** Following a diagnosis of diabetes mellitus Type I, approximately 33% of children develop symptoms of adjustment disorder.

31. **(E)** Tourette disorder is the most likely diagnosis because the boy's outbursts are consistent with vocal tics, and the report of "restless and jumpy" behavior is consistent with misinterpretation of motor tics. Tourette disorder most commonly develops in grade school-age boys, and the involuntary tics may be misinterpreted as purposefully disruptive behavior. It is not unusual for children with Tourette disorder to have difficulty with social and peer interactions. Of note, there is frequent comorbidity with ADHD. This boy does not suffer from conduct disorder or oppositional defiant disorder because he is polite and does not display hostile, destructive, or angry behaviors. The outbursts are not typical of panic disorder, in which there are discrete panic attacks, periods of intense fear, or discomfort with physical manifestations such as palpitations and subjective difficulty breathing. There is no evidence that this boy experiences distress and worry when separated from an important attachment figure as in separation anxiety disorder.

32. **(B)** Clonidine has become the first-line treatment for Tourette disorder. It has a limited side effect profile and helps control symptoms of a frequently associated comorbid disorder, attention-deficit/hyperactivity disorder (ADHD). Tricyclic antidepressants (TCAs) have been shown to be effective in the treatment of Tourette disorder, but other antidepressants such as bupropion, paroxetine, and venlafaxine are not known to be effective. High-potency antipsychotics such as haloperidol and pimozide were traditionally the first-line agents for Tourette disorder, but are more likely to cause significant side effects. Recently, the newer atypical (or second-generation) antipsychotics such as risperidone and olanzapine have also been used to treat the disorder.

33. **(A)** It is not unusual for parents of a seriously ill child to want to try to protect them from any further suffering or distress. Parents may end up treating such children as if they were younger than their actual age. When calling a parent's attention to the potential harm of such interaction, a clinician must be tactful and empathic. However, empathizing alone is not sufficient if your goal is to discuss parent–child interactions. Clearly having an ill child is tremendously overwhelming and anxiety provoking. By gently acknowledging this mother's distress, she will be more receptive to hearing feedback about her interactions with her child. Referring her to a parent support group might be useful following your initial discussion with her. Telling her she is treating her son like a baby is overly harsh and more likely to make her defensive rather that receptive.

34. **(C)** A psychiatric illness in a child or adolescent with a medical illness should be treated aggressively using the type of treatment most effective for the specific psychiatric illness. Effective treatment of a mental illness may positively affect a medical illness if improvement of psychiatric symptoms enables the child to more fully participate in treatment of the medical illness. In addition, emotional state is related to immune response. Although there is a specific stressor in this case, it is unclear whether the depressive symptoms would resolve if the leukemia goes into remission; in addition, given the impairment in this boy's functioning and that it is unclear if/when the leukemia would remit, not treating the depression would be inappropriate. Appropriate pharmacologic treatment should be avoided only if there are specific contraindications based on the medical treatment the child is receiving. In addition, the effectiveness of psychotherapy is related to the specific mental illness, not to the existence of, or lack of, a medical illness.

35. **(D)** It is not unusual for children with Tourette disorder to have comorbid psychiatric disorders. Obsessive-compulsive disorder is a very commonly associated disorder, often presenting in adolescence. Other anxiety disorders, attentional disorders, and learning disorders can be seen as well. Autistic disorders are not commonly associated with Tourette disorder. Mood lability can be an associated symptom, although the incidence of bipolar disorder is not particularly increased. Expressive language or separation anxiety disorders are also not increased in individuals with Tourette disorder.

36. **(B)** In Tourette disorder, both multiple motor tics and one or more vocal tics must be present at sometime during the illness. The motor and vocal tics do not need to occur concurrently. Onset is before the age of 18. The average age of onset is 7. Tics must be present nearly every day or intermittently for at least 1 year, with no tic-free period longer than 3 consecutive months. Vocal tics include various sounds such as grunts, yelps, coughs, and throat clearing, as well as words.

37. **(A)** This boy's history is typical of ADHD, combined type. He is fidgety and distractible in school as well as at home, and this is interfering with his ability to function. Increased energy and impulsivity can be a symptom of both ADHD and bipolar disorder, but the latter diagnosis is associated with inflated mood and grandiose ideation. This boy does not display excessive aggression, destruction of property, deceitfulness, theft, or serious violations of rules, as seen in conduct disorder. His behaviors are not negativistic, hostile, or defiant, so he does not suffer from oppositional defiant disorder. Disruptive behavior disorder not otherwise specified is a diagnosis reserved for cases in which there are conduct or oppositional defiant behaviors that do not meet the full criteria for conduct disorder or oppositional defiant disorder but cause significant impairment.

38. **(E)** Stimulant medications are the first-line treatment for ADHD but have been associated with an increased risk of developing tics. In general, if a child suffers from tics or has a family history of tics, stimulant medications should be avoided, and an alternate medication should be used to treat ADHD if necessary. Benzodiazepines, D_2 antagonists, MAOIs, and SSRIs are not known to exacerbate tics and are not used to treat ADHD.

39. **(C)** According to the *DSM-IV-TR*, in order to be diagnosed with a learning disorder, a person's achievement in reading needs to be substantially lower than the person's chronological age, measured intelligence quotient (IQ), and age-appropriate education. The learning disorder can be diagnosed regardless of whether the child has a below average IQ, average IQ, or above average IQ. It's the significant disparity between the achievement and IQ that is required.

40. **(D)** Approximately 50% of children with learning disorders have a comorbid psychiatric disorder. The most common comorbid conditions include ADHD, anxiety, and depressive disorders.

41. (B) Most children with enuresis are boys, and overall only approximately 20% have a comorbid mental disorder—girls with enuresis have a higher likelihood than boys.

42. (B) Of the choices provided, DDAVP is the treatment of choice for enuresis. DDAVP is a variation of the antidiuretic hormone vasopressin and is given intranasally. Benztropine is used to prevent extrapyramidal symptoms caused by neuroleptic use. Methylphenidate is commonly used in the treatment of attention-deficit/hyperactivity disorder. Paroxetine is a serotonin-specific reuptake inhibitor used to treat depression and anxiety. Trazodone is an antidepressant most often used for insomnia.

43. (B) The most common adverse effects of methylphenidate and other stimulant medications include insomnia, decreased appetite, weight loss, dysphoria, and irritability. Tremor, hypotension, weight gain, and liver toxicity are not side effects.

44. (E) Stimulant medications, such as methylphenidate, are effective in diminishing symptoms of ADHD in approximately 70% of patients.

45. (B) Atomoxetine is a nonstimulant, norepinephrine reuptake inhibitor which has been found to be helpful in treating both childhood and adult ADHD. Adderall is used to treat ADHD, but is a stimulant. Aripiprazole is a second-generation (atypical) antipsychotic, citalopram is an antidepressant, and valproic acid is a mood stabilizer used in bipolar disorder; none are used to treat ADHD.

46. (B) The clinician can be helpful to parents by explaining and normalizing the child's behavior. However, it is still important for the parent to respond to or correct this behavior. In the case of this young girl, jealousy of her younger sibling is entirely normal and is more difficult for her, since as a preschooler her language skills may not be developed sufficiently to articulate her distress. Once the mother accepts this child's behavior as understandable and in the normal range, she can respond in an empathic way while still setting limits on her aggressive behavior. Ignoring the behavior will not address the aggression and is not empathic. Under no circumstances is biting the child back helpful. Threatening to withdraw love is manipulative and anxiety-provoking to the child. By telling the child that she must love the baby, the mother is not truly empathizing with her and may elicit shame and further resentment toward the baby.

47. (B) A 37-month-old girl is a young preschool age child. At this stage, she should be able to state her age and gender and be involved in or have recently completed potty training. Although she has significant language, it would be very unusual for her to use her language spontaneously to identify and articulate her feelings about her younger sibling. Although a precocious 3-year-old may be able to count to 50, it would not necessarily be expected of her until she is 5. She is currently considered to be in the preoperational stage of cognitive development and cannot yet apply concepts of conservation of matter (concrete operations). Her gross motor skills and balance are likely not developed enough to ride a bicycle. She should be able to ride a tricycle, however.

48. (D) This patient's presentation is suspicious for autistic disorder. Of the choices provided, only language impairment is a required criteria for a diagnosis of autistic disorder. The language problem may involve a delay in speech, marked difficulty in beginning or sustaining a conversation, or stereotyped use of language. Attentional difficulties, impairment in motor skill development, or delay in potty training are not necessarily features of autistic disorder.

49. (D) Children with autistic disorder have more favorable prognoses if they are able to converse meaningfully with others rather than (verbally) interact inappropriately with others. It is not unusual for autistic children to be easily toilet trained, enjoy mechanical toys, be rigidly organized in their play, and be capable of memorizing or reciting poems, dialogue from a TV show or movie. These latter characteristics are not associated with a good prognosis.

50. **(A)** This girl likely has anorexia nervosa. Hypercholesterolemia is common in anorexia nervosa. Other findings associated with the starvation state are mild normocytic normochromic anemia and leukopenia. If vomiting is induced, hypokalemia, hypochloremia, and metabolic alkalosis may be seen. Hypercarotenemia, causing yellowing of the skin, may be seen if many carrots are eaten in an attempt to satisfy the appetite with a low-calorie food. TSH is not typically altered.

51. **(B)** While all of the choices are complications resulting from anorexia nervosa, a cardiac arrhythmia is considered a major complication and therefore alone justifies an inpatient admission. If the patient has multiple minor complications (eg, anemia, bradycardia, hypotension, lanugo), strong consideration for admission to the hospital should also be given.

52. **(E)** Stranger anxiety occurs as part of normal child development and, in fact, is evidence of the development of a secure bond of attachment. It does not suggest that a parent is inattentive; stranger anxiety usually appears by 7 to 8 months and generally resolves with time. Typically, stranger anxiety is stronger toward completely unknown persons than toward those who are more familiar. Autistic children often lack this developmental marker. Because stranger anxiety at this age is developmentally appropriate, this boy cannot be diagnosed with separation anxiety disorder and is not overly attached to his mother.

53. **(D)** This boy would be diagnosed with separation anxiety disorder. While an 8-month-old child would typically display stranger anxiety, an 8-year-old would not. This behavior would have normally gone away for most children by age 3 or 4. School age children are expected to be able to separate from the parent/caregiver in order to attend school and other activities. Individuals with agoraphobia often refuse to leave their home due to the fear of developing a panic attack. Obsessive-compulsive disorder is characterized by obsessions and compulsions; while it is an anxiety disorder the focus is not related to separation. Social phobia involves anxiety in a social or performance situation.

54. **(B)** Individuals who develop schizophrenia are more likely to have a parent with a psychotic or schizotypal disorder. Individuals who develop schizophrenia are much more likely to have a history of social withdrawal and introversion rather than extroversion. Recent stressors such as parental divorce or moving may contribute to the onset or exacerbation of some psychiatric disorders but not specifically schizophrenia in particular. Finally, recent drug use would be more likely to support a diagnosis of substance-induced psychosis.

55. **(D)** Very early onset of schizophrenia, before the age of 10, is rare and associated with a poorer outcome. A better prognosis is associated with an acute onset, more affective symptoms, older age at onset, good premorbid functioning, well-differentiated symptoms, and lack of a family history of schizophrenia.

56. **(C)** Children with ADHD often suffer from low self-esteem, while children with mania are more likely to be euphoric. Distractibility, impulsivity, motoric overactivity, and pressured speech may be seen in children with both disorders.

57. **(E)** If a school is unable to manage a child's behavioral or emotional difficulties despite added support and even special placement in a separate classroom, the most appropriate next step is therapeutic day school placement. Therapeutic schools are designed for students with psychiatric disorders that are severe enough that their home schools cannot keep the child or other students safe and manage the child in a learning environment. Home schooling, a parochial school, or a school for students with learning disabilities are not therapeutic in nature and do not have teachers and staff who are trained to work with students with emotional and behavioral disorders. Residential placement involves the child residing at the school while receiving therapeutic treatment and attending classes, and is reserved for students whose needs cannot be met by therapeutic schools.

58. **(E)** Valproic acid is an anticonvulsant which is also a mood stabilizer used to treat bipolar disorder. Duloxetine and bupropion are both antidepressants and not appropriate for treating mania as they may worsen the symptoms or promote rapid-cycling. Methylphenidate and mixed amphetamine salts are stimulants used in attention-deficit/hyperactivity disorder, and are contraindicated in mania because they may actually exacerbate mania.

59. **(D)** Typically, children are 7- or 8-year-old when they begin to understand the irreversibility of death. To understand that death is irreversible, children must have completed the cognitive stage of preoperational thought and developed the ability to have concrete thinking. Usually, this level of cognitive maturity is achieved between the ages of 6 and 10.

60. **(C)** This boy is displaying regression, a defense mechanism in which there is an attempt to return to an earlier developmental phase to avoid the tension and conflict at the present level of development (eg, distress over the grandmother's death). Acting out is a defense mechanism in which an unconscious wish or impulse is expressed through action to avoid an accompanying affect. Denial is a defense mechanism in which the awareness of a painful aspect of reality is avoided by negating sensory data. Repression is a defense mechanism in which an idea or feeling is expelled or withheld from consciousness. Somatization is the presence of physical symptoms that are a manifestation of emotional or psychological distress.

61. **(D)** Sedation is a frequent adverse effect of clonidine upon initiating treatment. With continued treatment, the sedation usually subsides. Dry mouth is a less common adverse effect. Hypotension is a possible side effect as clonidine is also used as an anti-hypertensive medication. The reduction in blood pressure usually does not result in significant symptoms, however. In general, nausea and tremor are not seen.

62. **(D)** Stimulants are the most commonly used medication in the treatment of ADHD, and although they can unmask tic disorders, ADHD treatment guidelines state that stimulants can still be used in individuals with tics. In fact, a recent study found that stimulants did not worsen tics in those with tic disorders. Antipsychotics and MAOIs are not used for ADHD. SSRIs are infrequently used to augment treatment in some cases and are not considered a first-line treatment. Although TCAs may be as effective as stimulants, their potential for inducing a cardiac arrhythmia or, less likely, sudden death preclude tricyclics from being used first line for ADHD.

63. **(D)** The finding of multiple fractures, especially when they are of different ages, is a red flag for physical abuse. Even though the boy may be scared to report what happened for fear of punishment, it is important to try to talk with him alone and find out as much as possible. Recommending extra vitamins or limited sports does not address the question of whether the boy is safe at home. It is not appropriate to refer the boy to an orthopedist or his pediatrician prior to investigating the possibility of physical abuse.

64. **(E)** In addressing the delicate task of helping a child stop or alter their method of self-soothing, sensitive and collaborative approaches are much more preferable to abrupt and harsh interventions. Encouraging a child to stop thumb sucking with a more flexible reward system that is enticing for the child engages the child in making choices about their own body, rather than imposing a harsh intervention. Both hot pepper sauce and a mouth appliance are punitive in nature. However, more passive approaches like ignoring or offering gum are also not likely to be successful. Because prolonged thumb sucking can result in significant dental problems, helping a child stop thumb sucking is eventually valuable.

65. **(D)** This teenager is likely suffering from panic disorder. Serotonin-specific reuptake inhibitors (SSRIs) such as sertraline are effective in the treatment of panic disorder. Antipsychotics, such as aripiprazole and risperidone, are not indicated for the treatment of panic disorder. Mood stabilizers, such as carbamazepine and valproic acid, are not effective in panic disorder.

66. **(E)** Although the symptoms that the patient describes are consistent with panic attacks, it is

important to rule out any medical causes that could be emulating that presentation (eg, metabolic, electrolyte, anemia). An ECG would be helpful if she reported cardiac symptoms as part of her presentation. This optional test can be done after the bloodwork is complete. An EEG and referral to a neurologist is not necessary unless one has suspicions of a seizure disorder. A pulmonary function test is used to diagnose asthma which is unlikely as the cause in this patient.

67. **(C)** Identification is the process of adopting other people's characteristics. Identification with a parent is important in personality formation. This girl's behavior may occur as an attempt to imitate the doctor because she admires her, or it may represent an effort to cope with anxiety about the doctor because she fears her. Displacement is a defense mechanism in which emotions are shifted from one idea or object to another that resembles the original but evokes less distress. Dissociation is a defense mechanism in which a person's character or sense of identity is temporarily but drastically modified in order to avoid emotional distress. Rationalization is a defense mechanism in which rational explanations are offered in an attempt to justify unacceptable attitudes, beliefs, or behaviors. Reaction formation is a defense mechanism in which an unacceptable impulse is transformed into its opposite.

68. **(A)** In all jurisdictions in the United States, clinicians are required to report all cases of suspected child abuse. The law does not leave the issue to the clinician's discretion or parental/guardian consent.

69. **(D)** Although all of the listed choices are possible outcomes associated with childhood abuse, depression is the most common one. In particular, abuse of a chronic nature can have a significant effect on personality development, and, in addition, predispose the child to significant psychopathology as an adult.

70. **(C)** This boy's history is most consistent with selective mutism. He does not speak at school but continues to talk at home. Consistent failure

to speak in a specific social situation despite speaking in other situations is not characteristic of dysthymic disorder, MDD, separation anxiety disorder, or social phobia.

71. **(C)** The mother is the most common perpetrator of intentionally producing physical or psychological symptoms in her child in order to assume the sick role by proxy. The victim is usually a preschool child, and an Axis IV listing diagnosis of physical abuse of a child may be appropriate.

72. **(A)** The case represents a child with conduct disorder. Individuals with conduct disorder are at increased risk of later development of antisocial personality disorder; in fact, *DSM-IV-TR* criteria for antisocial personality disorder require evidence of a conduct disorder before the age of 15.

73. **(C)** Disobedience toward authority figures is a characteristic of ODD. Aggression and violating rules are symptoms consistent with conduct disorder. If the hostile and negativistic behavior consistent with ODD occurs only in the context of a mood disorder, the child cannot be diagnosed with ODD. Reluctance to participate in tasks that require ongoing mental attention is a common symptom of attention-deficit/hyperactivity disorder (ADHD).

74. **(B)** Alexia is the inability to read. Agnosia is the inability to recognize objects despite intact senses. Anomia is the specific inability to name objects even though the object is recognizable and can be described by the patient. Aphasia is more global than alexia and is an abnormality in either the expression or the comprehension of language. Apraxia is an inability to perform learned motor skills despite normal strength and coordination.

75. **(A)** This patient's symptoms are consistent with obsessive-compulsive disorder (OCD). Cognitive behavioral therapy for OCD is the nonpharmacologic therapeutic treatment of choice. The CBT often involves exposure and response prevention to help extinguish compulsions. Family therapy can be helpful in

addressing family-related issues contributing to the child's symptoms. Group therapy can be part of an OCD treatment, particularly cognitive-behavioral group therapy. Short-term psychodynamic and supportive therapy are not considered adequate treatments alone, although they may be helpful in addressing related issues such as self esteem and relationships.

76. **(D)** The range of IQ for severe mental retardation is 25 to 39.

77. **(A)** The range of IQ for average (normal) intelligence is 90 to 110.

78. **(B)** The range of IQ for mild mental retardation is 55 to 70.

79. **(C)** The range of IQ for moderate mental retardation is 40 to 54.

80. **(F)** Palpitations, chest pain, shortness of breath, and diaphoresis commonly occur during panic attacks.

81. **(A)** Hypotension, bradycardia, and lanugo hair are classic sequelae of starvation seen in anorexia nervosa.

82. **(E)** Chapped hands and other dermatologic problems are often present in obsessive-compulsive disorder due to excessive washing with water or caustic cleaning agents.

83. **(J)** Trichotillomania is more common in girls, with the behavior peaking at around ages 5 to 8 and age 13. The repeated pulling out of hair results in decreased or complete loss of hair in a specific area. The scalp, eyebrows, and eyelashes are the sites most commonly involved.

Asperger disorder **(B)** is a pervasive developmental disorder characterized by impairments in social interactions and the development of stereotyped or repetitive patterns of behaviors, but without significant delay in language skills or cognitive function. Asperger occurs more commonly in males. Bulimia nervosa **(C)**, seen in 1% to 3% of adolescent girls and young women, is a bingeing and purging type of eating disorder. Hypochondriasis **(D)** is the preoccupation that one has a serious disease based on misinterpretation of symptoms, despite appropriate medical evaluation and reassurance. Pica **(G)** is the eating of non-nutritional substances such as dirt or paint. A *DSM-IV-TR* diagnosis of pyromania **(H)** requires several criteria, including deliberate and purposeful fire setting and tension or affective arousal before the act, which is not better accounted for by conduct disorder, a manic episode, or antisocial personality disorder. Eye tics such as blinking and eye rolling are the most common initial symptoms in Tourette disorder **(I)**. Facial tics such as grimacing or licking movements and vocal tics such as throat clearing or grunting are the next most common initial symptoms. Whole-body tics, such as body rocking or pelvic thrusting, and self-abusive tics, such as hitting, may develop later.

84–87. [84 (F), 85 (B), 86 (A), 87 (C)]. Selective mutism is rare, and children who suffer from it are only mute in certain situations (eg, school). It often involves a stressful life event such as parents' divorce and the children are mute by choice. Blurting out in class is a symptom of impulsivity that is often seen with ADHD. No language impairment is seen as part of ADHD. The boy in Question 86 who performs well in school but avoids social interactions is most likely to have Asperger disorder, because unlike those with autism, he has preserved expressive language; however, his use of it appropriately in social situations is severely impaired. Autistic children frequently display stereotyped and repetitive movements that are self-stimulating plus they also have impaired expressive language. In both Asperger disorder and autistic disorder, children have significant social difficulties. Children with expressive language disorder have an isolated language deficiency not associated with social or behavioral symptoms. Rett disorder is a pervasive developmental disorder only seen in girls, characterized by normal prenatal and perinatal development, followed by deceleration of head growth and loss of hand motor skills after 5 months, as well as loss of social skills, poor gait, and impaired language development.

88–93. [88 (D), 89 (B), 90 (A), 91 (C), 92 (E), 93 (D)] As children grow, they pass through different stages of development that represent emotional and cognitive maturation. A vital task of infancy is to establish a secure sense of trust that occurs in the relationship with one's responsive caregiver. Toddlers struggle with the increasing understanding that they are a separate being from their caregiver, and they practice separating and reuniting with their caregiver as a way to consolidate their sense of separateness and autonomy. Preschool children's identification with superheroes helps them cope with their own feelings of smallness and inadequacy (as compared to their parents) by identification with characters who are strong and powerful. This stage is also called the oedipal phase; at this time children experience longings toward the parent of the opposite sex and jealousy and hostility toward the same sex parent. School age children develop the ability to think more logically and concretely and thus can identify that equal amounts of liquid in two differently shaped containers hold the same amount. This phase of cognitive development is called concrete operations. In adolescence, one's cognitive abilities advance further, and one develops the ability to think in an abstract fashion (formal operations). Piaget identified and described concrete and formal operations.

94. **(C)** In differentiating substance abuse versus substance dependence, a clinician needs to assess different aspects of the person's substance use. Substance abuse relates to troublesome behaviors and consequences associated with the use, including a failure to meet work or school expectations (such as failing grades), putting oneself at risk (such as driving while using) or legal problems. Substance dependence reflects the person's physical and/or psychological dependency on the substance. This includes assessing tolerance, withdrawal, heavier use than intended, and displaying an ongoing desire or unsuccessful attempts to cut back on substance use. Neither using a substance alone nor the frequency used are considered criteria for abuse or dependence; however, using most days and using alone usually indicate the person's use is more extensive and potentially more concerning, prompting further questioning.

95. **(D)** This child fulfills the *DSM-IV-TR* criteria for conduct disorder, namely, three of the four following acts: aggression toward people and animals, destruction of property, deceitfulness, and serious violations of rules. There is nothing to suggest an autistic spectrum disorder, particularly because it would have likely been diagnosed much earlier; more importantly, his actions seem willful and not repetitive or stereotyped. A child with bipolar disorder may display impulsivity and aggressive behavior, however, the child maintains an overall sense of right and wrong and often experiences regret for the out-of-control behavior once symptoms are improved. Also, bipolar children have significant mood symptoms that underlie their behavior. Children with conduct disorder may also have a comorbid mood disorder, but mood symptoms are not necessarily part of the conduct disorder constellation. There is no evidence of psychotic symptoms, such as hallucinations or delusions that would be characteristic of childhood schizophrenia. Oppositional defiant disorder requires 6 months of negativistic, hostile, and defiant behavior directed mostly at authority figures. While it may be a premorbid condition of conduct disorder, it is not as severe.

CHAPTER 2

Adult Psychopathology
Questions

DIRECTIONS (Questions 1 through 120): For each of the multiple choice questions in this section select the lettered answer that is the one *best* response in each case.

Questions 1 and 2

A 22-year-old single, white man is referred to you for a 1-year history of strange behavior characterized by talking to the television, accusing local police of bugging his room, and carrying on conversations with himself. His mother also describes a 3- to 4-year history of progressive withdrawal from social activities. The patient dropped out of college in his final year and since then has been living in his room at home. Attempts to hold a job as a busboy at a local restaurant and as a night janitor have abruptly ended after disputes with the employers.

1. What is the prevalence of this patient's likely illness in the general population?

    (A) 0.1%
    (B) 0.5%
    (C) 1%
    (D) 3%
    (E) 5%

2. The patient's mother informs you that he has an identical twin brother. She is concerned about his also developing the same illness. What is the likely chance of the patient's twin also having the same illness?

    (A) 1%
    (B) 10%
    (C) 25%

    (D) 50%
    (E) 100%

Questions 3 and 4

A 40-year-old man with chronic schizophrenia comes for his regular outpatient medication management appointments. During his last visit, he reports that over the last week his intestines and heart have been removed. He has subsequently withdrawn and been staying in his basement apartment, avoiding friends and family members. When asked about his lack of getting out in the world, he responds, "What world? There is no world!"

3. Which of the following terms best describes this symptom?

    (A) Capgras syndrome
    (B) Cotard syndrome
    (C) folie à deux
    (D) Fregoli delusion
    (E) major depression

4. Upon returning for a follow-up visit 15 days later, the patient now claims that his mother and father have been recently replaced by "cyborg alien robots" that look identical to his parents. Which of the following terms best describes this symptom?

    (A) Capgras syndrome
    (B) Cotard syndrome
    (C) delusional disorder
    (D) folie à deux
    (E) Fregoli delusion

5. A 32-year-old woman 6 days postpartum is brought into the emergency room by her husband. She denies there is any problem, but he states that his wife has never acted like this, although her history is significant for a severe depression in her teenage years. He notes his wife has not been sleeping for the past several days, even while the newborn is. She has been notably irritable, and has been pacing in the middle of the night and weeping, while talking to no one in particular. Yesterday she began to ignore the infant, but today she volunteered that their child "is the Antichrist and must be destroyed." She admits to you that she wants to smother the infant in a humane way to prevent the apocalypse. Which of the following diagnoses should you most suspect?

(A) bipolar disorder
(B) delusional disorder
(C) major depressive disorder (MDD) with psychotic features
(D) schizoaffective disorder
(E) schizophrenia

Questions 6 through 8

An 18-year-old woman without prior psychiatric history has started her freshman year of college. She is brought to the emergency room after being found on the roof of her dormitory dressed only in her underwear, despite below freezing temperatures. She had been noted by campus police to be flapping her hands and climbing the banister on the roof, stating to an unseen other, "Lucifer, I hear you! I will do as you command—soar to my death to fulfill your prophecy!" She accused the policemen of being "Satan's horsemen" and "adulterers from the Court of King Herod." Her roommates confirm that for the past 5 weeks the patient has been acting bizarrely, and her speech has been disorganized. You plan to obtain collateral information from her family.

6. Which of the following features would you be most likely to find in her history?

(A) head trauma
(B) low intelligence
(C) neglectful mother

(D) physical or sexual abuse
(E) progressive social withdrawal

7. Plans are arranged for her admission to the psychiatric unit. Her physical examination is unremarkable, and her blood alcohol is undetectable. Her urine toxicology results come back positive for cannabis, however. Which of the following would be the most appropriate provisional diagnosis?

(A) brief psychotic disorder
(B) schizophreniform disorder
(C) schizophrenia
(D) substance-induced mood disorder
(E) substance-induced psychotic disorder

8. One year later this woman returns to your office with her mother for follow-up. Her symptoms remitted within a month after she stopped smoking marijuana. However, she has not done well in her freshman year, and for the past several months has continued to experience worsening social isolation and amotivation. While she has not used any substances since she last saw you, she reluctantly admits that occasionally she hears Lucifer communicating with her. She tries to ignore the communication, and has taken to arranging her books in a certain manner to prevent his controlling her thoughts. On her mental status examination she makes poor eye contact and her affect is notably blunted. Her mother notes that the patient now rarely calls home, though before she'd do so twice weekly. Which of the following is the most likely diagnosis?

(A) brief psychotic disorder
(B) schizophreniform disorder
(C) schizophrenia
(D) substance-induced mood disorder
(E) substance-induced psychotic disorder

9. A 42-year-old woman presents to a therapist with a history of dramatic mood swings since early adolescence, where she will quickly become deeply depressed for hours to days, usually in response to separation from a loved

one. She also admits to "rage attacks," where she will break items, scream, or scratch herself superficially on her arms. She binge drinks up to 1 to 2 pints of hard liquor at a time. She has had over 30 sexual partners, on many occasions without using contraception. Which of the following defense mechanisms does this patient most likely employ?

(A) altruism
(B) intellectualization
(C) splitting
(D) sublimation
(E) undoing

10. The family of a 26-year-old-schizophrenic patient brings him in for follow-up. He was initially diagnosed at age 25 after a psychotic break that, in retrospect, followed a protracted course of increasing isolation and amotivation. Despite difficulties, he was able to hold a full-time job in marketing after completing a double major by age 23. He reports intermittent hallucinations, but has been able to maintain his independent living and part-time employment when he is symptom-free. He is a disheveled man who articulates a multitude of delusional beliefs with a sophisticated vocabulary. Which of the following characteristics in this patient is most strongly associated with a better overall prognosis?

(A) age at presentation
(B) gender of patient
(C) insidious symptom onset
(D) predominantly positive symptoms
(E) premorbid functioning

Questions 11 and 12

A 36-year-old patient with no previous psychiatric history is brought to the emergency room by his family members. They are concerned that for the past month he has not been eating regularly, is moving very slowly, and has completely isolated himself in the apartment where he lives alone. They also note that 2 months ago he mentioned that he no longer enjoyed fishing, and that he felt like a burden on his fiancée. On mental status examination, he displays psychomotor retardation; he looks at you but rarely blinks. He responds in the negative to any question asked. On physical examination he appears in no acute distress, is afebrile, marginally hypotensive, and mildly tachycardic. He exhibits posturing and resists your motions with strength proportional to what you exert. He also crudely mimics your movements. His laboratory studies are unremarkable.

11. Which of the following diagnoses is most likely?

(A) hypothyroidism
(B) major depression, catatonic subtype
(C) malingering
(D) malignant catatonia
(E) schizophrenia, catatonic type

12. Recognizing the clinical situation in front of you, you admit the patient to the psychiatric ward for inability to care for self. Which of the following treatments would be best started immediately?

(A) amitriptyline
(B) electroconvulsive therapy
(C) lithium
(D) lorazepam
(E) sertraline

13. A 49-year-old bank teller with no known psychiatric history is referred to your office by her internist for an evaluation. For the past 2 months, she has been increasingly convinced that a well-known pop music star is in love with her and that they have had an ongoing affair. She is well-groomed, and there is no evidence of thought disorder or hallucinations. Her husband reveals that she has been functioning well at work and in other social relationships. Which of the following is the most likely diagnosis?

(A) brief psychotic disorder
(B) delusional disorder
(C) paranoid personality disorder
(D) schizophrenia
(E) schizophreniform disorder

Questions 14 and 15

A 46-year-old divorced, African-American woman with a history of major depressive disorder is admitted to your inpatient psychiatric unit following an intentional acetaminophen overdose. She has a history of multiple psychiatric hospitalizations with similar presentations. The patient reports a 3-week history of insomnia, difficulty concentrating, low energy, hopelessness, and a decreased appetite. She has been unable to work recently because of her depression and has lost interest in activities she once enjoyed. She has no history of a manic episode. Her past psychiatric history is significant for a prior episode of depression after the birth of her second child. She has undergone treatment with several adequate trials of medications, including augmentation with lithium, yet she has continued to have residual symptoms of depression. She has never been treated with psychotherapy. In the past she has experienced auditory hallucinations when her depression was most severe. Her medical history is significant for hypothyroidism, which is adequately managed with levothyroxine. She has required surgery to reduce a lower leg fractured in a suicide attempt where she jumped out of a window.

14. Which of the following factors would be most influential in your recommending electroconvulsive therapy (ECT) for this patient?

(A) concurrent thyroid dysfunction with adequate treatment

(B) history of associated psychotic symptoms with prior depression

(C) history of postpartum depression

(D) severe depression that has not responded to several medications

(E) treatment-resistant depression with recurrent suicidal ideation

15. The indications for ECT are discussed with the patient, as well as the risks, benefits, and side effects. She asks appropriate questions and consents to ECT. Further medical history is explored prior to beginning the procedure. Which of the following conditions would be a relative contraindication to proceed?

(A) coronary artery disease, with a myocardial infarction 2 years ago

(B) implanted pacemaker for periodic arrhythmia

(C) incidentally found frontal meningioma measuring 10 cm in diameter

(D) second trimester pregnancy

(E) traumatic brain injury sustained in teenage years

Questions 16 and 17

A 34-year-old white male is referred by his primary care physician for depression. Upon initial interview, he complains of feeling "blue." His mental status examination reveals a disheveled appearance, depressed mood, psychomotor retardation, and suicidal ideation without plan. His thought processes are significant for thought blocking and some slowing. Deficits with remote and short-term memory are noted. Judgment and insight are also impaired. Your provisional diagnosis is major depressive disorder.

16. Which type of sleep disturbance you would most expect to see in this patient?

(A) decreased response to sedative drugs

(B) early morning awakening

(C) increased rapid eye movement (REM) stage latency

(D) sleeping too deeply (difficulty being awakened)

(E) sleeping too lightly (awakened too easily)

17. Which of the following metabolic changes would be most likely found in this patient?

(A) decreased monoamine oxidase (MAO) activity

(B) increased catecholamine activity

(C) increased cortisol secretion

(D) increased sex hormones

(E) increased immune functions

Questions 18 and 19

A 35-year-old man is being successfully treated for major depression with paroxetine. He has missed his last two appointments, leaving messages telling you that "I've been spectacular!" His wife has since called you to report that her husband has been "very different." He has apparently been spending money on frivolous items, and when his wife went to the bank, she was told that their account was overdrawn. She states that one moment her husband is giddy and without notice he quickly becomes agitated and angry. She is able to convince her husband to see you in the office. During the interview, the patient questions your credentials and accuses you of being more loyal to his wife than to him. Most of the interview is spent interrupting the patient as you try to decipher his rapid speech. In his rant he threatens to cut the brake lines on his mother-in-law's SUV because he feels she has been intruding in his marriage.

18. Which of the following is the next most appropriate step?

   (A) Discharge the patient home as he refuses admission, but see him tomorrow.
   (B) Escort the patient (with police assistance as needed) to the nearest emergency room.
   (C) Inform the mother-in-law that she is in danger.
   (D) Inform the police that a threat has been made against the mother-in-law.
   (E) Tell the wife to have the mother-in-law stay with her.

19. After addressing the above situation, the patient is subsequently begun on valproic acid. Which of the following additional pharmacologic interventions would be the most appropriate?

   (A) Check a serum paroxetine level.
   (B) Cross taper the paroxetine to nortriptyline.
   (C) Discontinue the paroxetine.
   (D) Initiate bupropion.
   (E) Initiate lorazepam.

Questions 20 and 21

A new patient comes to your office for a psychiatric evaluation. His history suggests a pattern of subclinical depressions along with episodes of hypomania. He denies any drug or alcohol use, and he has no significant medical problems.

20. Which of the following diagnoses is most likely?

   (A) bipolar I disorder
   (B) bipolar II disorder
   (C) cyclothymic disorder
   (D) double depression
   (E) dysthymic disorder

21. The patient returns within 3 weeks, and he now describes symptoms consistent with a major depressive episode. Which of the following would be the most likely working diagnosis?

   (A) bipolar I disorder
   (B) bipolar II disorder
   (C) cyclothymic disorder
   (D) double depression
   (E) dysthymic disorder

Questions 22 and 23

A 26-year-old white female presents to the psychiatric emergency department in an acutely distressed, nervous state. She complains of terrible anxiety, and the emergency department staff is unable to calm her down or gain an adequate history from the patient. On physical examination, she is slightly diaphoretic, tachycardic, and her pupils are mildly dilated. She is on no medications.

22. Which of the following tests would most likely reveal a medical cause of her symptoms?

   (A) blood glucose
   (B) catecholamine metabolites
   (C) electrocardiogram (ECG)
   (D) thyroid function
   (E) urine toxicology

23. Which of the following substances would be most likely to appear on her urine toxicology results?

   (A) caffeine
   (B) cannabis
   (C) cocaine
   (D) heroin
   (E) LSD

Questions 24 through 26

A 46-year-old man is admitted to the hospital for elective cholecystectomy. On hospital day 4, he is noted to be afebrile, but acutely diaphoretic, tachycardic, hypertensive, tremulous, and agitated. He tears out his sutures and insists on leaving against medical advice (AMA). He is apparently hallucinating, judging from his insistence that he be allowed to "squash those bugs on the wall" (there are none).

24. Which of the following diagnoses is most likely?

(A) brief psychotic disorder
(B) conversion disorder
(C) delirium
(D) delusional disorder
(E) postoperative sepsis

25. Which of the following medications would be most appropriate to treat his condition?

(A) diazepam
(B) disulfiram
(C) oxazepam
(D) phenobarbital
(E) phenytoin

26. If untreated, what would be his most likely mortality rate?

(A) 5%
(B) 10%
(C) 30%
(D) 50%
(E) 60%

Questions 27 and 28

A 62-year-old woman presents to the nursing home where you work as a consulting psychiatrist. She has a history of a bilateral temporal lobectomy for intractable seizures. After a few weeks at the new facility, in addition to her short-term memory difficulties, the staff reports the following observations about the patient: She is extremely docile and displays very little emotion. She has a large appetite and compulsively puts both food and nonfood items in her mouth. She also displays sexual disinhibition, often walking out of her room without her pants on.

27. With which of the following clinical conditions is her behavior most consistent?

(A) Arnold-Chiari syndrome
(B) Klüver-Bucy syndrome
(C) Möbius syndrome
(D) Pick disease
(E) punchdrunk syndrome

28. Neuroimaging would most likely show damage to which temporal lobe structure?

(A) amygdala
(B) hippocampus
(C) inferior horn of the lateral ventricle
(D) insula
(E) superior temporal gyri

Questions 29 and 30

A 22-year-old woman presents with fatigue for 4 months. She also notes irritability and poor energy, with dismal sleep and poor concentration. She has maintained a rigorous exercise routine, as she states it makes her feel good to run off her boyfriend's cooking. Her PO intake has sharply dropped and she has lost a significant amount of weight, but she explains that she "hasn't been as hungry" due to increased stress. Her thyroid studies are normal, her CBC reveals anemia, and she is not pregnant.

29. Upon further questioning, which of the following qualities would you most expect to find in her social history?

(A) Her parents likely praise her successes.
(B) She has a legal history significant for reckless driving.
(C) She has aspired to be a model.
(D) She is of low socioeconomic status.
(E) She is a scholastically gifted perfectionist.

30. Which of the following diagnoses is most likely?

(A) anorexia nervosa
(B) bulimia nervosa

(C)   exercise-induced amenorrhea

(D)   obsessive-compulsive disorder (OCD)

(E)   psychogenic gastritis

31.   A 23-year-old college student has been suffering with frequent episodes of feeling "utter doom" for the past 3 months. During these periods, he also experiences tremulousness, sweating, dizziness, and tingling in his extremities. He reports having these attacks at least once a week and is now becoming fearful of attending classes lest he has an episode. Which of the following medications would be the most appropriate for immediate relief of his symptoms?

(A)   alprazolam (Xanax)

(B)   chlordiazepoxide (Librium)

(C)   divalproex sodium

(D)   fluoxetine (Prozac)

(E)   phenelzine (Nardil)

Questions 32 and 33

A 36-year-old graduate student comes to your office because of difficulty sleeping since breaking up with his fiancée 5 months ago. He is spending at least 2 hours in bed thinking about his ex-fiancée and what he could have done differently. His concentration is worsening and he's having difficulties completing his coursework. While he feels down, he is not suicidal, and he is seeking support of friends in the post-breakup period. He is attending most classes. He describes feeling tenser overall, especially when he is at a bar. He is having more trouble relaxing and has noted the new onset of low back and shoulder pain.

32.   Which of the following is the most likely diagnosis?

(A)   acute stress disorder

(B)   adjustment disorder

(C)   generalized anxiety disorder

(D)   major depressive disorder

(E)   normal reaction

33.   Seven months later, your patient's mood has worsened, and he feels worthless and hopeless that he will never find another mate. He has lost a few pounds and has not resumed dating, preferring to isolate himself in his studio apartment. He is still feeding his dog, but he has had to miss increasing amounts of work because he just can't get himself to get ready for class. Which of the following is the most likely diagnosis at this point?

(A)   acute stress disorder

(B)   adjustment disorder

(C)   generalized anxiety disorder

(D)   major depressive disorder

(E)   normal reaction

34.   A 21-year-old college student is brought to your office by her parents after completing her spring semester with uncharacteristically low grades. Her parents report that since the spring session ended 2 months ago their daughter has been staying in her room, but is irritable when they try to engage her in conversation. She is not interested in family barbeques or being a counselor for the park district soccer camp. After her parents leave the examination room, your patient discloses she has been feeling depressed since a month before final exams, and her concentration and sleep have been "dismal." She had suicidal thoughts after she got her report card back, but denies them currently. She also admits to drinking alcohol to make herself feel better, and her intake ranges from 3 to 4 beers or shots of liquor most days of the week. Aside from likely alcohol abuse, which of the following diagnoses is the most appropriate at this time?

(A)   acute stress disorder

(B)   adjustment disorder

(C)   amotivation syndrome

(D)   major depressive disorder (MDD)

(E)   substance-induced mood disorder

35. A 37-year-old woman, who works the night shift at a local grocery store taking inventory, reports that her childhood and college years were uneventful but happy. She spends most of her time alone when she is not at work. She does not venture out of her house and her social contacts are limited to work-related interactions with coworkers. She is an avid plant lover, and she spends most of her free time taking care of her indoor nursery. She reports that she is quite content with her life. Which of the following is the most likely diagnosis for this patient?

(A) agoraphobia
(B) autistic disorder
(C) avoidant personality disorder
(D) schizoid personality disorder
(E) schizotypal personality disorder

36. An 18-year-old, pregnant, human immunodeficiency virus (HIV)–positive white woman presents for the treatment of heroin addiction. She reports using heroin for the last 8 months with substantial (but unsuccessful) efforts to quit for the last 4 months. She is now homeless and has recently been arrested for shoplifting. Which of the following pharmacological therapies is most appropriate at this time?

(A) buprenorphine
(B) clonidine
(C) haloperidol
(D) hydrocodone
(E) methadone

37. A 47-year-old woman transfers care to your office. She has a long history of recurrent depression. She also has a history since her early twenties that is significant for intermittent command auditory hallucinations and persecutory delusions that are often present even when her affective symptoms are in remission. She holds a part time job and lives independently. She has been compliant with medications and has not been hospitalized since a suicide attempt over 7 years ago. Which of the following is the most likely provisional diagnosis?

(A) bipolar disorder with psychotic features
(B) major depressive disorder with psychotic features
(C) schizoaffective disorder
(D) schizophrenia
(E) schizophreniform disorder

38. A 42-year-old business executive presents for his first contact with a mental health provider. He reports that for the last 4 months he has been feeling depressed. His low energy level and poor motivation are affecting his job performance and the CEO of his company advised him to "take a couple of weeks off." The patient reports that he started feeling down when his wife discovered that he was involved in his third extramarital affair. Since then he has moved into a small apartment by himself. He is sleeping almost 12 hours every night, has a poor appetite, and is experiencing financial difficulty due to indiscriminate purchases. He laments the loss of his former self. He reports that he used to have periods of time when he only needed 4 to 5 hours of sleep, had large amounts of energy, and could "party all night and work all day." Which of the following diagnoses is most likely in this case?

(A) bipolar I disorder
(B) bipolar II disorder
(C) impulse control disorder, not otherwise specified
(D) major depressive disorder
(E) narcissistic personality disorder

39. A 52-year-old woman who has been treated with medication for 3 years for a chronic mood disorder reports that although she feels well, she wonders if her medication is causing side effects. She complains of dry mouth, trouble urinating, and occasional dizziness when she gets out of bed. Which of the following medications is she most likely being prescribed?

(A) divalproex sodium
(B) fluoxetine
(C) imipramine (Tofranil)
(D) lithium
(E) phenelzine

Questions 40 and 41

A 72-year-old man is brought in by his wife to your geriatric psychiatry clinic. The patient's wife is concerned about his progressive confusion over the last year. She is particularly distressed that he repeatedly asks the same questions throughout the day. She also notes that her husband has become increasingly unsteady on his feet and needs to use a walker when they go out. She wonders if these symptoms may be related to the meningitis he suffered from 3 years ago.

40. Which of the following would most likely be found in the additional history of this patient?

    (A) elevated opening pressure upon lumbar puncture
    (B) frontal release signs
    (C) history of incontinence
    (D) oculomotor difficulties
    (E) perseveration

41. Which of the following would most likely be found on neuroimaging with noncontrast computed tomography (CT) in this patient?

    (A) cerebellar atrophy
    (B) dilated lateral ventricles
    (C) focal subcortical hypointensities
    (D) frontoparietal atrophy
    (E) frontotemporal atrophy

Questions 42 through 44

A 69-year-old woman is brought to your geriatric psychiatric clinic by her husband. She denies anything is wrong, but he is concerned that for the past year or so she has been less able to recall things she reads about in her magazines. She used to be in charge of grocery shopping, but over the past year or so she's been leaving things off the list, and her husband has taken over the job since the patient can't seem to organize it anymore. She is no longer able to keep track of the couple's finances, and there have

been several occasions when her son found her wandering outside, a number of houses away. She's otherwise healthy, and takes a multivitamin daily. Her physical examination is unremarkable. Mental status examination reveals a healthy appearing woman who is cooperative with your questions, and laughs when she can't recall any of the three items you ask her to repeat. Her attention is intact. She has some difficulties naming objects. She states her mood as "good" and her affect is euthymic and full range.

42. Which of the following is the most appropriate provisional diagnosis?

    (A) age-related cognitive decline
    (B) delirium
    (C) dementia
    (D) major depression
    (E) normal pressure hydrocephalus

43. A workup is performed. Her laboratory values are unremarkable, and a CT scan of her brain demonstrates diffuse cortical atrophy and normal ventricles. Which of the following diagnoses is most likely?

    (A) Alzheimer dementia
    (B) dementia pugilistica
    (C) Lewy body disease
    (D) pseudodementia
    (E) vascular dementia

44. If the patient's CT scan revealed a preponderance of atrophy in the frontal and temporal regions, your provisional diagnosis would most likely be which of the following?

    (A) Alzheimer dementia
    (B) Binswanger disease
    (C) Lewy body disease
    (D) Pick disease
    (E) vascular dementia

45. A 48-year-old man has been drinking up to 6 beers per night during the week and up to 12 beers a night on the weekend. A year ago, he had his driver's license suspended for drunk driving. His marriage is failing because of these difficulties. Last month, he was diagnosed with a gastric ulcer as a result of alcohol consumption. He admits to an alcohol problem and has tried to stop on numerous occasions. He finds that he experiences insomnia if he does not drink for more than 2 days. Which of the following features of this case suggests alcohol dependence rather than alcohol abuse?

    (A) high quantity of alcohol consumed on a regular basis
    (B) history of drunk driving and license suspension
    (C) inability to stop drinking despite knowing the harmful effects
    (D) marital conflict due to drinking
    (E) sleep problems if no alcohol is consumed

46. A 26-year-old computer programmer without previous psychiatric history has been married for 4 years. His wife is expecting their first child. She reports that 3 months ago the patient became preoccupied with the idea that she became pregnant by another man. During this time, he began missing work and isolated himself in his bedroom. His affect has progressively become more blunted. Recently, he believes that his wife is carrying a child conceived by "extraterrestrial forces." He urged her to have an abortion and she refused. The patient denies any history of substance abuse and his recent medical evaluation was within normal limits. Which of the following is the most appropriate diagnosis?

    (A) brief psychotic disorder
    (B) delusional disorder
    (C) psychosis not otherwise specified
    (D) schizophreniform disorder
    (E) schizophrenia

47. A 27-year-old woman was involved in a train derailment 2 weeks ago. Since that event, she has experienced recurrent thoughts of the accident and has recurrent nightmares each night.

Lately, she has changed her commute to avoid the train, even though this adds 3 hours to her commute daily. When on the train she has an acute increase in her anxiety. She also often becomes "jumpy" whenever she hears the train going by her home. Which of the following diagnoses is the most appropriate for this patient?

    (A) acute stress disorder
    (B) adjustment disorder
    (C) generalized anxiety disorder (GAD)
    (D) posttraumatic stress disorder (PTSD)
    (E) major depressive disorder (MDD)

Questions 48 and 49

A 40-year-old woman with a 20-year history of schizophrenia presents to the psychiatric emergency department after a suicide attempt by carbon monoxide poisoning. She has ongoing command hallucinations to harm herself, and has acted on them at least 10 times since her initial diagnosis. She also has persistent delusions that she is responsible for world disasters, which is why she must eliminate herself as the source of pain and suffering in the world. She has been tried on both typical and atypical antipsychotics, though none have been effective in fully eliminating her psychotic symptoms. Her level of functioning remains poor, and she presently lives in a group home.

48. Which of the following is this patient's most likely lifetime risk of suicide?

    (A) 1%
    (B) 5%
    (C) 10%
    (D) 30%
    (E) 50%

49. Which of the following medications would be the most appropriate to prescribe for this patient?

    (A) clozapine
    (B) fluphenazine
    (C) haloperidol
    (D) lithium
    (E) ziprasidone

50. A 27-year-old internal medicine resident generally dislikes working in an outpatient clinic. Today, however, he is looking forward to his clinical work because one of his appointments is a follow-up visit for a single, attractive 31-year-old woman who is finishing her antibiotic regimen for treatment of pneumonia. The best psychodynamic term for this doctor's response to his patient is which of the following?

(A) countertransference
(B) empathy
(C) identification
(D) projection
(E) transference

Questions 51 through 53

A 31-year-old woman was admitted to a psychiatric unit after attempting suicide by overdose. She had recently broken up with her boyfriend of 4 months. She also admits to episodes of mood lability, marked by feelings of depression and anger directed toward the psychiatric resident who completed the rotation 5 days after her admission. When the resident left, she reported that she was having urges to cut her wrists. She has had numerous admissions for suicidal gestures and a lifelong history of tumultuous romantic relationships. As the patient nears her discharge date, she reports that "all the staff hates me except for Dr. Johnson." Dr. Johnson, a medical student, had a recent difference of opinion with the nursing staff regarding the patient's discharge.

51. Which of the following diagnoses is the most appropriate for this patient?

(A) borderline personality disorder
(B) cyclothymic disorder
(C) histrionic personality disorder
(D) major depressive disorder (MDD)
(E) schizoaffective disorder

52. Which of the following would be the most appropriate outpatient treatment for this patient?

(A) antidepressants
(B) benzodiazepines
(C) group psychotherapy
(D) individual psychotherapy
(E) mood stabilizers

53. In this patient, which type of psychotherapy would be the most efficacious?

(A) cognitive behavioral therapy (CBT)
(B) dialectical behavioral therapy (DBT)
(C) group therapy
(D) psychoanalysis
(E) psychodynamic therapy

Questions 54 and 55

A 34-year-old woman presents for the treatment of her severe, medication-refractory, major depressive disorder. She is referred to you by her outpatient psychiatrist because of your expertise in electroconvulsive therapy (ECT). After reviewing her past psychiatric history and interviewing the patient, you conclude that she would be appropriate for ECT.

54. In discussing the effects of ECT with the patient, which of the following should you tell her is the most likely side effect?

(A) amnesia
(B) aspiration
(C) cardiac arrhythmias
(D) convulsion fractures
(E) psychosis

55. For the best possible outcome, how many treatments is this patient likely to require?

(A) 2
(B) 4
(C) 10
(D) 15
(E) 20

Questions 56 and 57

A 38-year-old woman presents to your clinic telling you that she has had disturbing, recurrent thoughts about harming her 7-month-old infant. She imagines using a knife to stab her child, but she has no desire to hurt her child. As a result of having these distressing thoughts, she has removed all sharp objects from her kitchen. Because of this, she has not been able to prepare meals at home and has chosen to buy fast food or take-out for the family meals. She feels very anxious regarding these, although she has not shared these thoughts with her husband.

56. Which of the following diagnoses would be the most accurate for this patient?

    (A) impulse control disorder, not otherwise specified
    (B) obsessive-compulsive disorder
    (C) obsessive-compulsive personality disorder
    (D) schizophrenia
    (E) schizotypal personality disorder

57. Which of the following would be the most appropriate first-line pharmacotherapy for this condition?

    (A) lithium
    (B) lorazepam (Ativan)
    (C) fluvoxamine (Luvox)
    (D) haloperidol
    (E) nortriptyline (Pamelor)

Questions 58 through 61

A 72-year-old woman is brought to the emergency department from a nursing home for poor oral intake. She is afebrile, has a pulse of 95, and a blood pressure of 90/60. Mental status examination (MSE) reveals an awake and alert, but frail, malnourished and dehydrated woman who is oriented to person only. She reports that the president is Lyndon B. Johnson. She is easily distracted and cannot recall any of three items after a few minutes. She is irritable and swats at the staff when they try to insert an IV. The team starts IV fluids as blood and urine are sent to the laboratory; chest x-ray is unremarkable, as is the head CT. One hour later, she is calmer and reports the correct day, time, and place; she is less distractible.

58. Labs are remarkable for leukocytosis and dirty urinalysis. Aside from cystitis, which of the following is the most appropriate diagnosis for the patient?

    (A) amnestic disorder, not otherwise specified
    (B) cognitive disorder, not otherwise specified
    (C) delirium
    (D) dementia, not otherwise specified
    (E) major depressive disorder

59. The patient is subsequently admitted, but tries to hit several staff as they tend to her; she also repeatedly tries to get out of bed and demands to be let go. Which of the following would be the most appropriate immediate pharmacologic management for this patient?

    (A) diphenhydramine
    (B) haloperidol
    (C) lorazepam
    (D) phenobarbital
    (E) valproic acid

60. Which of the following would be the most appropriate long-term treatment of this patient?

    (A) antibiotic therapy
    (B) chest x-ray every 6 months
    (C) CT head every 6 months
    (D) indwelling Foley catheter
    (E) intravenous fluids

61. Which of the following is the most likely 3-month mortality of the diagnosis in Question 58?

    (A) 5%
    (B) 15%
    (C) 25%
    (D) 35%
    (E) 45%

Questions 62 and 63

You are a research psychiatrist conducting a double-blind, placebo-controlled trial of a new antidepressant. You have enrolled 200 patients in the study, all of whom meet the criteria for uncomplicated major depression. You plan to randomize 100 patients to a placebo medication and the other 100 patients to the experimental antidepressant.

62. Of the 100 patients taking the placebo, approximately how many patients would be expected to improve after 4 to 6 weeks?

(A) 5
(B) 10
(C) 30
(D) 50
(E) 70

63. Of the 100 patients taking the experimental antidepressant (assuming this drug is as efficacious as standard antidepressants), approximately how many patients would be expected to improve after 4 to 6 weeks?

(A) 10
(B) 30
(C) 50
(D) 70
(E) 90

Questions 64 and 65

Your patient is a 38-year-old divorced Catholic male with a month long history of depressed mood, anhedonia, initial insomnia, low energy, and poor appetite. He admits to suicidal ideation with a plan to overdose for the past several days, and he has gathered pills this morning. Upon further history, he admits to similar symptoms 5 years prior, also with a prior suicide attempt by overdosing. He drinks 1 beer weekly and denies illicit drugs. He is on no other medications except for a multivitamin. He is subsequently admitted after being medically cleared.

64. What percentage of patients with this illness eventually commit suicide?

(A) 1%
(B) 5%
(C) 10%
(D) 15%
(E) 20%

65. Which of the following characteristics of this patient is the number one predictor of a future completed suicide?

(A) age
(B) gender
(C) previous attempt
(D) relationship status
(E) religion

66. A 32-year-old single successful Wall Street executive tells you that on weekends he likes to visit a dominatrix. His regular, paid appointment with this person is described as humiliating and somewhat painful but also very sexually arousing. While he admits that this behavior "may be weird to some people," he enjoys it, can afford it, and it doesn't interfere with his work or other hobbies. Which of the following diagnoses is the most appropriate?

(A) fetishism
(B) frotteurism
(C) no diagnosis
(D) sexual masochism
(E) sexual sadism

Questions 67 and 68

A 28-year-old woman complains of falling asleep during the day. This problem has been occurring for 3 months and is now interfering with her work as a telephone operator as she falls asleep two or three times a day while speaking with customers. At times, she finds herself falling asleep at her desk, and she is awakened when her head hits the computer console in front of her. Oddly enough, she reports, this can happen when she becomes particularly stressed out, for example, if she is managing many calls. The patient also states that this disturbance has not improved despite her sleeping 8 hours each night.

67. Which of the following is the most appropriate diagnosis for this case?

(A) circadian rhythm sleep disorder
(B) dyssomnia, not otherwise specified
(C) narcolepsy
(D) nightmare disorder
(E) primary hypersomnia

68. Which of the following is the most appropriate pharmacotherapy for this condition?

    (A) bupropion (Wellbutrin)
    (B) fluoxetine
    (C) lorazepam
    (D) methylphenidate (Ritalin)
    (E) phenelzine

69. A 28-year-old woman presents for her annual gynecology appointment. She complains that in the week before her period, she often experiences marked anger and irritability and argues more with her boyfriend. She also reports diminished energy and concentration, and is sleeping more than is usual for her. These symptoms, in addition to breast tenderness and headaches, always remit in the week after her menses is finished. Which of the following is the most likely diagnosis?

    (A) dysthymic disorder
    (B) major depressive disorder
    (C) no diagnosis
    (D) premenstrual dysphoric disorder (PMDD)
    (E) premenstrual syndrome (PMS)

70. Mr P is a 37-year-old accountant who presents to the primary care clinic with complaints of insomnia. Upon further questioning, he admits that he has felt "blue" for 6 weeks since getting passed over for promotion. Since that time, he has had poor sleep, often awakening early in the morning. He also has had a decreased appetite with a 10- to 15-lb weight loss, poor energy, guilt over "not being good enough," and he has been distracted at work. He also admits to passive suicidal thoughts without a plan. Which of the following would be the likely course of this patient's illness if not treated?

    (A) 3 to 6 months
    (B) 3 to 7 months
    (C) 6 to 13 months
    (D) 9 to 15 months
    (E) 12 to 18 months

Questions 71 and 72

A 36-year-old man is brought to the emergency department in respiratory arrest. On examination, he is bradycardic and unresponsive. He has constricted pupils bilaterally. The team has difficulty establishing IV access, but is able to do so temporarily in the foot. There are no other obvious injuries on the patient, but no one is immediately available to provide collateral history. There is suspicion that the patient's condition may be the result of an overdose.

71. Which of the following drugs is most likely to cause this presentation?

    (A) alcohol
    (B) cocaine
    (C) heroin
    (D) inhalants
    (E) phencyclidine (PCP)

72. Which of the following would be most important to administer immediately?

    (A) acetylcysteine
    (B) deferoxamine
    (C) methadone
    (D) methylene blue
    (E) naloxone

73. A 25-year-old male veteran from Operation Iraqi Freedom/Operation Enduring Freedom presents to the mental health clinic at the urging of his wife. While stationed in Iraq on his third deployment, his unit was hit by a roadside bomb. He saw a fellow Marine killed, while he and several other members of the command sustained nonlethal injuries. Since that time, he has had chronic insomnia with ongoing nightmares of the event as well as occasional flashbacks. He describes always feeling "on edge," avoiding crowds, and becoming easily startled with loud noises. He admits to regular alcohol use, especially when his symptoms are worse. He reluctantly discloses to feeling detached from events with his family, preferring to isolate himself. Which of the following is the most appropriate treatment to begin for this patient?

(A) atypical antipsychotic
(B) benzodiazepine
(C) lithium
(D) serotonin-specific reuptake inhibitor (SSRI)
(E) valproic acid

74. A 40-year-old married woman is referred by her internist to a psychologist for further treatment. She presents an 8-month history of recurrent bouts of "terror," associated with chest pain, tachypnea, tremors, flushing, nausea, and fears of impending doom. These episodes last for approximately 15 minutes and do not have a particular trigger. As a result, she has had increasing difficulty traveling far from her home due to concerns over having further attacks in public. Despite adequate treatment with sertraline, she remains symptomatic and in significant distress. Which of the following psychotherapies would be the most appropriate for her condition?

(A) cognitive-behavioral therapy (CBT)
(B) eye movement desensitization and reprocessing (EMDR)
(C) insight-oriented therapy
(D) interpersonal psychotherapy
(E) supportive psychotherapy

Questions 75 and 76

You are treating a 48-year-old housewife on the inpatient medical unit for pyelonephritis; she has responded well to appropriate antibiotic therapy and has been afebrile for the last 24 hours. You inform her of likely discharge if she continues to improve. The next morning, however, she complains of feeling feverish and achy, and having dysuria again. The nursing staff reports that she has a sudden fever of 103°F. You treat the fever with acetaminophen and perform a physical examination, order chest x-rays, draw blood, and order a urinalysis with culture. While you are awaiting these results, the nurse informs you that she witnessed the patient dipping her thermometer into a hot cup of tea before her temperature was taken.

75. Which of the following diagnoses most likely accounts for this woman's behavior?

(A) conversion disorder
(B) factitious disorder
(C) hypochondriasis
(D) malingering
(E) somatization disorder

76. Which of the following is the most likely motivator of this patient's behavior?

(A) conscious desire to assume sick role
(B) conscious desire to avoid work
(C) unconscious desire to assume sick role
(D) unconscious desire to avoid work
(E) unconscious conflict producing symptoms

Questions 77 and 78

A 32-year-old man is brought to the psychiatric emergency department by the police after having been arrested for public nudity. On mental status examination, the patient cannot sit down and is only partly cooperative. He interrupts the interview several times demanding to be allowed to contact his lawyer, "because my rights given to me by God and ordained by the Jeffersonians and Washingtonians and Lincolnians have been infringed...and you, sir, are committing illegalities of the highest order." His speech is pressured. Collateral history from his sister indicates that this patient has been treated for at least two episodes of major depression in the past, one of which resulted in a suicide attempt. He is currently a computer programmer, but has been increasingly stressed at work. One month ago, his girlfriend broke up with him, and since then he has been increasingly irritable. Over the past 2 weeks he has maxed out his credit card from online gambling sites, which he has continued to visit over the past four consecutive nights. Laboratory tests show a negative drug screen and alcohol levels.

77. Which of the following is the most likely diagnosis for this patient?

(A) adjustment disorder
(B) bipolar disorder
(C) brief psychotic disorder
(D) cyclothymic disorder
(E) major depressive disorder (MDD)

78. Which of the following would be the most appropriate pharmacologic treatment for this patient?

    (A) aripiprazole
    (B) carbamazepine
    (C) lamotrigine
    (D) lithium
    (E) oxcarbazepine

79. A 68-year-old man without prior psychiatric history, but with a history of hypertension, hyperlipidemia, and arthritis is admitted for a new left middle cerebral artery stroke. Which of the following psychiatric symptoms would be most likely as a result?

    (A) anxiety
    (B) depression
    (C) mania
    (D) obsessions
    (E) panic attacks

80. A 45-year-old woman with no previous psychiatric history is admitted to neurology for treatment of an acute multiple sclerosis flare. She does not smoke, drink alcohol, or use other illicit drugs. She is started on appropriate therapy and by the third day her initial lower extremity weakness has resolved. However, she also begins to act strangely, and asks you to change her room to prevent the "ninjas outside from creeping in and stealing my soul." She also tells you the nurses have been poisoning her medicine, and that the president of the United States has ordered the nurses to make her death look like an accident. Which of the following diagnoses would be most likely?

    (A) adjustment disorder
    (B) bipolar disorder
    (C) psychotic disorder due to multiple sclerosis
    (D) schizophrenia
    (E) substance-induced psychotic disorder

81. A 42-year-old man presents with a chief complaint of impotence that has troubled him for the last year. Based on epidemiology of known causes in this patient's age group, which of the following is the chance that his problem is due to a psychological cause (rather than a medical cause)?

    (A) 10%
    (B) 30%
    (C) 50%
    (D) 70%
    (E) 90%

82. A 33-year-old male with a history of frequent fighting, aggression, impulsivity, and suicide attempts is referred to a research facility. He receives multiple tests and studies. Upon cerebrospinal fluid (CSF) analysis, which of the following metabolites would be most likely decreased compared to individuals without his problems?

    (A) dopamine
    (B) gamma-aminobutyric acid (GABA)
    (C) glutamate
    (D) norepinephrine
    (E) serotonin

83. A 38-year-old woman with multiple sclerosis of moderate severity has had symptoms of depression and memory loss increasing over the last year. On mental status examination, you notice a blunted affect and decreased speed of mental processing. A magnetic resonance imaging (MRI) examination is most likely to reveal which of the following?

    (A) global cerebral atrophy
    (B) multiple plaques in frontal white matter
    (C) normal brain
    (D) periventricular lacunar infarcts
    (E) ventricular enlargement

84. An 80-year-old widowed woman is admitted to the hospital for "confusion." Her primary medicine team has consulted a psychiatrist to help with the evaluation and management of her condition. On examination today she is somnolent, though earlier this morning she had been alert and aware. She is uncooperative, hostile, and clearly hallucinating. Her insight and

memory are poor. The primary team wishes to know if she is "delirious or demented." Which of the following signs/symptoms in this patient is the most specific for delirium?

(A) combativeness
(B) fluctuating consciousness
(C) poor memory
(D) psychosis
(E) uncooperativeness

85. A happily married graduate student comes to your clinic with complaints of insomnia. She has been unable to fall asleep because she ruminates about grades, money, her relationship, and her young children. During the day she is unable to concentrate because of these worries. She has always been concerned about these, but lately her worries have gotten out of control. She is unable to relax and feels constant tension in her muscles. While she denies symptoms of panic attacks, she has noticed an increase in headaches and gastrointestinal disturbances over the past few months, mostly when her stress level is high. She denies any problems with mood. She denies any recent stressors, changes to her routine, or changes to her husband's routine. Which of the following diagnoses is most likely in this patient?

(A) adjustment disorder
(B) generalized anxiety disorder
(C) obsessive-compulsive disorder
(D) panic disorder
(E) social phobia (social anxiety disorder)

86. You are a research psychiatrist who is studying signs and symptoms associated with certain psychiatric disorders, and notice a category of patients who have sensory gating deficits, short-term memory difficulties, and abnormalities in smooth-pursuit eye movements. Which of the following diagnoses is most likely to be found in this patient population?

(A) attention-deficit/hyperactivity disorder (ADHD)
(B) major depressive disorder (MDD)
(C) obsessive-compulsive disorder (OCD)
(D) posttraumatic stress disorder (PTSD)
(E) schizophrenia

87. A 23-year-old single medical student comes to your office complaining of difficulty sleeping. During the past year, he has been worrying excessively about a number of things, including his studies, his relationship with his parents, and that his girlfriend of 2 years is going to break up with him despite being happy with their relationship. He admits that he has difficulty controlling the time he spends worrying. He notes feeling irritable at times and has been experiencing muscle tension. Because of these symptoms, he has trouble with schoolwork and his grades have suffered. He does not endorse a depressed mood and asks, "Can you help me with my problems?" You diagnose him with generalized anxiety disorder, and prescribe a combination of psychotherapy and benzodiazepines. Three months later, the patient comes back to your office reporting that his mood has been down in the dumps, and he feels like he may never feel better. Recently, he has been thinking that life was not worth living anymore and has passive thoughts of suicide. When asked about specific suicidal plans, he reports ongoing thoughts of overdosing on pills. Which of the following would be the most appropriate next step?

(A) Call his parents and arrange a family meeting.
(B) Discontinue his benzodiazepine and have him return in 1 week.
(C) Refer the patient to the psychiatric emergency department.
(D) Prescribe an antidepressant and have him follow-up with you in 1 month.
(E) Schedule weekly outpatient visits.

88. A 36-year-old married white female presents to the emergency room with a 2-month history of depression, terminal insomnia, fatigue, decreased appetite, anhedonia, and excessive guilt. She reluctantly admits to suicidal ideation for the past week, with thoughts of "taking all of my medicines." After further questioning, she states that "I would never do it" as she is a devout Catholic who attends church regularly. Which of the following characteristics most increases this particular patient's risk of suicide?

(A) age
(B) gender
(C) marital status
(D) recurrent depression
(E) religion

Questions 89 and 90

A 29-year-old married white woman with a past medical history of recurrent migraines is brought to the psychiatric emergency department by her husband who reports that, despite feeling depressed 2 months ago and being compliant with prescribed treatment, she now has been acting bizarre for several days. On initial interview, the patient states, "I feel superbly supreme, and you have no idea what an amazing person I am! I am a direct descendant of Queen Elizabeth!" The patient is talking so rapidly that you cannot interrupt her. Her husband reports that the patient has not slept in over a week, and during the same time period, she has put a down payment for a car, has purchased a diamond tennis bracelet, and has booked an extravagant vacation.

89. Which of the following is the most likely diagnosis?

(A) anxiety disorder
(B) cognitive disorder
(C) mood disorder
(D) psychotic disorder
(E) somatoform disorder

90. You suspect a medication is the cause for her current condition, but neither she nor her husband recall the medication prescribed 2 months ago. Which of the following medications is the most likely etiology?

(A) amitriptyline
(B) clonazepam
(C) fluoxetine
(D) lithium
(E) venlafaxine

91. A 62-year-old male patient with chronic schizophrenia is brought into the emergency department by the police for trespassing. Upon interview, he tells the physician that over the past 3 weeks his television has been talking directly to him. Which of the following terms best describes this phenomenon?

(A) hallucination
(B) idea of reference
(C) illusion
(D) thought broadcasting
(E) thought insertion

92. A 45-year-old patient tells her doctor that after hearing that her husband died, she could not remember leaving her office and going home. In every other respect, her memory is intact. Which of the following types of amnesia is this an example of?

(A) continuous
(B) generalized
(C) localized
(D) retrograde
(E) selective

Questions 93 and 94

A 75-year-old man comes to your office complaining of poor sleep since his wife's death 1 month ago. Since that time, he has been unable to fall asleep, and he has felt "down." He is slightly more isolative now, as many of the activities he enjoyed doing were with his wife. His appetite is decreased, but he is still bathing and cooking. He sometimes feels guilty that she died before him, and is angry with the Lord that he is alive with no "soul mate" anymore. He sometimes hears the voice of his deceased wife encouraging him to move on.

93. Which of the following is the most appropriate diagnosis at this time?

    (A) adjustment disorder
    (B) bereavement
    (C) depressive disorder, not otherwise specified
    (D) major depressive disorder
    (E) schizophrenia

94. Which of the following would be the most appropriate treatment for this patient?

    (A) Hospitalize the patient immediately.
    (B) Prescribe an antidepressant.
    (C) Prescribe an antipsychotic.
    (D) Refer for brief supportive therapy.
    (E) Refer for cognitive behavioral therapy.

95. When asked about his level of education, a 48-year-old man with a history of schizoaffective disorder, depressed type, describes his high school grounds, friends he had at the time, clubs he joined, and his high school graduation ceremony. He concludes by saying, "And that was the end of my schooling." Which of the following terms does this response best demonstrate?

    (A) circumstantiality
    (B) loosening of associations
    (C) perseveration
    (D) pressured speech
    (E) tangentiality

96. In her psychiatrist's office, a patient suddenly lowers herself to the floor, begins flailing about wildly, then flings a garbage pail against the wall, and runs out of the office. Immediately afterward, she returns. She is alert and oriented, yet does not remember the incident. Which of the following is the most likely diagnosis?

    (A) complex partial seizure
    (B) jacksonian seizure
    (C) nonepileptic seizure

    (D) temporal lobe seizure
    (E) tonic-clonic seizure

97. A 26-year-old man newly diagnosed with narcolepsy explains that he has episodes of falling down without any loss of consciousness, precipitated by laughter or anger. Which of the following terms best describes this symptom?

    (A) catalepsy
    (B) cataplexy
    (C) hypersomnia
    (D) hypnagogic hallucinations
    (E) sleep paralysis

98. A 21-year-old man with newly diagnosed schizophrenia has been compliant with his medications and is less psychotic. At his next follow-up appointment, he is noted to be restless and constantly moving. He states that he feels as if he has to be moving all the time and is uncomfortable if he sits still. Which of the following side effects is he most likely experiencing?

    (A) akathisia
    (B) akinesia
    (C) dystonia
    (D) rabbit syndrome
    (E) tardive dyskinesia

99. A 21-year-old woman diagnosed with panic disorder without agoraphobia comes to the outpatient mental health clinic with increased frequency of panic attacks. As a result, she has been unwilling to leave her apartment for several weeks. She also complains of a new feeling, as if her surrounding environment is unreal and strange. Which of the following terms best describes this new symptom?

    (A) depersonalization
    (B) derealization
    (C) dereism
    (D) hypermnesia
    (E) paresthesia

Questions 100 and 101

A 60-year-old man with alcohol dependence is brought to the emergency department by his family after they notice a recent decline in his memory. On evaluation, the patient's remote memory is intact as verified by the family, but his recent recall is severely impaired. When his recent memory is formally tested, the patient provides verbose but erroneous answers in response to questions.

100. Which specific memory difficulties would be most likely demonstrated in this patient?

    (A) anterograde amnesia
    (B) astereognosis
    (C) dissociative amnesia
    (D) prosopagnosia
    (E) retrograde amnesia

101. Which of the following terms best describes the patient's answers in response to recent memory testing?

    (A) clang associations
    (B) confabulation
    (C) flight of ideas
    (D) hypermnesia
    (E) logorrhea

102. A 36-year-old man presents to the emergency department after being found without clothing in the street. He has multiple excoriations all over his body and states that bugs are crawling all over him. His toxicology screen is positive for cocaine. Which of the following terms best describes this particular physical symptom?

    (A) formication
    (B) gustatory hallucination
    (C) hypnagogic hallucination
    (D) hypnopompic hallucination
    (E) synesthesia

Questions 103 and 104

A 66-year-old college professor is seen for a regular checkup. On examination, he demonstrates flat speech with no melodic intonation. In addition, although demonstrating proper word choice and grammar, and eventually reaching a point, his answers are extensive with unnecessary detail.

103. Which of the following terms best describes his type of speech?

    (A) aphasia
    (B) aprosody
    (C) dysarthria
    (D) scanning
    (E) stuttering

104. Which of the following terms best describes the patient's thought process?

    (A) circumstantial
    (B) derailing
    (C) flight of ideas
    (D) loosening of associations
    (E) tangential

105. An 86-year-old woman with multiple medical problems and a recent hip fracture is admitted to the intensive care unit. While in the unit, she awakens at night and mistakes her intravenous (IV) pole for a family member coming for a visit. She calls the nurses to ask them to have the visitor leave until morning. Which of the following terms best describes this phenomenon?

    (A) hallucination
    (B) illusion
    (C) macropsia
    (D) micropsia
    (E) palinopsia

106. A 24-year-old graduate student in philosophy is referred by his student health center for a psychiatric evaluation. Although he claims to have had similar but attenuated symptoms since childhood, since beginning his thesis, he describes an acute worsening of fears that he will contract HIV. While he understands the modes and risks of contraction and practices safe sex, he is unable to "get rid of these thoughts." As a result, he feels compelled to wash his hands many times per day, even to the point of their becoming raw and bleeding. Despite his insight that his

concerns are irrational, he is not able to stop the behaviors. A positron emission tomography (PET) scan of this patient's brain would most likely demonstrate increased activity in which of the following structures?

(A) amygdala
(B) caudate nucleus
(C) cerebellum
(D) hippocampus
(E) parietal lobes

Questions 107 and 108

While interviewing a 78-year-old woman with dementia, Alzheimer type, you discover that, although she is able to recognize objects, she fails to provide an accurate name for many of them. When the patient is shown a pen, she responds, "that thing that you write with," and when shown a watch she replies, "the time teller."

107. Which of the following terms best describes this patient's answers?

(A) apraxia
(B) circumlocution
(C) clang association
(D) confabulation
(E) neologism

108. Which of the following language disorders is most appropriate for this patient's presentation?

(A) alexia
(B) anomia
(C) apraxia
(D) paralinguistic components of speech
(E) prosopagnosia

109. A 36-year-old woman presents with complaints of a depressed mood for the past month. She reports poor sleep, little appetite with weight loss, low energy, decreased concentration, and little libido. She admits to feeling hopeless and suicidal, although she denies a specific plan or intent. She is subsequently begun on paroxetine 20 mg at bedtime. Which of the following symptoms would be most likely to improve the earliest?

(A) decreased libido
(B) depressed mood
(C) hopelessness
(D) poor sleep
(E) suicidal ideation

110. A 35-year-old man complains to his therapist that his new partner enjoys sexual activity only when inflicting pain on him. This disturbs and frustrates the patient. Which of the following best describes the behavior exhibited by his partner?

(A) exhibitionism
(B) frotteurism
(C) sexual masochism
(D) sexual sadism
(E) transvestic fetishism

111. An anxious 23-year-old Asian male, university student presents to student health services claiming that his penis is shrinking into his abdomen. Despite reassurances from the staff and the physician, he remains convinced of this belief. Which of the following syndromes is this patient most likely suffering from?

(A) Capgras syndrome
(B) koro
(C) kuru
(D) taijin-kyofusho
(E) zar

112. A 21-year-old male college student is evaluated by his college student health center after being arrested for masturbating outside of a sorority window late at night. He admits to having watched a particular female student inside the building over a period of several months. Which of the following is the most likely diagnosis?

(A) exhibitionism
(B) hermaphroditism
(C) transsexualism
(D) transvestic fetishism
(E) voyeurism

113. During a shift in the psychiatric emergency room, you are asked to see a 75-year-old man whose family is concerned that he is unable to live by himself. During the interview you begin to suspect dementia as, although the patient smiles and is pleasant, he is not oriented to date, place, or time, does not know who the president is, and is unable to state where he lives. While you are performing a more detailed cognitive assessment, the patient stands uncomfortably close to you as you talk to him. Which of the following terms best describes this behavior?

(A) circumstantiality

(B) flight of ideas

(C) formication

(D) ideas of reference

(E) loss of ego boundaries

Questions 114 and 115

You are asked to see a 32-year-old man who was diagnosed with major depression 2 weeks ago and prescribed fluoxetine (Prozac). Once you enter the room and introduce yourself, you cannot get a question in as the man speaks rapidly about how terrific a doctor you are and how wonderful his life is. He tells you about the three cars he recently purchased. When you try to interrupt him, he says angrily, "You're just like my skinflint wife."

114. Which of the following terms would best describe this patient's affect?

(A) euphoric and bizarre

(B) euthymic

(C) expansive and irritable

(D) guarded and suspicious

(E) labile and dysphoric

115. Which of the following terms would best describe his speech?

(A) agitated

(B) hyperverbal

(C) pressured

(D) tangential

(E) uninterruptible

116. A 23-year-old white graduate student comes to the psychiatric emergency room complaining of anxiety. She has never been seen by a psychiatrist before and is not taking any medications. Her vital signs are notable for a heart rate of 100 beats/min. She is also slightly diaphoretic and has mildly dilated pupils. Given her present state, which area of this patient's brain would most likely demonstrate increased activity?

(A) amygdala

(B) basal ganglia

(C) hippocampus

(D) locus ceruleus

(E) thalamus

117. You are asked to give a psychiatric consultation on a 28-year-old woman with systemic lupus erythematosus who was admitted to the medical service. After you see her, one of your medical colleagues tells you that she will no longer speak to any of them because she "hates all of them" and now insists on seeing you because you are the "best doctor in the hospital." Which of the following terms best describes the patient's behavior?

(A) acting out

(B) externalization

(C) regression

(D) splitting

(E) sublimation

118. A 42-year-old woman with recurrent episodes of major depression is admitted to a medical unit after a car accident that rendered her unconscious. The patient regains consciousness after 3 days and corroborates that she was, indeed, on an antidepressant, but she says she also cannot remember which one. She is started on paroxetine (Paxil) for her depression. Two days after beginning this medication, she develops tachycardia, diaphoresis, and myoclonic jerks. The neurotransmitter most likely associated with the above reaction is synthesized in which of the following central nervous system structures?

(A) caudate nucleus
(B) locus ceruleus
(C) nucleus accumbens
(D) raphe nucleus
(E) substantia nigra

119. A 34-year-old man reveals to his doctor that he derives sexual satisfaction from rubbing up against women he doesn't know while on crowded subway trains. While he has not gotten in trouble as a result, he is increasingly distressed and worried about his behavior. Which of the following is the most likely diagnosis?

(A) exhibitionism
(B) fetishism
(C) frotteurism
(D) pedophilia
(E) voyeurism

120. You are asked to review neuropsychological testing for a 19-year-old patient who is failing classes at his local community college. His results indicate an intelligence quotient (IQ) of 55. Which of the following is the most appropriate diagnosis?

(A) mild mental retardation
(B) moderate mental retardation
(C) no diagnosis (normal intellectual functioning)
(D) profound mental retardation
(E) severe mental retardation

DIRECTIONS (Questions 121 through 145): The following group of numbered items are preceded by a list of lettered options. For each question, select the one lettered option that is *most* closely associated with it. Each lettered option may be used once, multiple times, or not at all.

Questions 121 through 130: Match each scenario with its most likely description.

(A) alcohol intoxication
(B) alcohol withdrawal
(C) amphetamine intoxication
(D) amphetamine withdrawal
(E) caffeine intoxication
(F) caffeine withdrawal
(G) cannabis intoxication
(H) cannabis withdrawal
(I) cocaine intoxication
(J) cocaine withdrawal
(K) hallucinogen intoxication
(L) inhalant intoxication
(M) opioid intoxication
(N) opioid withdrawal
(O) PCP intoxication

121. A 32-year-old single, male with injected conjunctiva can't concentrate at work, laughs readily at his coworkers' doodles, feels "relaxed," and speaks slowly while seemingly focused on the air in front of him.

122. A 45-year-old separated male admitted for depression and suicidal ideation is irritable, asks for extra food, and spends most of the first day sleeping. The chest pain he had on admission has subsided and he has no ECG changes.

123. After recess, a junior high school student smells "funny," is stumbling, feels dizzy and nauseated, yet remains smiling and says she feels "such a rush." By the middle of her next class she has a headache but otherwise feels like she did this morning.

124. A 17-year-old high school student attends a college fraternity party hosted by his elder brother. After several hours, he feels more courageous and approaches ladies he would normally be too shy to engage, his words are slightly slurred, and he has difficulties moving in a straight line. He is slightly flushed and notes mild memory problems for events earlier in the night.

125. A 27-year-old graduate student woke up late and skipped breakfast. She now has a massive headache and is irritable when she walks into her first morning class. She feels like falling asleep and as if she "has the flu" by the end of the morning.

126. A veterinarian technician is brought to the emergency department after attacking what he thought was a cougar (it was a housecat). In the emergency room he is febrile, appears panicked, has nystagmus, and demonstrates unexpected strength and rage.

127. A 35-year-old pilot is brought in for evaluation because he has not slept for days, and now he is anxious, tachycardic, tremulous, and unable to give coherent history. His pupils are dilated and his blood pressure is high, despite normal values 2 weeks ago on a flight physical.

128. A 54-year-old woman with arthritis complains of yawning, diarrhea, abdominal cramps, and nausea. Her pupils are dilated and she has notable piloerection.

129. A 23-year-old man is found unresponsive with slowed breathing. He has multiple scars on his arms and he has severe miosis.

130. On the third postoperative day your 63-year-old patient becomes agitated, demands you remove the snakes from his room, and asks why it's so loud at night (it's daytime). He is tachycardic, hypertensive, and tremulous.

Questions 131 through 136: Match each scenario with the most likely receptor responsible from the following list.

(A) 5-HT2A receptor
(B) alpha receptor
(C) beta receptor
(D) dopamine receptor
(E) histaminergic receptor
(F) muscarinic receptor

131. A 32-year-old man on clozapine experiences constipation.

132. A 29-year-old woman on quetiapine experiences dizziness on standing.

133. A 52-year-old man on risperidone experiences a milky discharge from his breasts.

134. A 41-year-old man on haloperidol experiences resolution of his auditory hallucinations and his delusions.

135. A 22-year-old woman on olanzapine experiences significant sedation and weight gain.

136. A 53-year-old man on quetiapine experiences improvement and stabilization of mood.

Questions 137 through 145: Match each scenario with its most likely defense mechanism from the following list.

(A) altruism
(B) denial
(C) displacement
(D) humor
(E) projection
(F) projective identification
(G) reaction formation
(H) rationalization
(I) splitting

137. A 37-year-old married male is just told by his wife that she has been having an affair. He immediately hugs her and tells her he loves her.

138. Your patient is angry with you and claims you are the worst doctor ever, as opposed to her former clinician, who actually listened to her.

139. Your borderline patient misses seven appointments in a row resulting in your terminating her treatment contract.

140. After slipping in front of your boss on a frozen puddle, you exclaim that "in a former life I was actually an elite figure skater!"

141. Your 69-year-old patient states he just has a bad cold after being diagnosed with metastatic lung cancer, and states all he needs is some hot tea and rest.

142. You argue with the boss at work, and when you come home you harshly groom your cat so that she actually wriggles away out of your arms.

143. A 68-year-old widow volunteers at the local veteran's nursing home.

144. After repeatedly failing to bring your portion of the group project to class, you accuse the group leader of forgetting to e-mail you a reminder.

145. After not matching into your chosen specialty, you say that it was full of boring nerds anyway and that you really have way too much personality to be part of them.

Answers and Explanations

1. **(C)** The patient's 3- to 4-year history of bizarre behavior, delusions, and decline in social functioning strongly suggest that he has schizophrenia. The prevalence of schizophrenia in the general population is approximately 1%. Schizophrenia is found in all societies and geographical areas around the world, and its prevalence is roughly equal.

2. **(D)** In twin studies, schizophrenia's monozygotic concordance is 47%, or approximately 50%, suggesting that there is a strong genetic component to the illness. The prevalence of schizophrenia in the following populations is as follows: 8% in the nontwin sibling of a schizophrenic patient, 12% in the child of one parent with schizophrenia, and 40% in the child of two parents with schizophrenia.

3. **(B)** Cotard syndrome describes nihilistic delusional content; in addition to lost possessions, patients may feel they have lost blood, heart, intestines, as well as that the world beyond them has been reduced to nothingness. This psychotic/delusional theme can be seen in many psychotic illnesses. Capgras syndrome is a delusion of doubles characterized by the belief that people have been replaced by identically appearing imposters. Folie à deux, or shared psychotic disorder, is when a similar delusion is aroused in one person by the close influence of another; both individuals are usually closely associated for a prolonged period of time. The Fregoli delusion is a variation of the delusion of doubles, and is the belief that familiar people assume the guise of strangers. While major depression can manifest with psychotic features, the prominence of psychosis with bizarre delusions makes this diagnosis less likely. Further, though nihilistic themes and negativism can be observed in depression, the delusions are usually nonbizarre.

4. **(A)** The belief that people have been replaced by imposters is the hallmark of Capgras syndrome. Delusional disorder is characterized by the presence of nonbizarre (potentially feasible) delusions. See explanations to Question 3 for further definitions.

5. **(A)** This woman's presentation is consistent with postpartum psychosis, also called puerperal psychosis, characterized by delusions and hallucinations within 1 week of delivery. She further exhibits insomnia, irritability, and mood lability. This, coupled with previous early depressive episodes, strongly suggests an episodic mood disorder. Though post-partum psychosis can be due to different etiologies, most cases eventually manifest as bipolar disorder. However, only a small fraction of women with bipolar disorder will manifest with psychosis. A less frequent underlying etiology is MDD. Primary psychotic illnesses, such as delusional disorder, schizoaffective disorder, and schizophrenia, are even rarer.

6. **(E)** Progressive social withdrawal is commonly seen as part of the prodrome of schizophrenia. All other choices—head trauma, low intelligence, a neglectful mother, and abuse—have not been proven in any conclusive way to be significantly linked to schizophrenia, although early theories held that a history of one or more was a predisposing factor.

7. **(E)** While her history strongly suggests a primary psychotic disorder such as brief psychotic disorder (lasting 1 day-1 month), schizophreniform disorder (lasting 1-6 months), or schizophrenia, the presence of cannabis on her toxicology screen precludes such a diagnosis at this time. Unless her symptoms persist after sobriety from cannabis is attained, her most appropriate diagnosis at this time is a substance-induced (specifically cannabis-induced) psychotic disorder.

8. **(C)** The patient meets Criteria A in *Diagnostic and Statistical Manual of Mental Disorders, Fourth Edition, Text Revision (DSM-IV-TR)* for schizophrenia: for at least 1 month she has exhibited hallucinations, delusions, and disorganized speech. Further her symptoms are occurring outside of an acute mood episode and are not due to a general medical condition. They have persisted for over a year, despite the patient maintaining sobriety from cannabis. Since her psychotic symptoms have lasted longer than 6 months, her most appropriate diagnosis is schizophrenia. Brief psychotic disorder is characterized by psychotic symptoms lasting 1 day to 1 month. Schizophreniform disorder refers to symptoms lasting more than 1 month but less than 6 in the absence of concurrent mood disorder, substance use, or a general medical condition.

9. **(C)** The patient meets the criteria for borderline personality disorder characterized by rapid mood swings, efforts to avoid abandonment, chronic feelings of emptiness, intense anger outbursts, impulsivity, fluctuations between idealization and devaluation, and recurrent self-mutilation or suicidality. Persons with this personality disorder commonly employ primitive defense mechanisms, such as denial, projective identification, and splitting. Splitting is dividing external objects (individuals) into "all good" or "all bad" categories. Altruism (living vicariously by helping others) and sublimation (gratifying urges in socially acceptable ways) are mature defenses, while intellectualization (using intellectual processes to avoid feelings) and undoing (acts performed to undo obsessional thoughts) are considered neurotic defenses.

10. **(E)** Good premorbid functioning portends a better prognosis for this patient. Other features of schizophrenia that predict a better prognosis include later age at presentation, female gender, acute and rapid onset of symptoms (as opposed to insidious onset), and the presence of mood symptoms. While predominantly positive symptoms also predict a more favorable prognosis, this patient has significant negative symptoms, as evidenced by his isolation and amotivation.

11. **(B)** This patient is presenting with several catatonic features, including negativism, psychomotor slowing, and echopraxia, with slight vital sign fluctuations. Catatonia is often underdiagnosed. While catatonia is considered a subtype of schizophrenia, it is found more frequently in affective disorders, especially major depression. This patient's history of isolation, anhedonia, psychomotor retardation, decreased appetite, and guilt (burden on fiancée) are more suggestive of major depression. Hypothyroidism should be ruled out, but catatonia is not a common presentation. There is no evidence to suggest that he is faking symptoms for secondary gain, as in malingering. Malignant catatonia would be correct if he had pronounced vital sign abnormalities, possibly with marked rigidity and elevations in CPK. Nothing in his history suggests the presence of a primary psychotic disorder, making a diagnosis of schizophrenia unlikely.

12. **(D)** The mainstay of treatment for catatonia is pharmacotherapy with benzodiazepines or electroconvulsive therapy. In this case, it is reasonable to attempt a trial of lorazepam and assess for response; if the patient begins to become unstable or requires high doses of lorazepam (>20 mg/d), or if his blood pressure/pulse do not tolerate the titration of lorazepam, ECT would be the appropriate course of action. Amitriptyline, sertraline, or lithium—depending on whether his diagnosis is unipolar or bipolar depression— would be appropriate maintenance therapy once the catatonia is treated.

13. **(B)** This woman's presentation is most consistent with a delusional disorder. Her fixed false belief is nonbizarre (ie, could potentially

happen), she has no other psychotic symptoms, her functioning is still good, and the delusion is isolated to one specific belief. She does not exhibit other psychotic symptoms, making brief psychotic disorder unlikely; further in brief psychotic disorder, symptoms must resolve within 1 month whereas her's have been occurring for at least 2 months. There is no evidence she has a paranoid personality disorder. Schizophrenia and schizophreniform disorder are unlikely since her symptoms are limited to one nonbizarre delusion, and she has no hallucinations, negative symptoms, nor impairment in functioning. In addition, the time course is insufficient for these diagnoses.

14. **(E)** This woman has a profound depression with many lifetime episodes, including several severe suicide attempts. This woman has not responded to several medications or augmentation strategies. The persistence of suicidality in light of the treatment resistance is the most pressing reason to pursue ECT. ECT can induce a rapid response, which would be paramount in this woman. Further, ECT has the best remission rates (up to 80%), markedly more than for medication alone. If her thyroid dysfunction were untreated, this would be a reasonable place to start, however her thyroid abnormality has been stabilized. Her prior history of psychotic symptoms does not necessarily imply she would be a good ECT candidate, but it is further evidence of the severity of her illness. Postpartum depression would spur the decision for ECT if she were currently in the postpartum state, acutely suicidal, and potentially a threat to her infant.

15. **(C)** There is no absolute contraindication to ECT. However, a space-occupying lesion can cause dangerous increases in intracranial pressure. Since ECT causes a temporary increase in cerebral perfusion and the skull is a fixed space (volume), the increase in blood volume causes increased intracranial pressure; a space-occupying lesion reduces the potential reserve the skull has to offset the increase in pressure. Due to the transient tachycardia that occurs with seizures, a recent MI (within 3 months) is

also a relative contraindication to ECT because of excess demands on the myocardium. After that time, however, cardiac risks of ECT are the same as those for general anesthesia. Pacemakers and a history of traumatic brain injury are not contraindications. Pregnancy is also not a contraindication to ECT, and the risks are the same as those of general anesthesia. With recent advances in anesthesia, fractures are uncommon since paralysis is attained for the duration of the induced seizure.

16. **(B)** While many sleep disturbances have been noted in depression (as described by the other choices), early morning awakening has been the most consistently linked with major depression. The decrease in REM sleep latency and slow wave sleep deficits often persist, even after treatment.

17. **(C)** Increased cortisol secretion in patients with depression is one of the earliest observations in biological psychiatry, and has been well borne out in subsequent studies. Levels of MAOs are unknown. Catecholamines, sex hormones, and immune function are decreased in depression.

18. **(B)** The most appropriate next step is to ensure the safety of the patient and others, and escorting the patient to the emergency room with police assistance guarantees this is preserved. Discharge is inappropriate at this time as the patient has made an active threat; while this patient is likely in a manic episode and the homicidal threat is related to the delusion of his mother-in-law, the threat must be taken seriously. States differ in the duty to warn, but at this time in order to maintain safety, admission is necessary. If on discharge the threat remains, the target and law enforcement may need to be notified. It would be inappropriate to have the wife stay with the mother-in-law as this would be putting her in harm's way.

19. **(C)** This patient is suffering from a manic episode, and given his antecedent treatment with an antidepressant, paroxetine, it is likely the antidepressant induced the manic switch. In addition to achieving mood stabilization through valproate, it is critical to stop the offending agent. While SSRIs are used in bipolar

patients with depressive episodes, their use is not recommended as monotherapy due to this potential to induce mania. Paroxetine levels are not used clinically. Nortriptyline would be less appropriate than paroxetine as tricyclic antidepressants are more likely than SSRIs to induce mania. Bupropion is also an antidepressant and would not be appropriate at this time. Lorazepam may help with agitation, but the more appropriate step is to stop the offending agent.

20. **(C)** Cyclothymia is characterized by episodic mood disturbances of hypomania and subclinical depression. Treatment is the same as for bipolar disorder. For a diagnosis of bipolar I, only a manic episode is necessary, though most patients will suffer from depressive episodes as well. Bipolar II disorder is characterized by major depressive episodes and hypomanic episodes. Dysthymic disorder is a chronic depression that does not meet severity for a major depressive episode; in dysthymia, symptoms persist for 2 years, with no more than 2 months of symptom- free periods. "Double depression" occurs when a major depressive episode is superimposed on dysthymic disorder.

21. **(B)** Bipolar II disorder is characterized by major depressive episodes and hypomanic episodes. See explanation for Question 20 for remaining definitions.

22. **(E)** In this young patient on no medications, a urine toxicology screen is most likely to determine the cause of her current state, probably due to a drug intoxication. Blood glucose is important to test as hypoglycemia can present with diaphoresis; however, it would be unlikely in this otherwise healthy woman. Catecholamine metabolites would be premature at this time. An ECG would be part of a workup to rule out any arrhythmias, but any abnormalities would not necessarily point to a specific etiology. Thyroid function tests are important, as thyrotoxicosis can manifest with panic-type symptoms, but again, in a healthy woman with acute onset of symptoms, the urine drug screen is more likely to yield an etiology.

23. **(C)** This patient is manifesting signs and symptoms of acute cocaine intoxication, including tachycardia, diaphoresis, and pupillary dilation. Caffeine is not routinely tested on urine tox screens and wouldn't cause such a severe reaction. Cannabis intoxication may present with anxiety and paranoia, as well as conjunctival injection, but it does not result in dilation of the pupils. Heroin and other opiatuse will usually present with sedation, respiratory depression, and constricted (pinpoint) pupils. LSD will often cause prominent hallucinations during intoxication.

24. **(C)** This patient has acute mental status changes, associated with vital sign abnormalities and hallucinations. This presentation is suspicious for acute delirium, specifically delirium tremens (DTs) due to alcohol withdrawal. DTs can be lethal. The likelihood for onset is highest in the third to fifth day after the last drink. While postoperative sepsis is another cause of delirium, lack of fever makes this less likely than alcohol withdrawal. Brief psychotic disorder, conversion disorder, and delusional disorder do not fit the acute onset of symptoms with alterations in the level of consciousness and vital sign abnormalities. In addition, conversion disorder does not usually manifest with hallucinations.

25. **(C)** Benzodiazepines are the mainstay of treatment for delirium tremens. Of the choices, only diazepam and oxazepam are benzodiazepines; diazepam is less ideal than oxazepam because it has active metabolites and undergoes extensive metabolism in the liver. Oxazepam and lorazepam are not dependent on liver function for their metabolism; they are therefore ideal to treat DTs in patients with underlying liver disease. Disulfiram is not appropriate in the acute treatment of DTs, but may have a role in sustained abstinence. Phenobarbital may be required to induce sedation in patients who develop seizures despite benzodiazepine treatment or those who require high doses of benzodiazepines (eg, enough to require intubation). Phenytoin does not have a role in acute DTs treatment.

26. **(C)** Delirium tremens, if untreated, has a mortality rate of close to 30%. Early recognition and treatment of alcohol withdrawal can prevent DTs in many cases.

27. **(B)** Klüver-Bucy syndrome presents with docility, lack of fear response, anterograde amnesia, hyperphagia, and hypersexuality. Arnold-Chiari syndrome describes a condition with hydrocephalus and cerebellar anatomic and functional abnormalities. Möbius syndrome is a congenital absence of the facial nerves and nuclei with resulting bilateral facial paralysis. Pick disease is a form of dementia, often indistinguishable from Alzheimer disease, in which the frontal and temporal lobes are preferentially atrophied. Punchdrunk syndrome describes an acquired movement disorder associated with traumatic damage to the substantia nigra, for example from boxing.

28. **(A)** Klüver-Bucy syndrome is most closely associated with severe damage to, or disconnectivity of, the amygdala bilaterally. The hippocampus, although important to short-term memory, is not directly involved with regulating aggressive drives, sexual behaviors, or fear responses. The lateral ventricle is a CSF-containing space that has no direct neuropsychiatric functional role. The insula, found deep within the central sulcus, is medial to the temporal lobe and not involved in Klüver-Bucy syndrome. Superior temporal gyri are more generally involved with processing complex auditory information such as the understanding of language.

29. **(E)** This patient is suffering from an eating disorder, possibly anorexia nervosa. Many patients with eating disorders have strong drives for perfection. Psychodynamically, patients often feel a lack of control and seek to control the one thing they perceive they can, that is, food. Further, patients also lack a sense of validation from caregivers. They don't characteristically have legal problems, and often are of a high socioeconomic status.

30. **(A)** While this patient's BMI is not given, and there is no data on the presence or absence of amenorrhea, this patient's most likely diagnosis is anorexia nervosa. She exhibits intense food restriction as well as compensatory behaviors of overexercising to make up for any caloric intake she may have had. Anemia is not uncommon in patients with anorexia, and fatigue is a frequent complaint. In bulimia, patients will engage in food binges, consuming large quantities of food and later feeling intense guilt and shame. Bulimic patients may also engage in compensatory mechanisms, such as laxatives, ipecac, self-induced vomiting, and overexercise to "make up" for the caloric intake. Exercise-induced amenorrhea is possible, but less likely given this patient's distorted necessity to compensate for any food intake. Many anorectic patients have obsessive-compulsive tendencies (perfectionism), but there is no indication that the patient has OCD. The presentation is not consistent with psychogenic gastritis.

31. **(A)** Benzodiazepines are effective in acutely stopping a panic attack such as described in the vignette. Alprazolam has the shortest half life as well as the most rapid onset of action, and is therefore the agent most likely to abort the panic attack. However, because of these same qualities, it also has significant abuse potential and requires at least BID (twice a day) dosing to prevent withdrawal symptoms. Librium is a longer acting benzodiazepine but does not have as rapid an onset of action. Depakote and phenelzine are not indicated for this patient in the absence of mood instability or psychosis, respectively. Fluoxetine and other serotonin reuptake inhibitors (SSRIs) are indicated for the treatment of panic disorder, but onset of symptom relief may take weeks. As such, many clinicians will start an SSRI but will also add an adjunctive benzodiazepine for the first few weeks of treatment, until the SSRI starts to take effect.

32. **(B)** At this time his diagnosis is most consistent with an adjustment disorder, specifically with anxiety. Adjustment disorder notes the onset of mood and behavioral changes following an acute stressor. The symptoms remit within 6 months after the stressor. In acute stress disorder, the patient is exposed to a traumatic event and experiences reexperiencing

(eg, flashbacks), numbing, and increased arousal symptoms for up to 1 month after the event. A breakup is not typically "traumatic" in the sense that life is not usually threatened. While this patient has an inability to relax an associated muscle tension, symptoms commonly associated with generalized anxiety disorder, his worries are limited to the recent relationship, and his symptoms have not been long-standing. The patient does not meet criteria for major depressive disorder at this time, but if his symptoms persist or worsen, this diagnosis should be considered. This patient's symptoms are more than what would be expected for a normal reaction—his sleep has been disrupted and it is starting to affect his schoolwork for the past 5 weeks.

33. **(D)** At this time the patient's condition has worsened, and he now has a pervasive depressed mood and disturbance in sleep, appetite, concentration as well as associated hopelessness and worthlessness. In addition to worsening self care, his symptoms are now significantly affecting his schoolwork and quality of life. He therefore now meets criteria for major depression and warrants appropriate treatment, whether with medication, therapy, or both.

34. **(E)** While this patient's symptoms are consistent with MDD, her ongoing alcohol use precludes the diagnosis at this time; therefore, substance-induced mood disorder is the most likely diagnosis. If she remains sober for a period of time and her depressive symptoms continue, she would then be diagnosed with MDD. Amotivation syndrome is a controversial syndrome associated with cannabis use, and is not appropriate in this case given the lack of cannabis use. In acute stress disorder, the patient is exposed to a traumatic event and experiences reexperiencing (eg, flashbacks), numbing, and increased arousal symptoms for up to 1 month after the event. Adjustment disorder is characterized by the onset of mood and behavioral changes following an acute stressor.

35. **(D)** Persons with schizoid personality disorder are reclusive and do not mind the lack of social interaction. Agoraphobia is tied to the fear of having panic symptoms in public. Such symptoms are not mentioned in this case. Autistic disorder is a pervasive developmental disorder. Patients have pronounced deficits in language, communication, and socialization, which are not evident in this case of a woman who had uneventful but happy formative years. Persons with avoidant personality disorder are shy and fearful of social rejection. However, their lack of socialization is distressing to them. Schizotypal individuals can have schizoid features but they also have bizarre thinking.

36. **(E)** Methadone maintenance is the most appropriate pharmacological therapy for treatment of heroin addiction, even in pregnancy. Methadone maintenance, especially when combined with psychosocial services and obstetric monitoring, significantly improves neonatal outcomes and obstetric outcomes for heroin-addicted women. The lowest effective dose should be used, and no withdrawal to abstinence should be attempted during pregnancy. There are no known teratogenic effects from methadone. Women may require higher doses of methadone in the third trimester due to increased metabolism of the drug at that time. Buprenorphine is a partial opiate agonist that has a role in maintenance treatment, but its safety during pregnancy and breastfeeding has not been definitively established. Clonidine can be used to treat hypertension and other symptoms during acute opiate withdrawal. While haloperidol (a first-generation antipsychotic) may be used safely in pregnancy, it has no use for the treatment of heroin dependence unless agitation from acute withdrawal is problematic. Hydrocodone is a narcotic analgesic which may decrease opiate withdrawal symptomatology, but is not appropriate in this case.

37. **(C)** This patient exhibits episodic mood symptoms as well as chronic psychotic symptoms outside of those mood episodes, making her most likely diagnosis schizoaffective disorder. There is no evidence of prior manic episodes, making bipolar disorder unlikely. If the hallucinations and delusions only occurred in the context of her depressive episodes, the most

likely diagnosis would be major depression with psychotic features. While schizophrenia would be on the differential, her affective (depressive) symptoms are prominent. Schizophreniform disorder is characterized by symptoms of schizophrenia which last from 1 month to 6 months, so this is not appropriate given the chronicity of her symptoms.

38. **(B)** This patient's history is consistent with a mood pattern defined by periods of hypomania (symptoms of mania not severe enough to cause occupational dysfunction or psychiatric hospitalization) and currently a major depressive episode. Hypomania with major depression defines bipolar II disorder. In bipolar I disorder, the mania is more severe causing notable occupational dysfunction, psychotic symptoms, or hospitalization. While this patient is in the midst of a major depressive episode, his history of hypomania indicates a bipolar diagnosis; this is an important distinction because improper treatment with antidepressants can precipitate a manic episode. This patient does display impulsivity but an impulse control disorder can be diagnosed only after the exclusion of a major mental illness such as bipolar disorder, which may have impulsive features. Narcissistic personality disorder is an Axis II diagnosis characterized by a pervasive pattern of grandiosity, need for admiration, and lack of empathy.

39. **(C)** Dry mouth, dizziness (associated with hypotension), and urinary hesitancy are due to anticholinergic and antiadrenergic effects of tricyclic antidepressants (TCAs) such as imipramine. Divalproex sodium is a mood stabilizer that may cause gastrointestinal upset but is otherwise commonly associated with sedation and tremor at higher doses. Fluoxetine, a serotonin-specific reuptake inhibitor (SSRI), is most often associated with gastrointestinal upset, sexual dysfunction, and activation/agitation. Lithium is another mood stabilizer, used in bipolar disorder, most often associated with polyuria, polydipsia, tremor, and mental confusion at higher doses. Phenelzine, a monoamine oxidase inhibitor (MAOI), can be associated with hypotension but is less likely to have anticholinergic effects.

40. **(C)** This patient likely has normal pressure hydrocephalus (NPH), one of the few potentially reversible causes of dementia. The classic triad of NPH is confusion, gait apraxia, and incontinence. Elevated opening pressure is not found in NPH (thus the "normal pressure" part of the diagnosis). Frontal release signs and perseveration are nonspecific findings common in demented patients but not specific to NPH. Oculomotor difficulties are a part of the Wernicke-Korsakoff syndrome.

41. **(B)** In NPH, CT scan commonly reveals dilated ventricles thought to be the result of increased pressure waves impinging within the ventricular system. Cerebellar atrophy is seen most often in congenital disorders and alcoholism. Hypointensities found in subcortical areas are often indicative of lacunar strokes. Frontoparietal atrophy is seen in Alzheimer dementia. Frontotemporal atrophy is found in Pick disease, an uncommon type of dementia.

42. **(C)** This patient is most likely suffering from dementia, characterized by progressive impairment of cognitive function in the absence of delirium. Memory impairment and loss of function in at least one other cognitive domain are hallmarks. While some loss of cognitive function is expected with age, it is too severe and this patient is no longer able to function independently. Delirium is characterized by acute mental status change with deficits in attention (ie, fluctuating levels of consciousness). There is no indication of depression or the gait apraxia and urinary incontinence characteristic of normal pressure hydrocephalus.

43. **(A)** The most common type of dementia is Alzheimer type, which demonstrates diffuse atrophy. Dementia pugilistica (punchdrunk syndrome) is a type of dementia seen following repeated head trauma over years (as in boxers) and is characterized by emotional lability, dysarthria, and impulsivity. Lewy body disease is clinically similar to Alzheimer, but also

includes hallucinations, parkinsonian features, and extrapyramidal signs. Pseudodementia refers to a condition where the patient demonstrates symptoms consistent with memory difficulties, but in the absence of a dementia; it is often seen in depression. Patients with pseudodementia usually have more depressive symptoms, have more insight into their symptoms than demented patients, and will often have a history of depression. Vascular dementia (formerly multi-infarct dementia) is the second most common type of dementia, and involves small widespread lacunar infarcts. It is seen in those with hypertension or other cardiovascular disease.

44. **(D)** Pick disease is a dementia characterized by preferential atrophy of the frontotemporal region, as opposed to the parietotemporal distribution seen in Alzheimer disease. Binswanger disease refers to subcortical arteriosclerotic encephalopathy, and is characterized by multiple small infarcts in the white matter with sparing of the cortical regions. The other definitions are given in the explanation for Question 43.

45. **(C)** The patient's inability to quit drinking regardless of a desire to quit or knowledge of its negative aspects best differentiates dependence from abuse. Neither dependence nor abuse is determined based on quantity of alcohol consumed. The patient's history of drunk driving and marital problems are both consequences of his ongoing alcohol use, which, according to the *DSM-IV-TR*, are consistent with abuse. The patient's statement that he cannot sleep when he tries to quit drinking does imply physiologic dependence but the alcohol dependence criteria can be met with a "without physiologic dependence" qualifier.

46. **(D)** This patient would meet the criteria for schizophrenia except that the duration of his illness has been less than 6 months. Brief psychotic disorder may present with psychosis but the duration of the disturbance must be 1 month or less. This patient's delusions are too bizarre to meet the criteria for delusional disorder, and the age of onset for delusional disorder is usually

middle age. Psychosis, not otherwise specified, is reserved for cases of psychosis in which the etiology is not known or full criteria for another psychotic disorder are not met.

47. **(A)** This patient has symptoms consistent with PTSD or acute stress disorder (ie, traumatic event, intrusive memories of trauma, avoidance of reminders, hypervigilance), but the fact that the trauma was only 3 weeks prior means that she would be diagnosed with acute distress disorder. If her symptoms persist after 4 weeks, then she would be diagnosed with PTSD. Adjustment disorder most often represents a change in mood, anxiety, or conduct that happens after a nontraumatic event. In GAD, there is no associated trauma, and the symptoms of anxiety last for at least 6 months. The patient has no evidence of a primary depressive illness such as MDD.

48. **(C)** The lifetime incidence of suicide in patients with schizophrenia is approximately 10%, compared with less than 1% in the general population.

49. **(A)** Clozapine, the first atypical antipsychotic, has been shown to decrease suicidality in schizophrenic patients and is particularly effective in treatment-refractory patients, such as the one in this example. Because of possible side effects (potentially deadly agranulocytosis), it requires regular blood monitoring. None of the remaining antipsychotics, such as fluphenazine, haloperidol, or ziprasidone, have been shown to be effective in treatment-refractory schizophrenia or to decrease suicidality. While lithium has also been shown to decrease suicidality, its use is not indicated in this case given lack of any affective symptoms.

50. **(A)** Feelings and attitudes originating from the clinician, evoked by the patient, are called countertransference. Transference denotes feelings and attitudes about the physician coming from the patient. Empathy is the ability of the clinician to psychologically "put himself in his patient's shoes" and thereby understand his patient's thinking, feelings, or behavior. Identification is a defense mechanism

characterized by the unconscious incorporation of someone else's traits into one's own manner—for example, adolescents having hairstyles similar to admired rock stars. Projection is a primitive defense mechanism whereby one assigns emotions to another person in an attempt to psychologically defend against (cover up) the presence of those emotions within oneself; for example, the doctor in the case may tell his fellow resident that he believes that his female patient is attracted to him, when in actuality he is attracted to her.

51. **(A)** This patient displays symptoms of fear of loss and abandonment, intense interpersonal relationships, recurrent suicidal behavior or threats, affective instability, and difficulty controlling intense anger, consistent with borderline personality disorder. Patients with cyclothymia often present with similar symptoms, namely their prominent mood instability and impulsivity. In this case, the other criteria for borderline personality disorder are met. Patients with histrionic personality disorder, like those with borderline personality disorder, may display excessive emotionality and attention seeking, but their core symptoms center around superficial seductiveness and theatricality. While patients with borderline personality disorder may have depressive symptoms that develop into MDD, this patient's depressive symptoms are fleeting and in response to stressors such as perceived abandonment. Although this patient appears paranoid that "all the staff hates me," there is no other evidence for a primary psychotic illness such as schizoaffective disorder.

52. **(D)** Individual psychotherapy and steady social support represent the best long-term method for the management of borderline personality disorder. Antidepressants, neuroleptics, and mood stabilizers have all been shown to have some efficacy in treating target symptoms in some borderline patients. Benzodiazepines may treat anxiety in these patients, but they have particular abuse liability in these impulsive patients.

53. **(B)** Psychotherapy is the mainstay of borderline personality disorder treatment. Of the available types of therapy, dialectical behavioral therapy has shown to be particularly effective with borderline individuals, especially when used in conjunction with groups. DBT is an offshoot from cognitive behavioral therapy and focuses on mindfulness and distress tolerance. CBT is often a short course of therapy focused on dysfunctional thoughts with their resulting behavioral and emotional manifestations. Group therapy is a component of DBT, but should be used in conjunction with, not in place of, individual therapy. Psychoanalysis and psychodynamic therapies utilize psychoanalytic principles and focus on formative childhood experiences and the recurrent patterns of behaviors in interpersonal relationships, unresolved feelings, and building of ego defenses. While these therapies may be of benefit, the regression and intense emotions evoked may be too difficult for the patient to handle.

54. **(A)** Amnesia is a common side effect of ECT, presenting in the form of short-term memory deficits. Aspiration, fractures, and arrhythmias are rare side effects. Psychosis can be improved, rather than worsened, with ECT; in fact, ECT is a treatment of choice in patients with major depression with psychotic features.

55. **(C)** For major depression, 6 to 12 sessions are generally optimal for a good risk-benefit ratio of positive treatment effects versus memory impairment (which is more likely with greater than 20 treatments). For catatonic conditions, two or four ECT treatments may be effective. When ECT is used for psychosis or mania, 20 or more treatments may be necessary for a positive response.

56. **(B)** This patient has recurrent thoughts (or obsessions) that are distressing to her. They are conceived as a product of her mind and not as implanted messages, as may occur in schizophrenia. She attempts to ignore or suppress her symptoms by not explaining to her husband how she feels and by getting rid of all the knives in her kitchen. Obsessions are the mental acts, whereas compulsions are physical actions performed to decrease anxiety associated with

the obsessions. Impulse control disorder, not otherwise specified, is appropriate for patients with the acting of impulses that are not as ego-dystonic (disturbing) as in this case, and that do not have an obsessional, non-enacted (thinking) component. Obsessive-compulsive personality disorder is a pervasive character style marked by a pattern of preoccupation with orderliness, perfectionism, and mental and interpersonal control. These individuals are often described as "control freaks" by laypersons and are noted to be particularly inflexible. Schizophrenia is an inappropriate diagnosis because this patient has fair insight regarding her obsessional thinking; she does act on her thoughts and they are disturbing to her. She is not delusional, hallucinating, or disorganized, and therefore is not psychotic. There is no mention of a history of odd beliefs or strangeness prior to the birth of her child, which would be consistent with schizotypal personality disorder.

57. **(C)** Fluvoxamine and other serotonin-specific reuptake inhibitors (SSRIs) (eg, paroxetine, fluoxetine, sertraline, citalopram) are known for their antiobsessional effects as well as for their antidepressant and antianxiety effects. Patients may require higher doses than those needed for depression. Lithium is a mood stabilizer used for bipolar disorder. Lorazepam, a benzodiazepine, may decrease anxiety but has no direct antiobsessional effects. Haloperidol is a typical high-potency neuroleptic that may be useful in severe forms of OCD in which there is a psychotic component. However, it does not ameliorate purely obsessional thinking. Because of the importance of serotonin in the treatment of obsessive-compulsive disorder, nortriptyline and most other tricyclic antidepressants (TCAs) have not proven efficacious for OCD.

58. **(C)** This patient's presentation and MSE are most consistent with delirium, as evidenced by a fluctuating mental status with attentional deficits. Any number of medical conditions can cause delirium, and the elderly are particularly prone. This woman is elderly, dehydrated, and with an active infection; any one of these can increase the risk of delirium. Urinary tract infections are a frequent cause

of altered mental status in the elderly. A chest x-ray can also elucidate the presence of infection, and a head CT can rule out acute intracranial pathology, both of which can cause delirium. Amnestic disorder is not likely given this patient's shifts in attention and memory fluctuations. Cognitive disorder, not otherwise specified, is reserved for cases presenting with cognitive deficits which do not meet criteria for dementia and delirium, such as traumatic brain injury. Although this patient would be likely to have dementia as she came from a nursing home, her fluctuating mental status is indicative of a delirium. Dementias are diagnosed in the context of a relatively stable set of deficits on MSE, and the underlying causes are rarely associated with acute medical insults. Importantly, however, the presence of dementia does predispose a patient to a delirium. Major depressive disorder can cause cognitive deficits on MSEs that are reversible with antidepressant treatment. These "pseudodementias," like dementia, most often present with a more stable MSE than is illustrated in this case.

59. **(B)** Polypharmacy can worsen delirium. Antipsychotics such as haloperidol can be used to calm an agitated patient with delirium. Anticholinergic agents like diphenhydramine should be avoided as they can worsen or cause delirium, and sedating medications should be used at lowest possible doses. In cases of delirium with very severe agitation, phenobarbital may be used, but this would not be the appropriate management in this case. Valproic acid, an anticonvulsant and mood stabilizer used in bipolar disorder, is not indicated in this patient.

60. **(A)** The definitive treatment for delirium is to treat the underlying cause, in this case, treatment of the urinary tract infection with antibiotics. Mental status needs to be monitored carefully as some antibiotics can also worsen delirium. Scheduled chest x-rays or CT scans have no role in treatment of this patient's condition and carry unnecessary radiation exposure. An indwelling Foley catheter would increase the risk of developing a urinary tract infection, and unless there is indication, should be avoided. Any associated electrolyte abnormalities that

may have resulted from the patient's poor PO intake need to be corrected, but intravenous fluids will not, by themselves, treat the infection.

61. **(C)** Delirium carries a high-mortality rate and is a poor prognostic sign. The 3-month mortality rate of patients who have had one episode of delirium ranges from 23% to 33%. The 1-year mortality may be as high as 50%.

62. **(C)** About one-third of all patients with depression respond to the surprisingly powerful placebo effect. However, this response is not as well-sustained as in patients placed on antidepressant medications.

63. **(D)** Standard antidepressant therapies, including SSRIs and TCAs, have a positive response in 65% to 75% of patients.

64. **(D)** This patient likely has major depressive disorder. The rate of completed suicide in patients with major depression is approximately 15%. Approximately two-thirds of patients with major depression will have some degree of suicidal ideation, and at least 30% of patients with major depression will attempt suicide. Screening for suicide should be performed in any patient with depression, and studies have shown that asking about suicide does *not* plant the thought in patients; most patients who have attempted suicide have seen a doctor within 4 to 6 weeks of the attempt.

65. **(C)** The number one predictor of a completed suicide is a previous attempt. Older single (or divorced) males are more likely to attempt. Religion, good support, and children can be protective factors. Concurrent substance abuse and anxiety disorders can increase the risk of suicide.

66. **(C)** There is no evidence of occupational or social dysfunction or marked distress caused by this patient's activities. Virtually all *DSM-IV-TR* diagnoses are qualified by these criteria. If the patient did describe such concerns, the diagnosis would most likely be sexual masochism, in which patients are aroused by psychologically or physically punishing acts by another person (or fantasies of punishment). In sexual sadism, the patient is aroused by giving such punishment (or fantasies of giving it) to others. Fetishism involves sexual arousal connected to nonliving objects. In frotteurism, the patient is sexually aroused by touching or rubbing up against a nonconsenting person.

67. **(C)** Narcolepsy is a disorder often affecting persons in their teens or twenties. It is a disorder of REM sleep mechanisms, characterized by cataplexy (sudden loss of muscle tone following intense emotion), hypnopompic or hypnagogic hallucinations, or sleep paralysis (an inability to perform voluntary movements either at sleep onset or awakening that can be terrifying). Circadian rhythm sleep disorder is a disorder caused most often by sleep scheduling changes such as jet lag or night-shift work. Dyssomnia, not otherwise specified, is reserved for sleep disturbances of unknown cause or causes associated with environmental disturbances such as those that produce prolonged sleep deprivation. Restless legs syndrome falls under this category. Nightmare disorder is diagnosed in the absence of other predisposing mental illness (eg, PTSD) in which the patient has repeated nightmares causing significant distress. Primary hypersomnia is excessive daytime drowsiness or hours spent sleeping at night that is not better accounted for by an identifiable environmental or medical cause, substance abuse, or mental disorder (eg, major depression); it is not associated with specific stigmata of narcolepsy such as cataplexy or sleep paralysis.

68. **(D)** Methylphenidate, a stimulant, has been shown to be useful in inhibiting the onset of narcoleptic episodes, likely owing to the capacity for the drug to enhance CNS arousal mechanisms that inhibit REM-related mechanisms. Antidepressant treatment with tricyclic antidepressants has been found to be useful in combination with methylphenidate in some patients with narcolepsy. However, the efficacy of bupropion, fluoxetine (a serotonin-specific reuptake inhibitor), and phenelzine (a monoamine oxidase inhibitor) has not been well-studied.

Benzodiazepine regimens are not particularly effective for narcolepsy.

69. **(D)** This patient's symptoms fit *DSM-IV-TR* criteria for PMDD. The remittance of symptoms in the week after menses is typical of PMDD. In adults, dysthymic disorder is characterized by subthreshold depressive symptoms, for more days than not, over a 2-year period. Her symptoms are not severe enough nor of sufficient duration (2 or more weeks) to diagnose MDD. Her symptoms are more disruptive and cause more distress than purely PMS.

70. **(C)** This patient is displaying symptoms consistent with major depressive disorder, single episode. The average untreated depressive episode lasts anywhere from 6 to 13 months; with treatment, the duration decreases to approximately 3 months. Treatment can also decrease the risk of recurrence in the future.

71. **(C)** Heroin overdose is most likely to have caused the clinical situation described, including the decreased level of consciousness, respiratory depression, and pinpoint pupils. Many IV heroin users have scarred veins. Alcohol intoxication and PCP may cause coma but both are associated with nystagmus rather than pupillary size changes. Cocaine use causes pupillary dilatation, not constriction, and is usually associated with agitation in large amounts. Inhalants may rarely cause coma but are not classically associated with pupillary constriction.

72. **(E)** Naloxone is used to reverse the acute effects of opiate overdose by blocking CNS opioid receptors. Acetylcysteine is administered in acetaminophen overdose and deferoxamine is used in iron overdose. Methadone is used for the long-term maintenance of opiate addiction and would only worsen the symptoms of heroin overdose. Methylene blue is used to treat methemoglobinemia.

73. **(D)** This patient is suffering from symptoms of post-traumatic stress disorder (PTSD), an anxiety disorder consisting of reexperiencing symptoms (eg, nightmares, flashbacks,

intrusive thoughts), increased arousal (eg, hyperstartle, hypervigilence, irritability), and avoidance/emotional numbing. The best studied and most efficacious medications are considered to be the SSRIs. Antipsychotics, including the atypicals, should not be used as monotherapy, although may be used in conjunction, especially if there are associated psychotic symptoms. Benzodiazepines should be avoided in this patient population not only because of the significant comorbidity with substance addiction but also as they have not been found to be particularly effective. Mood stabilizers, such as lithium and valproic acid, are occasionally used in addition to SSRIs in order to target the mood lability or aggression sometimes seen in PTSD, although they are not believed to be as effective as SSRIs.

74. **(A)** This is an example of a case of panic disorder with agoraphobia inadequately treated with appropriate medication, namely sertraline. Many mental illnesses, including anxiety disorders, are best treated with a combination of pharmacology and psychotherapy. The best-studied psychotherapy for panic disorder is CBT. EMDR is a specific therapy that has been developed for PTSD. Insight-oriented therapy is a long-term dynamic therapy. Although it may be useful in some cases of panic disorder, it has not been as validated as CBT. Interpersonal therapy addresses relationships as a contributor of depression and is used to treat individuals with major depression. The purpose of supportive psychotherapy is to strengthen the patient's defense mechanisms in order to return them to a previous level of functioning. It has not been adequately studied for panic disorder.

75. **(B)** This case depicts a patient who is feigning or producing symptoms of an illness to gain gratification by assuming the sick role. Factitious disorder is sometimes referred to as Munchausen syndrome; when caretakers intentionally cause illness in their charges, such as children, the disorder is called factitious disorder (or Munchausen syndrome) by proxy. In conversion disorder, patients present with neurologic symptoms that are not physiologic. In hypochondriasis, a patient believes that he or

she has some particular medical diagnosis despite reassurances to the contrary; it is the worry about the illness that causes much of the distress. There is little reason to believe this act could help her achieve financial or other material gain as in malingering. Patients with somatization disorder tend to have clusters of subjective symptoms over time affecting multiple organ symptoms or anatomic parts that do not correlate to any specific medical diagnosis.

76. **(C)** Patients with factitious disorder have an unconscious desire to assume the sick role. Their symptom production is fully conscious. In malingering, both symptom production and the desire for secondary gain (work avoidance) are conscious. In conversion disorder, the symptom production is due to unconscious conflicts.

77. **(B)** This patient meets criteria for a current manic episode with symptoms of psychomotor agitation, pressured speech, grandiose delusions, flight of ideas, and history of excessive spending as evidenced by his credit card debt. His history of good premorbid functioning and a remitted major depression are also consistent with a diagnosis of bipolar disorder. Adjustment disorders can present following an identifiable stressor and may manifest with mild mood, anxiety, or behavioral disturbances, but not overt mania. Brief psychotic disorder is characterized by psychotic symptoms lasting 1 day to 1 month, but which are not better accounted for by another mood disorder with psychotic features (such as bipolar disorder) or psychotic disorder. Cyclothymia is incorrect as this patient has had both manic and depressive episodes, whereas in cyclothymia the highs do not exceed a hypomanic episode, and the lows do not extend to a major depressive episode. The patient's current manic episode rules out major depressive disorder; in fact, although he may have future major depressive episodes, he should never be diagnosed with MDD.

78. **(D)** Lithium and valproic acid are considered first-line mood stabilizers. They are both indicated in the treatment of acute mania as well as prevention of future mood episodes. Carbamazepine and oxcarbazepine are both effective mood stabilizers, but are usually not first-line. While antipsychotics such as aripiprazole can be used in bipolar disorder, their side effect profile presents a fairly high level of risk that is less with a different mood stabilizer. Lamotrigine and lithium are both indicated in the treatment of acute depressive episodes of bipolar disorder.

79. **(B)** Classically, infarcts of the left frontal hemispheres (part of left middle cerebral artery distribution) present with depression, whereas those of the right frontal hemisphere present with euphoria, inappropriate indifference, or mania (although recent research tends to refute this). Obsessive-compulsive behaviors present occasionally after diffuse bilateral frontal injury. Anxiety and panic symptoms have not been described as having any particular association with left middle cerebral artery strokes, although such comorbid cases may exist.

80. **(E)** This woman has developed psychosis marked by hallucinations, delusions, and paranoia. She was most likely given high-dose steroids to treat her acute multiple sclerosis flare, and the steroids induced a psychotic state. High-dose steroids can cause mood disturbance in many patients, and florid psychosis in a smaller subset. The symptoms usually entirely remit once steroids are stopped or tapered appropriately. While most symptoms occur at high doses, such as with IV steroids, steroid psychosis can occur in patients treated with chronic lower level oral steroids as well. Her psychotic symptoms rule out an adjustment disorder, and her age and lack of psychiatric history would not be consistent with a first episode of bipolar disorder or schizophrenia. While multiple sclerosis can, by itself, produce depression and affective lability, it does not usually cause psychotic symptoms.

81. **(E)** About 90% of cases of impotence in the age group 30 to 50 have a psychological etiology. After 50, the etiology becomes increasingly medically-related to causes such as medications, diabetes, hypertension, and alcoholism.

82. **(E)** The serotonin metabolite designated 5-hydroxyindole acetic acid (5-HIAA) measured in the CSF has been shown to be lower in postmortem analysis of victims of suicide and patients with impulsivity and violence or aggression when compared with control groups. No such associations have been established with the other neurotransmitters listed.

83. **(B)** Depression is the most common presenting psychiatric symptom in patients with multiple sclerosis. It may present during the course of mild progressive cognitive decline that is consistent with a subcortical dementia (slowing of mental processing, motor difficulties, blunted or inappropriate affect, with relative preservation of language-dependent skills). Neuroimaging of these patients usually shows diffuse white matter plaques affecting the frontal lobes. Cerebral atrophy and ventricular enlargement are associated with the most common form of cortical dementia, Alzheimer disease. Periventricular white-matter changes are observed in vascular dementia (formally multi-infarct dementia).

84. **(B)** The patient appears to be suffering from delirium. Although aggressiveness or combativeness, memory deficits, psychotic symptoms, and uncooperativeness may be seen in either delirium or dementia, a fluctuation in the level of consciousness (ie, from alertness to somnolence) with deficits in attention are the hallmarks for delirium. Attention is usually intact in dementia. Further, the acute onset of symptoms is more suggestive of delirium. It is important to remember that having dementia predisposes patients to delirium, and so the two may be seen in the same patient.

85. **(B)** This patient is suffering from generalized anxiety disorder. Her symptoms include ruminations about many aspects of her life, despite there not being any disruption in those areas. She also has physical symptoms associated with anxiety. There is no particular stressor to qualify for adjustment disorder. Her ruminations may have an obsessional quality, but they are not limited to a specific thought nor associated with any compensatory compulsions,

therefore making obsessive-compulsive disorder unlikely. She does not have specific panic attacks or fears of future attacks consistent with panic disorder. Her anxiety is not related to fears of humiliation or scrutiny in a performance situation, which would be consistent with social phobia (social anxiety disorder).

86. **(E)** There are a number of stigmata associated with schizophrenia that are not included in *DSM-IV-TR* diagnostic criteria. These include soft neurologic signs such as short-term memory deficits, unstable smooth-pursuit eye movements, and decreased ability to habituate to repeated sensory stimuli (sensory gating abnormalities). In addition, patients with schizophrenia have difficulty in conceptualizing complex visual compositions. Patients with ADHD, MDD, OCD, and PTSD have also demonstrated short-term memory difficulties, but not the other signs mentioned.

87. **(C)** The most appropriate next step is to send the patient to the psychiatric emergency department. This patient is experiencing an acute episode of major depression and, because of his suicidal ideation with active plan and means to overdose, he should be referred to the emergency department for further assessment while ensuring his safety. Stopping his prescription will not address the immediate danger to self, and having him follow up in 1 week or for weekly outpatient visits are also inappropriate given the safety concerns. While his parents may be called for collateral information in the future, the more pressing step is to ensure the patient's safety. Although he will likely require an antidepressant in the long term, this will not resolve his acute suicidality, and is therefore inappropriate as the next immediate step.

88. **(D)** The woman presents with a classic presentation for major depressive disorder. Having a depressive disorder significantly increases one's risk for suicide. Many other factors also increase the risk for completed suicide such as white race, male gender, older age, single/divorced, and having poor social support.

89. (C) The presentation exemplifies a manic episode, with symptoms that include inflated self-esteem and grandiosity, pressured speech, a decreased need for sleep, and an impulsive shopping excursion without considering possible consequences. The most likely diagnosis is a mood disorder, as this patient has a history of depression and now is manic. However, before diagnosing bipolar disorder type I, the contribution of mania induced by an antidepressant must be ruled out. If this manic episode occurred because of an antidepressant, a more appropriate diagnosis would be substance-induced mood disorder. Anxiety disorders and cognitive disorders do not present with the classic signs of mania. While this patient has psychotic symptoms (grandiose delusions), a psychotic disorder such as schizophrenia cannot be diagnosed as there is no indication of prominent psychotic symptoms (hallucinations, disorganized thought processes and speech) in the absence of mood symptoms. Her primary symptoms do not involve physical or somatic symptoms which would be seen in a somatoform disorder.

90. (A) This patient was most likely prescribed an antidepressant since her initial presentation was for a depressive episode 2 months ago. Since she also has migraines, and tricyclic antidepressants are often used in their treatment, this was most likely the agent she has been taking. While all antidepressants have the potential to induce a manic switch in susceptible patients, the rate is slightly higher for tricyclic antidepressants than for serotonin-specific reuptake inhibitors or serotonin-norepinephrine reuptake inhibitors, such as fluoxetine or venlafaxine, respectively. Benzodiazepines (eg, clonazepam) are not known to cause mood switches into mania, and mood stabilizers such as lithium are a treatment for bipolar disorder.

91. (B) The specific phenomenon described here is an idea of reference. The patient interprets an event as relating to him, even though it clearly does not. A hallucination is a perception in the absence of a clearly defined stimulus, whereas an illusion is a misinterpretation of an evident stimulus (for instance, IV tubing appearing like snakes). Thought broadcasting is a delusional belief that one's thoughts can be heard or somehow known by others without direct communication. Thought insertion is another delusion where the patient believes thoughts from some external entity are placed in his mind.

92. (C) The choices in this question describe different patterns of amnesia. Localized amnesia refers to memory loss surrounding a discrete period of time, typically occurring after a traumatic event; in this case, the patient's amnesia results from learning of her husband's death. Rarely, a patient may forget his or her entire preceding life (generalized amnesia) or forget all events following a trauma, except for the immediate past (continuous amnesia). Retrograde amnesia is any amnesia for events that come before a traumatic event. Selective amnesia involves the inability to recall certain aspects of an event, though other memories of the event may be intact.

93. (B) This patient is suffering from bereavement. His wife has died within the last 2 months, and his symptoms include an appropriately depressed mood, although he is still able to function and is taking care of his basic needs. It is not uncommon to have auditory or visual hallucinations of the deceased during the grieving period. Also, many individuals experience survivor's guilt as part of their grieving. While this patient had a significant stressor (death of wife), his symptoms are better accounted for by bereavement rather than adjustment disorder. If he had suicidal ideation, severe loss of functioning, significant distressing auditory hallucinations or other symptoms of psychosis, a diagnosis of major depression with or without psychotic features would be more appropriate. Besides the hallucinations relating to the deceased wife, there is no other evidence of a primary psychotic illness such as schizophrenia. Strict *DSM-IV-TR* criteria limit bereavement symptoms to 2 months after death, but many clinicians argue that grieving can take up to a year, especially after a longstanding significant relationship.

94. **(D)** The most appropriate treatment at this stage is support. If symptoms persist, and he begins to experience loss of functioning or significant distress, an antidepressant may be warranted. Hospitalization would be indicated if this patient had active thoughts of suicide and was at risk of harming himself or others. At this time, he is experiencing survivor's guilt but is not actively suicidal. There is no indication for an antipsychotic, and cognitive behavioral therapy is not indicated in this case.

95. **(A)** Circumstantiality involves a circuitous, over-inclusive answer that only eventually gets to the point as the patient demonstrates in this example. Loosening of associations is a response composed of a series of disconnected ideas. The pointless repetition of a word, phrase, or idea is perseveration. Pressured speech is a continuous, usually rapid, uninterruptible stream of ideas that may make sense but is often hard to follow. While this patient's speech may be pressured, this is unable to be determined by the vignette alone. Tangentiality occurs when the patient strays off the point entirely, never returning to the original intention of the answer. Generally, the speech of a schizophrenic or schizoaffective patient may demonstrate any of these characteristics.

96. **(C)** A pseudoseizure (nonepileptic seizure) is a psychogenically-induced behavior that resembles epileptic activity externally, but the EEG is entirely normal. Although the syndrome may in some cases be motivated by secondary gain (as in malingering), it most often occurs in reaction to stress or in a setting of personality disorder, severe affective disorders, or conversion reactions. The other choices, which each represent true epileptic seizures, rarely, if ever, include the purposeful, complex activity as is seen in this case. Not uncommonly, patients with pseudoseizures also have a concurrent seizure disorder, and it is quite difficult to sort out the genuine seizures from the pseudoseizures. Diagnosing a pseudoseizure often requires demonstrating a normal EEG at the time of the pseudoseizure. The prognosis for pseudoseizures is quite poor, with frequent exacerbations.

97. **(B)** Narcolepsy is a sleep disorder characterized by the tetrad of hypersomnia (excessive daytime somnolence), cataplexy (transient loss of motor tone associated with strong emotions, as demonstrated in this case), sleep paralysis (total or partial paralysis in sleep–wake transition), and hypnagogic or hypnopompic hallucinations (vivid dream-like hallucinations occurring in the wake/sleep transition). Catalepsy is a state of immobility sometimes seen in catatonic states.

98. **(A)** All of the choices are possible side effects, either short term or long term, of antipsychotic medication. Akathisia is the subjective sensation of motor and mental restlessness. Akinesia is a dysfunction of slowed or absent movement that can be associated with pseudoparkinsonism in the setting of neuroleptics. A dystonia, like akathisia and akinesia, can occur acutely and involve muscle rigidity and spasticity. Rabbit syndrome is a late-onset side effect that involves fine, rhythmic movements of the lips. Tardive dyskinesia is another late-onset neurologic effect of neuroleptics and can include tongue and lip movements, as well as choreoathetoid movement of the trunk or limbs.

99. **(B)** Both depersonalization and derealization can be seen in anxiety disorders, especially during panic attacks as in panic disorder. Derealization is the sense that one's surroundings are strange or unreal, and depersonalization is the feeling that one's identity is lost or the feeling of being unreal or strange. Dereism is simply mental activity not in accordance with reality. Hypermnesia is an abnormal recall of details. Paresthesia is an abnormal sensation such as tingling or prickling.

100. **(A)** This patient is likely suffering from Wernicke- Korsakoff syndrome, a complication of long-term alcoholism, manifesting as anterograde amnesia, the loss of immediate or short-term memory; patients are unable to form new memories. Retrograde amnesia, in contrast, is the loss of remote or previously formed memories. Astereognosis is the inability to recognize an object by touch despite tactile sensation being intact. Dissociative amnesia is the loss

of memory for a period of time without the loss of ability to form new memories. It is usually associated with emotional trauma and is not due to drugs or a medical condition. Prosopagnosia is the inability to remember faces despite being able to recognize that they are faces.

101. **(B)** Confabulation is the fluent fabrication of fictitious responses in compensation of a memory disturbance, classically seen in dementias or Korsakoff syndrome. Clang associations are the use of words based on sound and not with reference to the meaning; this may be seen in manic or psychotic states. Flight of ideas is another form of thought process in manic patients, where thoughts and speech shift rapidly from one idea to another, although the relationship between the themes can sometimes be followed. Hypermnesia is the ability to recall detailed material that is not usually available to recall. Logorrhea is uncontrollable or excessive talking sometimes seen in manic episodes.

102. **(A)** Formication is a particular type of tactile hallucination in which one has the sensation of bugs crawling on or under the skin. It can be seen in cocaine intoxication and in alcohol withdrawal. Gustatory hallucinations are taste without stimulus. Hypnagogic and hypnopompic hallucinations are not tactile hallucinations but hallucinations experienced in the transition state from wakefulness to sleep and sleep to wakefulness, respectively. Synesthesia is a secondary sensation of an actual perception (eg, the sensation of a color associated with a taste); it is usually secondary to neurologic disease or hallucinogen use, most notably LSD.

103. **(B)** All of these terms are used to describe speech. Prosody describes the melody, rhythm, or intonation of speech that carries its emotional quality. The lack of this type of emotional variation is called aprosodic speech. Aphasia is the inability to communicate by speech or language. Dysarthria is poor articulation, often due to a neurologic injury such as a stroke. Scanning speech is irregular pauses between syllables, which also breaks the fluidity but

does not cause the repeating of sounds or syllables. Stuttering is the disturbance of the fluidity of speech as in repeating sounds or syllables or using broken words.

104. **(A)** Circumstantial speech is the overuse of detailed information providing extraneous detail in a digressive manner in order to convey an idea. Derailment refers to the abrupt interruption of an idea and then, after a period of time (a few seconds), beginning a new topic. This is usually without the patient's being aware of the switch in material. In flight of ideas, there are rapid and frequent changes in ideas or topics, but the connections may still be recognizable. In loosening of associations, the logical connections between ideas are completely lost; although proper grammar and words may be used, the speech is not logical or goal directed. Tangential speech quickly moves off topic but can be followed, although the patient never arrives at the point that is trying to be made.

105. **(B)** An illusion is a misperception of an actual stimulus, and a hallucination is the perception in the absence of a stimulus. Macropsia and micropsia are the misperceptions of objects being larger or smaller than they actually are. Palinopsia is the persistence of a visual image after the stimulus has been removed.

106. **(B)** This patient suffers from obsessive-compulsive disorder (OCD), an anxiety disorder characterized by recurrent obsessions (eg, fear of contracting HIV) and/or compulsions (eg, frequent hand washing), which cause significant distress or impairment in functioning. The neurophysiologic nature of this illness can be demonstrated through neuroimaging, which shows increased activity (metabolism) in the caudate nucleus, frontal lobes, and cingulum. These differences are actually reversed after adequate pharmacologic or behavioral therapy. The other areas of the brain are not believed to be as involved in OCD.

107. **(B)** Circumlocution is the substitution of a word or description for a word that cannot be recalled or spoken. Apraxia is the inability to

perform previously learned motor skills. Clang association is the use of words based on sound and not with reference to the meaning, commonly seen in mania. Confabulation is the fluent fabrication of fictitious responses in compensation of a memory disturbance, such as dementia. A neologism is a novel word used by patients, often in psychotic disorders (eg, schizophrenia).

108. **(B)** Anomia is an inability to name objects, not solely due to an aphasia. Apraxia is the inability to perform previously learned motor skills. Both anomia and apraxia are common components of dementias. Alexia is the inability to read. Paralinguistic components of speech refer to nonverbal communications such as facial expression and body movements. Prosopagnosia refers to the inability to recognize faces despite perception of all the components.

109. **(D)** While antidepressants such as paroxetine help all the symptoms of depression, some respond quicker to medications. Sleep, energy, and appetite changes are the first to respond, followed later by libido, hopelessness/helplessness, and suicidal ideation. Because of the differential response times, it is important to monitor a suicidal patient as the energy and motivation may improve before the depression and suicidality, and therefore, the patient may have the energy to commit suicide.

110. **(D)** Sexual sadism and sexual masochism are, respectively, the derivation of sexual pleasure from causing or receiving mental/physical abuse. Exhibitionism is exposure of the genitalia in public to an unwilling participant, and usually occurs in men. Frotteurism, the rubbing of genitals against another to achieve arousal and orgasm, is also usually seen in men and performed in crowded places. Transvestic fetishism is arousal by cross-dressing.

111. **(B)** Koro, taijin-kyofusho, and zar are all examples of culture-bound delusions. Koro is the worry that the penis is shrinking into the abdomen and is found in South and East Asia. Taijin-kyofusho is the belief that one's body is offensive to others, and zar is the delusional belief of possession by a spirit. Capgras syndrome is the delusional idea that imposters have replaced once familiar persons. Kuru is a slowly progressive neurologic disease leading to death, thought to be caused by an agent similar to Creutzfeldt-Jakob disease.

112. **(E)** Voyeurism is deriving sexual pleasure from watching another person or persons involved in the act of undressing or other sexually oriented activity. Exhibitionism is another paraphilia involving exposing one's genitalia to an unsuspecting audience. Hermaphroditism is not a paraphilia, but is a rare disorder in which one possesses both male and female sexual characteristics. Transvestic fetishism involves being dressed in clothing of the opposite sex for sexual excitement. It is often present in heterosexual men and differs from transsexualism in that the person is usually comfortable and content with his gender identity. It is, however, possible to see these disorders concomitantly.

113. **(E)** Loss of ego boundaries is commonly manifested as inappropriate conversational distance. Circumstantiality is manifested by speech and thoughts with identifiable connections between thoughts, but which drift off the point and ramble, eventually coming back to the point. Flight of ideas is the rapid flow of poorly connected speech and thoughts. Formication is the sensation that bugs are crawling on one's skin, often in drug intoxication or withdrawal. Idea of reference is the inaccurate belief that others are focusing on or referring to the patient in some positive or negative way.

114. **(C)** This is a typical presentation for mania, an episode that seems to have been at least partially induced by treatment with an antidepressant (all antidepressants can induce or exacerbate mania). This patient's affect, like that of many patients with mania, is expansive and irritable. He is to a lesser extent guarded and suspicious but this does not adequately capture the full picture of his mania. His affect would not be considered euthymic. While he is labile, he is not dysphoric, and while he is euphoric, he is not bizarre.

115. (C) Although the other choices might explain some of his speech characteristics, pressured speech (speech that is rapid and uninterruptible) is the best description of his speech pattern. Hyperverbal speech is at a rapid rate but remains interruptible. Tangentiality refers to thought process, not speech.

116. (D) The locus ceruleus is the "alarm" center of the brain and is hyperactive in anxiety states. It is the location of most of the norepinephrine-containing neurons in the brain. The amygdala and hippocampus, both part of the limbic system, are involved in fear/anger responses and memory formation, respectively. The basal ganglia coordinate motor activity, while the thalamus is the brain's relay center.

117. (D) Splitting is a primitive defense mechanism, manifested by viewing others as either all good or all bad. It is common in patients with borderline personality disorder although there is no other evidence of borderline pathology in this case. Acting out represents the enactment of a behavior originating from a conflict; the behavior relieves the sense that the conflict exists at all. Externalization represents the tendency to project one's own internal characteristics onto others. Regression is a return to patterns of relating, thinking, or feeling that had come before one's current developmental stage; for example, many medical students who return home act as if they are teenagers with regard to their parents or other hometown friends. Sublimation is the channeling of drives or conflicts into goals that are gratifying but socially acceptable (eg, individuals afraid of blood and hospitals who become hospital workers or physicians).

118. (D) This patient's reaction to paroxetine is consistent with serotonin syndrome, a potentially life-threatening condition caused by the interaction of a serotonin-specific reuptake inhibitor (SSRI), such as paroxetine, with a monoamine oxidase inhibitor (MAOI), which results in increased amounts of both catecholamines and indolamines. Features of mild serotonin syndrome include tachycardia, flushing, fever, hypertension, ocular oscillations, and myoclonic jerks. Severe serotonin syndrome may result in severe hyperthermia, coma, autonomic instability, convulsions, and death; therefore, clinicians must wait at least 14 days after discontinuing an MAOI before starting a serotonergic agent. Most serotonin in the CNS is synthesized in the dorsal and medial raphe nucleus of the brain stem. The caudate nucleus is located in the brain stem and concerned with memory formation. The nucleus accumbens is located in the striatum and thought to be involved with sensations of reward and pleasure, as well as addictive behaviors. The locus ceruleus synthesizes norepinephrine, and the substantia nigra synthesizes dopamine.

119. (C) Paraphilias encompass a wide variety of maladaptive sexual behaviors and fantasies. Frotteurism is the syndrome of recurrent, intense sexual fantasies and behaviors involving touching or rubbing against a nonconsenting adult. Exhibitionism involves revealing one's genitals to unsuspecting strangers. Fetishism is sexual urges or fantasies involving an inanimate object. Pedophilia involves sexual fantasies and behaviors concerning children. Voyeurism involves secretly watching someone engaged in disrobing, nudity, or sexual behavior.

120. (A) An IQ of 55 places this patient in the mild mental retardation (MR) category. Average IQ is 100, and a standard deviation of 15 is utilized; therefore, most of the population falls within 2 standard deviations. As such, the lower end of "normal" IQ is 70. IQs of 50 to 69 are classified as mild MR; between 35 and 49 as moderate MR; between 20 and 34 as severe MR; and less than 20 as profound MR.

121–130. [121 (G), 122 (J), 123 (L), 124 (A), 125 (F), 126 (O), 127 (C), 128 (N), 129 (M), 130 (B)] In acute alcohol intoxication **(A)**, as blood concentration of alcohol increases, there is worsening motor performance, incoordination and judgment errors, mood lability, nystagmus, slurred speech, potential blackouts, altered vital signs, and possibly death. Alcohol withdrawal **(B)** can start hours after the last drink, and is characterized by autonomic instability (sweating, tachycardia), tremors, insomnia, nausea/emesis, transient hallucinations or illusions, psychomotor agitation, anxiety, and seizures. Delirium tremens can develop, and can be deadly. Amphetamine intoxication (C) is characterized by both behavioral and physiological changes. Patients may experience euphoria, interpersonal sensitivity, anxiety, tension, or anger, impaired judgment, and impaired social and occupational functioning. Further, they may have tachycardia or bradycardia, pupillary dilation, insomnia, blood pressure changes, sweating or chills, nausea or vomiting. Chronic use may result in dry skin, acne-like lesions, or chronic nose bleeds. Amphetamine withdrawal (D) is characterized by fatigue, vivid dreams, sleep disturbances, increased appetite, and psychomotor retardation or agitation. A caffeine intoxication syndrome (E) is possible, especially in individuals who consume a large amount or who are unaccustomed to it. In studies, participants report symptoms of jitteriness, diuresis, irritability, insomnia, psychomotor agitation, and nausea. Caffeine withdrawal (F) can occur when people abruptly stop their accustomed intake. Symptoms include headache, sleepiness, irritability, concentration problems, vomiting, and muscle aches/stiffness. Cannabis intoxication (G) includes increased heart rate for several hours, posture-dependent changes in blood pressure, injected conjunctivae, a "high" with mild euphoria, feeling of relaxation, perceptual changes (time distortion, intensified ordinary experiences), and increased sociability. There is evidence of a mild cannabis withdrawal (H) syndrome lasting several weeks, characterized by decreases in mood and appetite, with increases in irritability, anxiety, and tension. Cocaine intoxication (I) is similar to amphetamine intoxication. At higher doses, signs of toxicity may develop and include seizures, chest pain, hyperpyrexia, and death. Susceptible users may also experience paranoia, ranging from mild hypervigilance to frank paranoia and persecution. Cocaine withdrawal (J) is characterized by onset of dysphoric mood, hypersomnia, increased appetite, and fatigue. Hallucinogens include substances such as LSD, mescaline, and ecstasy. They primarily affect perceptions and in intoxication (K) can result in mood changes, paranoia, ideas of reference, depersonalization,

hallucinations, and synesthesia. Autonomic symptoms may also occur, and include blurry vision, tachycardia, sweating, tremors, and pupil dilation. Inhalants have become increasingly common drugs of abuse. Signs and symptoms of intoxication (L) are inhalant specific, but generally include rapid onset of effects, dizziness, nausea, then slowing, ataxia, slurred speech, and disorientation. Bronchospasm may also occur. Intoxication usually improves within an hour of abstinence because the substances are usually volatile hydrocarbons. Treatment of inhalant withdrawal is supportive. Opiates can be illegal or prescription, such as narcotic analgesics. Symptoms of acute intoxication (M) include pupillary constriction (can be dilation once anoxic brain injury has occurred from respiratory depression), drowsiness, slurred speech, and possibly pulmonary edema. At higher doses, coma or death with respiratory depression may occur. Opiate withdrawal (N) is characterized by dysphoria, nausea, vomiting, muscle aches, lacrimation, rhinorrhea, piloerection, sweating, diarrhea, yawning, fever, and insomnia. Phencyclidine (PCP) (O) and other dissociative anesthetics can induce vertical or horizontal nystagmus (rotary with ketamine), hypertension (at least mild, but hypertensive crisis can occur), tachycardia, ataxia, numbness and high pain tolerance, ataxia, hyperacusis, hyperthermia, muscle rigidity, seizures including status epilepticus, and death. The presence of nystagmus helps to distinguish PCP intoxication from other forms of psychosis. Behavioral manifestations can be severe, and severe agitation, rage, and panic coupled with disinhibition may cause a dangerous clinical situation.

131–136. [131 (F), 132 (B), 133 (D), 134 (D), 135 (E), 136 (A)] Blockade at the 5-HT2A (serotonin) receptor (A) is thought to improve cognitive and affective symptoms in schizophrenia and other psychotic disorders. Blockade at the alpha-1 receptor (B) is responsible for the dizziness, sedation, and orthostatic hypotension associated with many of the atypical antipsychotics. The antipsychotics are not known to affect beta receptors (C). Blockade at the dopaminergic D2 receptors (D) in the mesolimbic and mesocortical areas of the brain are responsible for reducing the positive psychotic symptoms in schizophrenia. Blockade of the D2 receptor in other pathways is responsible for some undesirable side effects: blockade in the nigrostriatal pathway is associated with movement disorders such as extrapyramidal symptoms, whereas blockade in the tubero-infundibular pathway is responsible for the prolactinemia seen with antipsychotics. Blockade at the histamine-1 receptor **(E)** is believed to contribute to sedation and cause weight gain. By blocking muscarinic-1 receptors **(F)**, antipsychotics cause anticholinergic side effects of sedation, dry mouth, and constipation.

137–145. [137 (G), 138 (I), 139 (F), 140 (D), 141 (B), 142 (C), 143 (A), 144 (E), 145 (H)] Defense mechanisms are conceptualized as the mind's (mostly unconscious) way of dealing with distressing wishes/drives/thoughts. They can be subdivided into immature, neurotic, or mature defenses. The lower functioning defense mechanisms are as follows: Denial **(B)** is when an individual refuses to accept reality because it is too distressing; splitting **(I)** is also an immature defense where the person sees others or other situations as "all good or all bad" and is unable to tolerate positive and negative aspects to be present within one entity; displacement **(C)** is the channeling of one's unacceptable wishes or feelings into less anxiety producing ones—for instance, jerking the dog's leash harshly when one was really upset at having been woken up by a spouse (truly being angry with the spouse); in projection **(E)** one's unacceptable ideas or thoughts are seen as coming from another (for instance, a cheating husband accuses his wife of being unfaithful); projective identification **(F)** can be thought of as a self-fulfilling prophecy, wherein the patient's unacceptable feelings are projected to another, but the other (eg, therapist) acts in such a way that they become true—for instance, a patient views the world as full of unloving people (she hates herself), then acts to push her therapist to the breaking point where he terminates her care, therefore confirming her belief that the world is full of unloving people. Examples of neurotic defenses are as follows: rationalization **(H)** is the process of "making excuses" or cognitively reframing a situation to make it less anxiety or distress provoking; reaction formation **(G)** describes the process of turning unacceptable drives and desires into their opposite. The following are mature defense mechanisms: altruism **(A)** involves acceptable actions that serve others and bring pleasure to the individual; humor **(D)** involves expressing unpleasant thoughts or feelings in a way that, brings enjoyment and pleasure to others.

CHAPTER 3

Somatic Treatment and Psychopharmacology
Questions

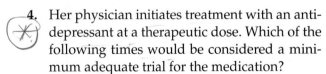

Questions 1 and 2

A 32-year-old man is admitted to a general hospital after ingesting an unknown quantity of phenelzine in a suicide attempt. After gastric lavage and administration of a charcoal slurry, he is transferred to the medical intensive care unit for monitoring. Twenty-four hours later, he begins to see horses running in the hall and pulls out his intravenous (IV) lines.

1. Which of the following treatments would be the most important at this time?

    (A) chlorpromazine
    (B) cyproheptadine
    (C) lorazepam
    (D) meperidine
    (E) phenytoin

2. Twelve days after his suicide attempt, he receives venlafaxine (Effexor) to treat his depression. One hour after ingestion of the venlafaxine, he becomes tachycardic and diaphoretic and develops myoclonic jerks. Which of the following conditions has he developed?

    (A) acute dystonia
    (B) akathisia
    (C) neuroleptic malignant syndrome
    (D) opisthotonos
    (E) serotonin syndrome

Questions 3 and 4

A 24-year-old woman presents to her primary care physician for a regular checkup. During the examination, her doctor notes a 15-lb weight gain. The patient complains that she always feels tired during the day despite sleeping from 8 PM to 9 AM daily. On further questioning, the physician learns that the patient feels sad and empty, often thinks about death, cannot concentrate at work, and lacks the energy to care for her two children. However, her mood picks up when her physician questions her about her children.

3. Which of the following medications would be most effective in treating her illness?

    (A) fluoxetine
    (B) nortriptyline
    (C) phenelzine
    (D) sertraline
    (E) trazodone

4. Her physician initiates treatment with an antidepressant at a therapeutic dose. Which of the following times would be considered a minimum adequate trial for the medication?

    (A) 1 week
    (B) 2 weeks
    (C) 6 weeks
    (D) 3 months
    (E) 6 months

Questions 5 and 6

While on call in a general hospital, you are called at 4:30 AM to evaluate a patient who wants to be discharged. Upon arriving on the floor, the nurse tells you he just pulled out his third IV of the day and started to swing the IV pole in the air while yelling profanities. He tells a nurse's aide he must capture the tiger that is loose in the parking lot. You quickly look at his chart and see that he is a 55-year-old man with a history of alcohol dependence, admitted 36 hours earlier for abdominal pain, nausea, and vomiting. His transaminases were elevated on admission, but his hepatitis profile is still pending. He is scheduled for upper endoscopy in the morning.

5. Which of the following should be the initial medication given at this time?

    (A) chlordiazepoxide
    (B) chlorpromazine
    (C) disulfiram
    (D) haloperidol
    (E) oxazepam

6. You speak briefly with this patient and are able to settle him down. His temperature is 102.1°F, pulse is 130 beats/min, and blood pressure is 220/120 mm Hg. Which of the following is the most appropriate medication and route of administration to give?

    (A) haloperidol intramuscularly (IM)
    (B) haloperidol intravenously (IV)
    (C) labetalol IV
    (D) lorazepam IM
    (E) lorazepam IV

7. A 32-year-old single woman presents to the emergency department escorted by her family after she revealed to them her suicide plan to take a full bottle of acetaminophen and drink a bottle of wine. She states that she cannot handle work any longer because her boss is trying to have her fired and her coworkers are helping him find fault in her work. She claims they have even tapped her phone and are having her followed. She reports difficulty falling asleep and poor concentration at work. She has lost 10 lb over the past 2 months, in

part because she is worried that her food may be poisoned. Upon interview, she displays poor eye contact, psychomotor retardation, and a tearful and constricted affect. Which of the following is the best medication regimen for this patient?

(A) clozapine
(B) fluoxetine and risperidone
(C) fluoxetine and clonazepam
(D) fluoxetine monotherapy
(E) risperidone monotherapy

8. A 40-year-old woman with bipolar disorder presents to the emergency room 2 weeks after starting a new medication. She reports that she was doing "well" until she got a viral gastroenteritis and was unable to eat for several days. While the viral symptoms resolved, she now complains of nausea and vomiting, ataxia, and tremor. Which of the following studies should be ordered first?

(A) carbamazepine level
(B) depakote level
(C) head CT
(D) lithium level
(E) urine toxicology screen

9. A 25-year-old man presents to the emergency department accompanied by his family who report that the patient has not left his bedroom in 3 weeks. They report that he spends his day reading science fiction novels that they provide for him. On examination, you find him to be malodorous and disheveled. He is guarded when you speak with him. He does not make eye contact and he avoids looking at the television in the waiting room because, he says, he wants to prevent intruders from controlling his thoughts. After completing the examination, you admit him to the inpatient psychiatric unit and begin aripiprazole. After 1 week, he is no longer afraid to look at the television but he spends much of the day pacing the floor, stating that he feels restless. After reducing the aripiprazole to the lowest dose you feel he needs, he still paces the halls. Which of the following is the most appropriate next step?

(A) Add benztropine.

(B) Add diphenhydramine.

(C) Add lorazepam.

(D) Add propranolol.

(E) Discontinue aripiprazole and try another antipsychotic.

10. A 35-year-old woman presents to the office stating that she is depressed. She was laid off from her work 5 weeks ago, and is having trouble finding a new job. She describes feeling very low, with feelings of hopelessness about the future and difficulty getting herself up and dressed in the morning. She has lost 5 lb. She is sleeping poorly. She reports one previous episode of depression. Additionally, she describes a period about a year ago in which she stayed up for several days in a row planning a big party for her husband's birthday; at that time, others commented that she was talking quickly and acting "like the energizer bunny." Which of the following medications would be the most appropriate treatment for her depression?

(A) bupropion

(B) fluoxetine

(C) lamotrigine

(D) valproic acid

(E) venlafaxine

Questions 11 and 12

A 33-year-old mentally retarded male resident of a group home presents to the emergency department escorted by staff members who believe he has become confused and disoriented over the past few days. He has been a resident there for several years without incident, but last week his thioridazine was changed to haloperidol because of concerns about the long-term use of high doses of thioridazine. On examination, you find him to be disoriented to place and time; he is diaphoretic with a temperature of 105.8°F, has a heart rate of 130 beats/min and a respiratory rate of 20 breaths/min. His extremities are stiff. Routine laboratories reveal a white blood cell (WBC) count of 15,000/mL, blood urea nitrogen (BUN) 75 mg/dL, creatinine 1.2 mg/dL, and creatinine phosphokinase 2300 Iμ/L.

11. Which of the following is the most likely serious complication this patient may experience?

(A) diffuse intravascular coagulation

(B) myocardial infarction

(C) pulmonary embolism

(D) respiratory failure

(E) rhabdomyolysis

12. Which of the following long-term side effects of high-dose thioridazine most likely led his physician to switch to haloperidol?

(A) agranulocytosis

(B) hyperprolactinemia

(C) priapism

(D) retinal pigmentation

(E) tardive dyskinesia

Questions 13 and 14

A 45-year-old unemployed investment banker presents to your office accompanied by his wife. He has been out of work for 1 month because he is afraid to take the train into work. He never had difficulty traveling until 2 months ago, when on a train during a family vacation, he suffered chest pain, shortness of breath, nausea, and a fear of dying. These symptoms lasted about 15 minutes. A workup by a cardiologist was negative. However, these symptoms have continued, also accompanied by intense fear and a feeling of being detached from himself. He has had approximately two attacks per week but also has severe anxiety when just thinking about returning to work as he is afraid he will die on the train. He tells you that he could not have come to see you without his wife's help.

13. Which of the following medications would be the most appropriate first choice for this patient?

(A) bupropion

(B) buspirone

(C) fluoxetine

(D) propranolol

(E) trazodone

14. The patient is anxious about waiting until the medication takes effect, and asks if you can give him something that will provide more immediate relief. You decide to prescribe a benzodiazepine in the interim. Which of the following medications would be the most potent?

(A) alprazolam
(B) chlordiazepoxide
(C) clonazepam
(D) diazepam
(E) oxazepam

Questions 15 and 16

A 22-year-old single male college music student reluctantly presents to your office at the request of his parents. His parents are worried because he has not been eating, talks constantly, and never seems to sleep. The patient states he has never felt better, that he's been composing several songs a day, and requires only several hours of sleep to function. He believes he will be the next great rock star and wants to finish the interview in order to get back to writing, but he cannot stay focused long enough to answer any of your questions. He does not have any prior or family psychiatric history and denies using any substances abuse.

15. You decide to begin a trial of lithium. Before initiating treatment, which of the following would be the minimum laboratory information that should be obtained?

(A) complete blood count (CBC)
(B) fasting glucose and lipid panel
(C) liver function tests
(D) serum ammonia
(E) serum creatinine, BUN and electrolytes, thyroid studies

16. One week after starting the lithium, the patient sprains his ankle while exercising. His primary care doctor examines him and tells him to use over-the-counter ibuprofen, which he will have to take for more than 1 week. Which of the following would be the most appropriate course of action?

(A) Continue ibuprofen at the prescribed dose.
(B) Decrease the dose of ibuprofen.

(C) Increase the dose of ibuprofen.
(D) Stop the lithium.
(E) Switch from ibuprofen to aspirin.

Questions 17 and 18

A 9-year-old boy is brought to the physician because his parents have received a note from his second-grade teacher complaining that he is disruptive in class. His teacher believes he could achieve better grades if he could sit still and pay attention. His parents report he has always been an active child but does have difficulty getting along with other children in the neighborhood. In the examination room, the boy seems unable to sit still and has difficulty completing a task you have assigned. You decide to prescribe him methylphenidate.

17. Which of the following is the most common side effect of this treatment?

(A) daytime drowsiness
(B) decrease in systolic blood pressure
(C) difficulty falling asleep
(D) increase in appetite
(E) slowed growth

18. Which of the following symptoms would most likely be exacerbated by the medication?

(A) bedwetting
(B) myopia
(C) poor impulse control
(D) reading difficulties
(E) tics

19. An 8-year-old boy is brought to your office by his mother because of his "compulsions," which have worsened over the past year. She first noticed them last year when several times a day he would repeatedly blink his eyes and frown while clearing his throat. He continues to do this despite trying not to, and, in addition, he often sticks out his tongue and smells his shirt while speaking with classmates. These behaviors have resulted in his being teased and losing friends at school. Which of the following agents would be the most effective to treat his disorder?

(A) alprazolam
(B) amitriptyline
(C) clonidine
(D) haloperidol
(E) paroxetine

20. A 45-year-old man with a history of hypertension, myocardial infarction, and chronic insomnia is referred to you by his primary care physician for evaluation of his major depressive episode. He has been treated for 3 months with fluoxetine 60 mg daily, with no improvement. He has no history of prior major depressive episodes. Which of the following would be the most appropriate next step in his treatment?

(A) Add lithium.
(B) Add thyroid hormone (T3).
(C) Switch to citalopram.
(D) Switch to nortriptyline.
(E) Switch to venlafaxine.

Questions 21 and 22

You have been treating a 55-year-old man with schizophrenia for 20 years with haloperidol and benztropine. Generally, he has done well and has not required major medication changes or hospitalizations. About 2 years ago, you noticed some lip smacking and tongue protrusions that did not bother him; however, now he also has odd, irregular movements of his arms which make it difficult for him to eat.

21. Which of the following conditions is most likely the cause of these symptoms?

(A) anticholinergic toxicity
(B) Huntington disease
(C) Meige syndrome
(D) Sydenham chorea
(E) tardive dyskinesia

22. Which of the following medications may best improve these symptoms?

(A) benztropine
(B) clozapine
(C) levodopa
(D) olanzapine
(E) trihexyphenidyl

23. A 24-year-old married secretary has complained of dizziness, palpitations, and sweaty palms for the past 10 months. She also occasionally has extreme muscle tension in her neck that occurs both at work and at home. She has difficulty falling asleep and feels "edgy" most of the day. In addition, she has had difficulty concentrating at work resulting in her making mistakes. She has gone to a local emergency room three times because of the palpitations but "nothing was found." Her family practitioner placed her on a hypoglycemic diet and referred her to a neurologist who found no focal abnormalities. She tells you she has many worries about her family but does not feel particularly depressed. Which of the following medications would provide the most immediate relief of her symptoms?

(A) bupropion
(B) buspirone
(C) clomipramine
(D) fluoxetine
(E) lorazepam

24. A 22-year-old woman is admitted to a psychiatric unit after a serious suicide attempt. She has had many suicide attempts in the past with varying severity. Her arms are scarred from prior attempts at hurting herself. She had been a good student until high school, when she took up with a "fast" crowd, began abusing alcohol and marijuana, and ran away from home several times. She has had several intense, stormy relationships with men. Outpatient treatment has mostly consisted of her complaints to her therapist about her family. She usually calls her therapist daily about different crises; however, her therapist was on vacation during her most recent crisis. She describes feelings of hopelessness and helplessness; she is sleeping poorly and has lost some weight. Which of the following medications would be most helpful for this patient?

(A) clonazepam
(B) fluoxetine
(C) haloperidol
(D) lithium
(E) ziprasidone

25. A 30-year-old woman, 10 weeks pregnant with her first child, presents to your office stating that she is depressed and is having doubts about becoming a mother. She has been experiencing daily emesis and is having trouble functioning at work. She reports that she was depressed throughout her 20s, but discontinued her antidepressants when she became pregnant because of concerns about harming her child. She would like your help in evaluating risks and benefits of restarting sertraline, which worked well for her in the past. Which of the following risks would be most likely to occur?

    (A) Epstein anomaly
    (B) gestational diabetes
    (C) infant developmental delay
    (D) neural tube defects
    (E) persistent pulmonary hypertension of the newborn

26. A 19-year-old woman is admitted to an inpatient psychiatric facility for her eating disorder. She weighs 82 lb and stands 5 ft 6 in tall. She began dieting in high school to lose unwanted 5 lb. Encouraged by compliments on her figure, she continued to lose another 10 lb. Her eating habits are ritualized: She cuts her food into small pieces and moves it around on her plate. She has an intense fear of being overweight. Which of the following medications would be the most useful for this patient?

    (A) cyproheptadine
    (B) fluoxetine
    (C) no medication
    (D) olanzapine
    (E) topiramate

27. A 36-year-old man with his first episode of major depression has been treated for 8 months with paroxetine and is currently in remission. Because of sexual dysfunction, he decided to stop taking the medication 3 days ago without first informing you. Yesterday, he became acutely irritable and even had a crying spell. He also complains of body aches, chills, and general lethargy. Which of the following steps would best alleviate his symptoms?

    (A) Restart paroxetine.
    (B) Start acetaminophen.
    (C) Start bupropion.
    (D) Start valproic acid.
    (E) Start venlafaxine.

28. A 20-year-old woman is started on lamotrigine for bipolar depression. Two months later, she comes back reporting that her symptoms are unchanged, despite her being compliant with the medication. You double check her medication list and discover that she was recently started on new medication(s). Which of the following medications would be most likely responsible for the lack of efficacy?

    (A) drospirenone and ethinyl estradiol
    (B) ibuprofen
    (C) lithium
    (D) valproic acid
    (E) ziprasidone

Questions 29 and 30

A 65-year-old man presents to your office on a referral from his primary care physician for evaluation of depression. He feels depressed and hopeless and has lost his appetite. He no longer enjoys seeing his grandchildren. It takes him several hours to fall asleep at night, and he stays asleep for only about 3 hours. He occasionally does not buy food because he is concerned about going broke; however, his family informs you that he is financially well-off. In addition, the patient feels significant guilt about becoming a burden on his family. His height is 6 ft with a weight of 155 lb, much less than his usual 175 lb.

29. Which of the following medications would be the most appropriate immediately in treating his insomnia?
    (A) bupropion
    (B) diazepam
    (C) diphenhydramine
    (D) fluoxetine
    (E) trazodone

30. Which of the following side effects of this medication would be the most important to educate the patient about?

(A) anorgasmia
(B) gynecomastia
(C) impotence
(D) premature ejaculation
(E) priapism

Questions 31 and 32

A 57-year-old man with bipolar disorder, whom you have treated successfully for 20 years with lithium 300 mg tid, is admitted to the general hospital with chest pain.

31. Which of the following findings would be most likely seen on his electrocardiogram (ECG)?

(A) first-degree atrioventricular (AV) block
(B) PR interval prolongation
(C) QT interval prolongation
(D) sinoatrial block
(E) T-wave depression

32. The patient is determined to have suffered a myocardial infarction (MI) and quickly undergoes angioplasty. He is eventually stabilized and discharged from the hospital on propranolol, topical nitroglycerin, hydrochlorothiazide, and aspirin, in addition to his lithium. Prior to his MI, his lithium level was usually 0.8 to 0.9 mmol/L. Now it is 1.3 mmol/L on the same dose. Which of the following is the most likely cause for this change?

(A) aspirin
(B) decreased fluid intake
(C) hydrochlorothiazide
(D) nitroglycerin
(E) propranolol

Questions 33 and 34

A 47-year-old male novelist has fears of contamination from anything he believes is "dirty." In restaurants, he uses his own plastic utensils that he carries with him. Elsewhere, he wears gloves or uses paper towels to avoid touching "dirty objects." Upon returning home, he then proceeds to wash his hands 10 times before going about his activities. If he accidentally touches anything prior to the completion of washing his hands, he experiences anxiety and is then unable to perform his usual nightly tasks. As a result of these symptoms he remains unable to have a meaningful social life.

33. Which of the following medications is the most effective treatment for his condition?

(A) clomipramine
(B) clonazepam
(C) nortriptyline
(D) olanzapine
(E) phenelzine

34. After 12 weeks of a therapeutic dose of the medication, the patient no longer needs to wash his hands quite so often but still has significant distress when he touches "dirty things." Which of the following treatments would be the most appropriate next step?

(A) Add buspirone.
(B) Add lithium.
(C) Add risperidone.
(D) Change to risperidone.
(E) Refer for cingulotomy.

Questions 35 and 36

A 21-year-old college student has been experiencing auditory hallucinations with commands telling him to hurt himself for more than a year. He has had trials with the following agents since that time: quetiapine 400 mg bid for 2 months, then haloperidol 10 mg bid for 6 weeks, then olanzapine 30 mg daily for 2 months. Despite a minor reduction in the voices, he remains isolated from family and friends.

35. Which of the following agents would be the most appropriate to begin?

(A) aripiprazole
(B) clozapine
(C) perphenazine
(D) risperidone
(E) ziprasidone

36. Which of the following receptors is most likely responsible for the above medication's efficacy?

(A) D_2

(B) D_3

(C) D_4

(D) 5-hydroxytryptamine-1 (5-HT$_1$)

(E) 5-hydroxytryptamine-3 (5-HT$_3$)

37. A 65-year-old man with major depression and hypertension presents to the emergency department because he fell to the ground after arising from a chair. He has no significant cardiac history and his ECG, electrolytes, and neurologic examination are unremarkable. His family reports that his physician recently started a new antidepressant but they do not know its name. Which of the following antidepressants is most likely responsible for his presentation?

(A) bupropion

(B) fluoxetine

(C) imipramine

(D) mirtazapine

(E) nortriptyline

38. A 21-year-old woman with a history of bulimia nervosa presents to the emergency department with her parents. She returned from college last week, and since that time, has been staying up very late, calling friends around the world and "talking nonsense" about an internet start-up that she is planning. She asks you to hurry up with your interview, since she has work to get back to. Her parents report that she failed several classes because she has not been going to class or turning in assignments. She is not taking any medications and her toxicology screen is negative. On mental status examination, her speech is pressured and her thought process is tangential. You decide to admit her to the hospital. Which of the following medications would be the most appropriate to begin?

(A) citalopram

(B) lamotrigine

(C) olanzapine

(D) topiramate

(E) valproic acid

39. A 28-year-old woman whom you are treating for bipolar disorder informs you that she is 3-week pregnant and is anxious about the baby's health. She is currently prescribed lithium 300 mg bid, and she has not had a manic episode in 3 years. What would be best to advise her regarding the use of lithium during pregnancy?

(A) Lithium is highest risk during the third trimester of pregnancy.

(B) Lithium increases the risk of neural tube defects.

(C) Lithium causes developmental delay in exposed infants.

(D) Lithium increases the risk of cardiac malformation.

(E) Lithium increases the risk of cleft lip and palate.

40. You are called to consult on an 85-year-old surgical patient who has become combative, yelling, punching staff, and pulling out her IVs. She demands to leave but is too weak to get out of her hospital bed. Which of the following would be the most appropriate intervention at this time?

(A) diphenhydramine

(B) donepezil

(C) lorazepam

(D) orientation to her surroundings

(E) risperidone

Questions 41 and 42

A 67-year-old woman presents to your office for evaluation of a 20-lb weight loss over a 4-month period and insomnia for the past 4 weeks. Her daughter informs you that her mother no longer enjoys any of her hobbies and has been speaking lately about dying. They have already consulted an internist who performed an extensive medical workup, including chemistries, blood count, thyroid studies, gastrointestinal imaging, and endoscopy, all of which were normal.

41. You would like to begin an antidepressant medication but would like to minimize adverse side effects while "exploiting" other side effects.

Which of the following agents would be the most appropriate?

(A) bupropion
(B) fluoxetine
(C) mirtazapine
(D) nortriptyline
(E) sertraline

42. Upon further history, you learn that she has had several failed trials of antidepressants and would like to start a tricyclic antidepressant. Which of the following conditions would most preclude using such an agent?

(A) estrogen replacement therapy
(B) lacunar infarcts
(C) left bundle branch block on ECG
(D) treatment with amlodipine
(E) urinary retention

Questions 43 and 44

A 72-year-old man is admitted to a general hospital's intensive care unit because of altered mental status. His medical workup has revealed pneumonia and congestive heart failure (CHF). On the second hospital day, he is agitated and pulls out his IV access. He also has been noted to speak out loud with no one in the room. His level of consciousness seems to wax and wane. He does not have a psychiatric history and is not allergic to any medications. Besides his CHF and pneumonia, he does not have other comorbid conditions.

43. Which of the following agents would be the most appropriate to administer for his agitation?

(A) chlorpromazine
(B) haloperidol
(C) lorazepam
(D) risperidone
(E) thioridazine

44. Which of the following agents would be the most appropriate to give in order to minimize the patient's risk of falling?

(A) haloperidol
(B) perphenazine
(C) quetiapine
(D) risperidone
(E) thioridazine

Questions 45 and 46

A 32-year-old man presents to your clinic after losing his job because he was intoxicated while working. He has been drinking daily since he was 16 years old. He was able to complete college and went to work full-time right after graduation, but has lost several jobs since. After the loss of his last job, his wife threatened to leave him if he does not get help.

45. Which of the following medications would be most useful as a behavioral modifier to decrease his alcohol use?

(A) acamprosate
(B) disulfiram
(C) flumazenil
(D) naloxone
(E) naltrexone

46. Further history reveals that he does not have a mood disorder. He tells you that often he simply cannot control his craving to have another drink. Which of the following agents would be most likely to decrease his cravings for alcohol?

(A) bupropion
(B) disulfiram
(C) flumazenil
(D) naloxone
(E) naltrexone

Questions 47 and 48

A 36-year-old woman is referred to you by her primary care physician for management of anxiety and fear that has persisted for several months. She reports that she was raped and held hostage on a boat for several days by two armed men. During this, she experienced intense fear for her life. Since then, she has had intense stress whenever she is near the water and has frequent nightmares. She cannot recall details of the ordeal but tries to avoid driving her car within sight of the ocean, which has been difficult because of the location of her home. She feels detached from her husband and family and has abandoned plans to pursue her career as a painter. She has difficulty falling asleep and is easily startled by phone calls. As a result of her experience, she no longer goes to public places alone.

47. Which of the following medications would be most helpful in treating the symptoms she is experiencing?

    (A) alprazolam
    (B) carbamazepine
    (C) fluoxetine
    (D) naltrexone
    (E) thioridazine

48. She is treated with the appropriate medication and has a significant reduction in most of her symptoms. However, she continues to experiences frequent, intense nightmares, resulting in her having poor sleep and fatigue the next day. Which of the following agents would be the most beneficial in reducing these symptoms?

    (A) lorazepam
    (B) naltrexone
    (C) olanzapine
    (D) perphenazine
    (E) prazosin

49. You have been asked to evaluate an 80-year-old male nursing home resident because of a change in mental status. The nursing staff reports that he has been a patient there for about a year without any problems until about 1 month ago when he began having difficulty sleeping. The staff physician prescribed lorazepam 2 mg at bedtime; however, he was

still unable to sleep. He started wandering during the day and has since been restricted to his room. Because he remains agitated during the day, they have been giving him lorazepam 2 mg every 6 hours for agitation. His other medications include hydrochlorothiazide 25 mg/d, digoxin 0.125 mg every other day, diltiazem 240 mg sustained release daily, and transdermal nitroglycerin 0.4 mg/h as needed. His electrolytes are normal except for a potassium level of 3.4 mmol/L. A recent digoxin level is not available. Which of the following interventions should be considered first?

    (A) checking the hydrochlorothiazide level
    (B) monitoring orthostatic vitals
    (C) replacing the potassium
    (D) stopping the room seclusion
    (E) tapering the lorazepam

Questions 50 and 51

A 64-year-old man, accompanied by his wife, presents to your office complaining of memory loss. He is a retired stockbroker who can no longer recall stock quotes like he did several years ago. His wife has become both concerned and annoyed because he seems to immediately forget whatever she tells him. These memory problems have slowly progressed over several years. Recently, he had difficulty getting dressed, and more than once, he put his underwear on over his pants. His wife has also noted that he speaks much less during dinner than he once did. He does not have any other significant medical illnesses.

50. Which of the following medications would be most likely to improve his condition?

    (A) aspirin
    (B) donepezil
    (C) fluoxetine
    (D) pemoline
    (E) trazodone

51. Upon further questioning, his wife reports that he does not sleep well at night and wanders around the house aimlessly. Subsequently, he sleeps for a large part of the day. Which of the

following medications would be the most useful to control this behavior?

(A) haloperidol

(B) lorazepam

(C) trazodone

(D) triazolam

(E) quetiapine

Questions 52 and 53

A 25-year-old man is brought into the emergency department lethargic and stuporous. He responds only to painful stimuli, wakes up briefly and yells, then goes back to sleep. Ambulance personnel report that they found him near a house known for drug trafficking. There is no evidence of physical injury.

52. Which of the following medications should he receive first?

(A) dextrose and flumazenil

(B) dextrose, flumazenil, and naloxone

(C) dextrose, flumazenil, naloxone, and thiamine

(D) dextrose and naloxone

(E) dextrose, naloxone, and thiamine

53. The patient is subsequently treated and a urine toxicology screen is positive for the presence of opioids. When he is more alert, he informs you that he has been using intravenous (IV) heroin daily for several weeks. His last use was about 8 hours ago. His heroin use escalated from snorting to IV use after he no longer felt a good "high" from snorting. He has never detoxified before. He has no comorbid medical conditions and he does not use alcohol. Which of the following medications would be the most appropriate to detoxify this patient?

(A) buprenorphine

(B) chlordiazepoxide

(C) clonidine

(D) naloxone

(E) propranolol

54. A 45-year-old woman presents to your practice with complaints of depression. Her mother passed away 6 months ago from lung cancer and her father died 4 years ago from the same disease. She has seen therapists to help with her grief but she continues to have ongoing sadness, terminal insomnia, low energy, poor appetite, and difficulty concentrating. She has passive thoughts of suicidal but no plan or intent. She denies prior suicide attempts. In addition, despite several attempts to quit smoking, she still smokes two packs of cigarettes a day and has had worsening asthma as a result. She has no additional medical problems. Which of the following medications would be the most appropriate to use in this patient?

(A) bupropion

(B) buspirone

(C) imipramine

(D) phenelzine

(E) trazodone

55. A 52-year-old man who has poorly controlled diabetes is referred to you for evaluation of medication noncompliance. You learn that he cannot fall asleep at night and has no energy during the day. His appetite is gone and he does not enjoy activities as he once did. Overall he feels depressed. Additionally, he has been experiencing chronic pain in his feet, deemed to be due to neuropathic pain, which is not relieved by analgesics. Which of the following medications would be the most useful in treating this patient's symptoms?

(A) alprazolam

(B) amitriptyline

(C) bupropion

(D) citalopram

(E) duloxetine

56. A 47-year-old woman presents to your office for psychiatric care because she has just relocated to your town. She has a history of bipolar disorder, but her prior psychiatrist recently stopped her lithium because she developed thyroid autoantibodies. She complains of being irritable and not able to sleep for several weeks. She tells you that her thoughts are racing and you have a difficult time redirecting her answers. However, she believes her biggest problem is her facial pain, which was diagnosed as trigeminal neuralgia and has not improved with analgesics. Which of the following medications would be the most appropriate in treating this patient's symptoms?

(A) amitriptyline
(B) carbamazepine
(C) fluoxetine
(D) gabapentin
(E) lithium

57. A 33-year-old woman with a history of schizophrenia has recently started treatment with olanzapine. She has tolerated the medication well and is living in a group home, anticipating moving into her own apartment. She no longer hears voices and no longer has a desire to hurt herself. Which of the following side effects would be most likely to interfere with her compliance?

(A) agranulocytosis
(B) development of cataracts
(C) galactorrhea
(D) increased excitability
(E) weight gain

58. A 42-year-old male with schizophrenia is being treated for an acute exacerbation of his auditory hallucinations. As is his pattern, he responds very favorably to medications while hospitalized, but when he is discharged forgets to take them regularly. This results in a cycle of subsequent worsening of his psychosis and rehospitalization. He is currently taking risperidone 5 mg/d orally, and he is tolerating it well with good efficacy. Which of the following would be the most appropriate next step in his treatment?

(A) continue the current regimen
(B) switch to clozapine
(C) switch to haloperidol
(D) switch to olanzapine
(E) switch to risperidone long-acting injection

Questions 59 and 60

A 50-year-old man who has felt depressed for several months, presents to your office for evaluation. He has had poor sleep, a decreased appetite with weight loss, no interest in his hobbies, and cannot concentrate during your cognitive examination. He has passing thoughts of dying but no active plan or intent. He reluctantly admits to frequently hearing voices telling him that he is going to die soon. You subsequently decide to start an antidepressant and risperidone at 0.5 mg bid.

59. Which of the following side effects of risperidone would be the most likely?

(A) agranulocytosis
(B) anticholinergic side effects
(C) leukocytosis
(D) orthostatic hypotension
(E) weight loss

60. As his dose of risperidone is increased, the risk of which of the following side effects will also increase?

(A) agranulocytosis
(B) anticholinergic effects
(C) extrapyramidal symptoms
(D) leukocytosis
(E) weight loss

61. A 33-year-old married female with a history of postpartum psychosis, likely due to bipolar disorder, has been stable since being maintained on risperidone for the past several years. Her son is doing well, and the patient and husband wish to have another child. For the past year she has been attempting to conceive without success. She is on no other medications besides the psychotropic, and she has not been using birth control. She has no other medical problems, and she is currently asymptomatic, without depression or psychotic symptoms.

She drinks 1 to 2 glasses of wine per week, denies illicit drugs, and does not use tobacco products. Involvement of which of the following brain pathways is most likely responsible for her infertility?

- (A) locus ceruleus
- (B) mesocortical tract
- (C) mesolimbic tract
- (D) nigrostriatal tract
- (E) tuberoinfundibular tract

Questions 62 and 63

A 19-year-old college student presents to the office at the urging of her friends, who are concerned about her well-being. For the past several months, she has been increasingly preoccupied with her weight and body image, and has been regularly cancelling plans with friends because she does not want to eat with other people. She states that she is "fat" and would like to lose 10 lb. When queried further, she admits that she is bingeing and throwing up almost every day. She denies any laxative use, and she has not been restricting her eating. She is 5 ft 4 in and weighs 110 lb. Her potassium is 3.4; other electrolytes are within normal limits. You replete her potassium and refer her for psychotherapy.

62. Which of the following would be the most effective medication for her condition?

- (A) bupropion
- (B) fluoxetine
- (C) lamotrigine
- (D) lithium
- (E) mirtazapine

63. You later learn that she was treated in high school for the same symptoms with sertraline and citalopram, both at high doses for over 3 months each, but with little improvement in her symptoms. Which of the following medications would be the most appropriate next step?

- (A) bupropion
- (B) lithium
- (C) paroxetine
- (D) topiramate
- (E) valproic acid

64. A 45-year-old female executive who travels often to Europe from the United States presents to your office complaining of significant insomnia and daytime fatigue after arriving in Germany. Which of the following medications would be the most appropriate treatment for her complaints?

- (A) amitriptyline
- (B) diphenhydramine
- (C) quetiapine
- (D) temazepam
- (E) zolpidem

Questions 65 and 66

A 60-year-old man presents to your office complaining of the sudden onset of palpitations, sweating, shaking, shortness of breath, choking, and feeling that he is "going crazy." These symptoms last 5 to 10 minutes and have occurred several times per week for the last 3 months. He denies any particular stressor or event which provokes the attacks, although he is "constantly" afraid of having future episodes. He has recently been seen by his cardiologist who has ruled out a cardiac etiology.

65. Which of the following is the most appropriate medication to treat this patient's disorder?

- (A) bupropion
- (B) imipramine
- (C) phenelzine
- (D) quetiapine
- (E) sertraline

66. If the patient's symptoms were due to a cardiac etiology and he subsequently became depressed, which medication would pose the highest risk?

- (A) amitriptyline
- (B) bupropion
- (C) methylphenidate
- (D) sertraline
- (E) venlafaxine

67. A 33-year-old woman with a diagnosis of chronic paranoid schizophrenia has been maintained on haloperidol since she was diagnosed at age 24. In your office, she says she has not had her menstrual period in several months, has diminished sex drive, has been discharging milk from her breasts, and has pain during sexual intercourse. Which of the following would most likely be increased in this patient?

(A) adrenocorticotropic hormone (ACTH)

(B) dopamine

(C) norepinephrine

(D) prolactin

(E) serotonin

68. A 24-year-old man is hospitalized because he has been hearing voices for 6 months telling him to kill himself and now fears that he may act on them. He lost his job 2 months ago and on mental status examination appears unkempt and disorganized, with a flat affect. He is begun on aripiprazole, and his symptoms eventually decrease enough for him to be discharged. On a follow-up visit to your office, he reports that his hallucinations have improved but that he "can't sit still" and feels like he needs to be constantly in motion. The patient intermittently stands up and walks around your office as you interview him. Which of the following conditions account for his new complaints?

(A) acute dystonic reaction

(B) akathisia

(C) manic episode

(D) neuroleptic malignant syndrome

(E) tardive dyskinesia

69. A 55-year-old man with a long history of major depression presents to your office after multiple failed antidepressant trials. Since the age of 20, he has had adequate trials of nortriptyline, phenelzine, fluoxetine, sertraline, bupropion, mirtazapine, venlafaxine, and duloxetine, with minimal response. Other psychiatrists have suggested ECT in the past, but he is concerned about memory loss. He would like to try transcranial magnetic stimulation (rTMS), and wants to know more about side effects. Which

of the following side effects do you inform him is the most likely?

(A) headache

(B) hearing loss

(C) memory loss

(D) seizures

(E) tooth pain

70. You have been treating a 33-year-old woman with bipolar disorder for 4 years. In preparation for a planned pregnancy, you have agreed to taper her medications but see her frequently in case of a manic episode. Six weeks into her pregnancy, she presents to your office with pressured speech and the belief that her baby is Jesus Christ. Her husband says he is concerned because she has stopped taking her prenatal vitamins and is acting bizarrely. Which of the following treatments would be the safest to treat her symptoms?

(A) carbamazepine

(B) diazepam

(C) divalproex sodium

(D) electroconvulsive therapy (ECT)

(E) lithium carbonate

71. You are the consult-liaison psychiatrist on call for the trauma surgery team. You are asked to evaluate a man who was hit by a car and severely injured. He is unable to give a history, but an acquaintance who accompanied the patient to the hospital reports that he is a daily, heavy drug user. On examination, the patient is noted to have track marks on his arms. Which of the following classes of drugs do you tell the surgeons is the most dangerous if abruptly withdrawn?

(A) cannabinoids

(B) hallucinogens

(C) opiates

(D) sedative-hypnotics

(E) stimulants

Questions 72 and 73

A 44-year-old man with a history of chronic, severe alcoholism is brought to the emergency room. You get a report from a family member that he "has been living off booze and drugs and nothing else for weeks." The emergency department nurse is about to go in to draw blood from the patient and offer him food.

72. Which of the following is the most appropriate next step in the treatment of this patient?

   (A) Administer lorazepam.
   (B) Administer thiamine.
   (C) Listen for a cardiac murmur.
   (D) Obtain liver function tests.
   (E) Obtain a vitamin B_{12} level.

73. After he is admitted to the medicine service, which of the following medications would be the most appropriate to initiate?

   (A) acamprosate
   (B) clonidine
   (C) disulfiram
   (D) lorazepam
   (E) naltrexone

DIRECTIONS (Questions 74 through 83): The following group of numbered items are preceded by a list of lettered options. For each vignette, select the one lettered option that is *most* closely associated with it. Each lettered option may be used once, multiple times, or not at all.

Questions 74 through 81

For each vignette, choose the medication most likely to be associated with the side effect.

   (A) carbamazepine
   (B) clozapine
   (C) divalproex sodium
   (D) haloperidol
   (E) lithium
   (F) paroxetine
   (G) perphenazine
   (H) pimozide
   (I) ziprasidone

74. A 14-year-old boy being treated pharmacologically for Tourette disorder is additionally started on citalopram and has an increase of 11 msec in his QTc values on ECG.

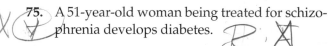

75. A 51-year-old woman being treated for schizophrenia develops diabetes.

76. An 11-year-old girl being treated for major depressive disorder reports frequent suicidal ideation.

77. A 34-year-old woman being treated for bipolar I disorder develops acute pain in her abdomen and is diagnosed with pancreatitis.

78. The WBC count of a 27-year-old man being treated for treatment refractory schizophrenia drops to 3000/mL.

79. A 42-year-old man stops his antidepressant. Two days later, he experiences a feeling of hopelessness, has difficulty sleeping, and feels quite anxious.

80. A 36-year-old woman being treated for bipolar disorder finds herself urinating very frequently.

81. Several months after starting on a new antipsychotic, a 32-year-old patient's total cholesterol increases from 200 to 250 mg/dL.

Questions 82 and 83

For each vignette, choose the medication most appropriate to prescribe.

   (A) alprazolam
   (B) citalopram
   (C) divalproex sodium
   (D) fluoxetine
   (E) haloperidol
   (F) lithium
   (G) clozapine
   (H) paroxetine
   (I) risperidone
   (J) sertraline
   (K) trazodone

82. A 34-year-old man with schizoaffective disorder has been noncompliant with medications in the past. You want to be able to give him a depot injection of an antipsychotic.

83. You are treating a 45-year-old veteran with a history of alcoholism for posttraumatic stress disorder (PTSD) and he asked you for something to help him sleep.

DIRECTIONS (Questions 84 through 105): For each of the multiple choice questions in this section, select the lettered answer that is the one *best* response in each case.

Questions 84 and 85

A 28-year-old single woman presents with 8 weeks of depression, insomnia, low energy and fatigue, distractibility, and poor appetite. She has not prior psychiatric history and no family psychiatric history. After further history and laboratory evaluations are completed, she is begun on sertraline, which is eventually increased to 100 mg/d. After 2 months on that dose, the patient reports that she feels "back to normal" and asks when she can stop the medication.

84. How long should you recommend her to continue the medication?

   (A) 1 month
   (B) 2 months
   (C) 4 months
   (D) 10 months
   (E) 2 years

85. She returns for a follow-up visit 1 month later. Her symptoms have continued to remain in remission, although she describes recent conflict with her boyfriend due to having "little sex drive." The patient states that it has gotten to the point where she has decided to stop the medication unless something can be done. She is willing to switch to another medication despite the risk of relapse. Which of the following agents would be the most appropriate choice?

   (A) bupropion
   (B) citalopram
   (C) clomipramine
   (D) fluoxetine
   (E) fluvoxamine

Questions 86 and 87

You are treating a 28-year-old man with a 6-year history of schizophrenia who lives with his parents. The patient has had a number of debilitating side effects, such as severe extrapyramidal symptoms, from traditional antipsychotics including haloperidol. His family is worried about weight gain, which the patient experienced on olanzapine. Despite the numerous medications, his psychotic symptoms continue. You discuss clozapine with the patient and his family and they agree to try the medication. You have initiated treatment slowly and he has shown some improvement; however, he has been producing a large amount of saliva and drool soaking his shirts.

86. Which of the following is the most appropriate next step?

   (A) Add amantadine.
   (B) Add propranolol.
   (C) Add propylthiouracil.
   (D) Discontinue clozapine.
   (E) Increase the dose of clozapine.

87. In addition to the above, the patient complains of palpitations. An ECG reveals sinus tachycardia, which is consistent with prior ECGs performed over the past month. Which of the following is the most appropriate next step?

   (A) Add benztropine.
   (B) Add labetalol.
   (C) Add lorazepam.
   (D) Add propranolol.
   (E) Discontinue clozapine.

88. A 21-year-old single female college student is brought to the university health service by her roommates. She makes it clear to you that she does not think there's anything wrong with her, but her roommates tell you that they "can't deal with her anymore" because she never sleeps and "never shuts up." The patient insists this is because she has discovered an important mathematical proof that she must finish writing. She's convinced that the university will immediately grant her tenure as soon as they see the

proof, although she has trouble staying on topic when you ask questions about it. She has not seen a psychiatrist before, and a urine toxicology screen, which she consents to "to prove I'm not crazy," is negative. Which of the following is the most appropriate agent for initial and maintenance treatment of this patient?

(A) haloperidol
(B) lamotrigine
(C) lithium
(D) lorazepam
(E) olanzapine

89. A 34-year-old electrical engineer complains to his doctor that he has been feeling depressed for several months after the breakup of his marriage. Since that time, he has had significant insomnia, difficulty concentrating, has lost 25 lb in the last 3 months because his appetite isn't the same, feels fatigued, has significant feelings of guilt regarding the separation, feels hopeless and helpless, and has felt suicidal without a specific plan. A diagnosis of major depressive disorder is made and he is begun on an antidepressant. Which of the following symptoms would be expected to take the most time to improve?

(A) decreased appetite
(B) decreased concentration
(C) decreased energy
(D) insomnia
(E) suicidality

90. A 56-year-old man with a history of cirrhosis, hepatitis C, and alcoholism wishes to quit drinking but wants to detox first. Which of the following medications would be the most appropriate drug to use in this patient?

(A) alprazolam
(B) chlordiazepoxide
(C) clonazepam
(D) diazepam
(E) lorazepam

91. The patient is a 59-year-old female with chronic schizophrenia, undifferentiated type, as well

as poorly controlled diabetes mellitus, obesity, hyperlipidemia, and hypertension. She has been treated for over 35 years with various first-generation antipsychotics, and although she is on an adequate dose, she still has residual psychotic symptoms and has now begun to develop involuntary blinking and tongue rolling movements. She is agreeable to switching to a second-generation antipsychotic. Which of the following medications would be the most appropriate for this patient?

(A) aripiprazole
(B) clozapine
(C) olanzapine
(D) quetiapine
(E) risperidone

92. Jane is a 20-year-old woman who has been using cocaine regularly for more than 3 years. Over the past 12 months, she finds that she has had to use increasing amounts of cocaine in order to obtain the same level of "high." Which of the following terms best describes this effect?

(A) abuse
(B) addiction
(C) dependence
(D) tolerance
(E) withdrawal

93. A 35-year-old single man presents to your office complaining of insomnia. He reports that he is able to fall asleep at night, but stays asleep for only 2 or 3 hours, then wakes up frequently throughout the night. He is exhausted and would like something to help him sleep. Other than feeling frustrated and fatigued during the day, he denies other depressive symptoms or any past psychiatric history. Which of the following medications would be the most appropriate for this patient?

(A) amitriptyline
(B) ramelteon
(C) trazodone
(D) zaleplon
(E) zolpidem

94. A 42-year-old married, pregnant woman with a history of hypertension, myocardial infarction, degenerative disc disease, and major depression with psychotic features is being considered for electroconvulsive therapy (ECT) after failing multiple antidepressant and antipsychotic trials. Which of the following conditions would be a relative contraindication to ECT?

    (A) degenerative disc disease
    (B) hypertension
    (C) pregnancy
    (D) psychotic depression
    (E) recent myocardial infarction

95. You are called to consult on a 70-year-old woman, hospitalized in the ICU after a myocardial infarction. The patient is yelling at staff, pulling out her IV and trying to get out of bed. She refuses to take any medication by mouth. Her ECG shows a QTc of 460. Which of the following medications would be best to help her agitation?

    (A) diazepam IV
    (B) haloperidol IV
    (C) lorazepam IV
    (D) olanzapine IM
    (E) risperidone Consta IM

96. A 30-year-old woman with no previous psychiatric history presents to your office asking for help in managing performance anxiety. She loves to act and sing in her community theatre, but she becomes terrified when getting on stage in front of crowds. As a result, her voice shakes and she has been unable to get "good parts." Which of the following medications would be the most appropriate to prescribe?

    (A) buspirone
    (B) fluoxetine
    (C) fluvoxamine
    (D) lorazepam
    (E) propranolol

97. A 23-year-old patient with schizophrenia who was recently started on risperidone complains that he cannot sit still and feels constantly restless. The nursing staff has noted that he often paces. Which of the following side effects is the patient most likely experiencing?

    (A) acute dystonia
    (B) akathisia
    (C) neuroleptic malignant syndrome
    (D) parkinsonism
    (E) tardive dyskinesia

98. A 29-year-old woman with a history of seizures is diagnosed with bipolar disorder, most recent episode depressed, and started on lamotrigine. Which of the following side effects would be the most important about which to educate the patient?

    (A) acute dystonia
    (B) akathisia
    (C) aplastic anemia
    (D) rash
    (E) renal failure

99. A 19-year-old man with bipolar disorder is brought in to the emergency room by the police. He is grandiose and delusional, as well as agitated and combative. He is given an intramuscular injection of haloperidol. After 30 minutes, the patient is found arching forward. On physical examination, stiffness of the neck and back muscles are noted. Which of the following terms best describes this side effect?

    (A) laryngospasm
    (B) oculogyric crisis
    (C) opisthotonos
    (D) pleurothotonos
    (E) torticollis

100. The patient is a 59-year-old woman with a past medical history of hypercholesterolemia, diabetes, and diabetic neuropathy, who presents to her primary care doctor with the chief complaint of "headaches." Upon further interview, she states her symptoms began after the death of her husband 5 months ago. Since that time, she has felt "empty," with poor sleep, fatigue, decreased concentration, and wishes she "would die so I can join him." Her review of systems is remarkable for ongoing "sharp pins

and needles" in her extremities. Her physical examination is unremarkable and her blood sugars have been relatively well-controlled. Which of the following would be the most appropriate treatment for her symptoms?

(A) bupropion
(B) duloxetine
(C) fluoxetine
(D) mirtazapine
(E) reassurance

101. A 44-year-old married male patient with a history of recurrent major depressive disorder presents to a psychiatrist after stopping his sertraline 1 month ago. Although it has been effective in the treatment of his depression, he has had increasing difficulty maintaining an erection, and this has caused friction and conflicts with his wife. He is concerned, however, that he will have a relapse of his depressive symptoms if not medicated. Which of the following would be the most appropriate pharmacologic treatment for this individual?

(A) Begin mirtazapine.
(B) Begin paroxetine.
(C) Begin venlafaxine.
(D) No medication.
(E) Restart sertraline.

102. A 58-year-old man with atrial fibrillation, hypercholesterolemia, and hypertension is sent to you by his primary care physician for help in managing his anxiety. He reports that for many years he has worried "about everything," and that he occasionally has to stay home from work because he becomes so fearful. He often has difficulty falling asleep and not uncommonly gets tension headaches when particularly stressed. His medications include warfarin, atorvastatin, and hydrochlorothiazide. He does not drink alcohol or caffeine. Which of the following medications would be the most appropriate to treat this patient's symptoms?

(A) bupropion
(B) buspirone
(C) citalopram

(D) clonazepam
(E) venlafaxine

103. A 40-year-old man is started on fluoxetine for major depressive disorder. He notes improvement in his mood, but has difficulty sleeping. Trazodone is subsequently added to his regimen. Three days later, he calls complaining of a painful erection that has not subsided after several hours. Which of the following best describes this patient's condition?

(A) erectile dysfunction
(B) nymphomania
(C) parapraxis
(D) priapism
(E) satyriasis

104. A 35-year-old married female is being followed by a psychiatrist for her first episode of major depression. She is prescribed citalopram 40 mg daily and has been in remission for 3 months. She now complains of the new onset of decreased libido which is causing her a moderate amount of distress. Which of the following would be the most appropriate to add to her current regimen?

(A) bupropion
(B) desipramine
(C) lithium
(D) tranylcypromine
(E) venlafaxine

105. A 41-year-old woman presents to your office asking for help in managing her binge eating. She eats large amounts of junk food three or four times a week, hides food, and subsequently feels guilty about her actions. Her BMI is 31. After performing a thorough history and physical examination, you decide to prescribe topiramate. Which of the following side effects do you tell her is most likely?

(A) improved attention
(B) pancreatitis
(C) polyuria
(D) renal stones
(E) weight gain

DIRECTIONS (Questions 106 through 109): The following group of questions are preceded by a list of lettered options. For each question, select the one lettered option that is *most* closely associated with it. Each lettered option may be used once, multiple times, or not at all.

Questions 106 through 109

For the following vignettes, choose the correct term from the list below.

- (A) abuse
- (B) amotivational syndrome
- (C) cannabis
- (D) dependence
- (E) formication
- (F) inhalants
- (G) intoxication
- (H) post-hallucinogen perception disorder
- (I) tolerance
- (J) withdrawal

106. A 45-year-old man with chronic cocaine dependence presents to the emergency department with complaints of bugs crawling on his skin.

107. A 16-year-old boy is brought to you by his mother. She states that despite having a high IQ he doesn't complete his homework, has been failing in school, and has stopped going out with friends. He admits to smoking two to three joints of marijuana daily.

108. A 21-year-old man is brought into the emergency department by the police after getting arrested for stealing gasoline. The patient feels disconnected from reality and frightened. On physical examination, he is noted to have a rash around his mouth.

109. A 54-year-old man with opiate dependence relapsed on heroin after several months of sobriety. While he began using $10 to $20 per day at first, he quickly increased his use to $50 to $60 per day because "I don't get high now unless I use more."

DIRECTIONS (Question 110): Select the lettered answer that is the one *best* response in this case.

110. A 27-year-old man with paranoid schizophrenia notices the development of breasts, a decreased libido, and not ejaculating when he has an orgasm. He is currently being treated with risperidone. Which of the following dopaminergic pathways is most likely responsible for these side effects?
- (A) extrapyramidal
- (B) mesocortical
- (C) mesolimbic
- (D) nigrostriatal
- (E) tuberoinfundibular

DIRECTIONS (Questions 111 through 121): The following group of questions are preceded by a list of lettered options. For each question, select the one lettered option that is *most* closely associated with it. Each lettered option may be used once, multiple times, or not at all.

Questions 111 through 121

For the following vignettes, choose the correct side effect from the list below.

- (A) agranulocytosis
- (B) akathisia
- (C) blepharospasm
- (D) constipation
- (E) galactorrhea
- (F) gynecomastia
- (G) neuroleptic malignant syndrome
- (H) obstructive jaundice
- (I) opisthotonos
- (J) orthostatic hypotension
- (K) pigmented retinopathy
- (L) pseudoparkinsonism
- (M) rabbit syndrome
- (N) retrograde ejaculation
- (O) tardive dyskinesia
- (P) torticollis

111. A 35-year-old man with chronic schizophrenia taking thioridazine notices that, if he urinates after masturbating, his urine appears cloudy.

112. A 46-year-old Caucasian woman with schizoaffective disorder, bipolar type has been managed for many years on risperidone 3 mg twice daily orally. She denies any complaints but on mental status examination is noted to have repetitive, rapid movements of her mouth (but not tongue) with smacking of her lips.

113. A 22-year-old African-American man on clozapine for 3 months reports a sore throat and fever. A CBC is obtained with a WBC count of $1000/\text{mm}^3$ with 1% granulocytes.

114. A 43-year-old man with schizophrenia is on haloperidol. He is noted to have a flexed posture, festinating gait, resting tremor, and bradykinesia.

115. The same 43-year-old man was continued on haloperidol despite his side effects and after several years developed choreoathetoid movements of the trunk and limbs along with lip smacking and tongue movements.

116. A 21-year-old man with psychosis was started on haloperidol at high doses. Eight days into his treatment, he developed fever, generalized rigidity, diaphoresis, and altered mental status.

117. A 36-year-old man with schizoaffective disorder, depressed type has been receiving fluphenazine decanoate 50 mg intramuscularly every 2 weeks. While his symptoms are well-controlled, he has recently noticed a white discharge from his nipples, bilaterally.

118. A 26-year-old man being treated with high-dose thioridazine is found on ophthalmologic examination to have peppery pigmentation of the retina. Despite discontinuation of the medication, the pigmentation continues and the patient eventually suffers total blindness.

119. A 22-year-old man complains of severe restlessness and agitation after starting on aripiprazole. He complains that he cannot sit still and paces constantly.

120. A 26-year-old patient with schizophrenia is started on chlorpromazine. After 1 week, he complains of flu-like symptoms. A CBC is obtained and is normal. After another week, the patient develops a yellowish color to his skin and sclera.

121. A 45-year-old patient with schizophrenia is started on a high dose of chlorpromazine. The next day, he complains of being light-headed every time he stands. On examination, he is noted to have a significant decrease in blood pressure and an increase in heart rate.

DIRECTIONS (Questions 122 and 123): For each of the multiple choice questions in this section, select the lettered answer that is the one *best* response in each case.

122. You are called in the middle of the night by the surgical service to see a 52-year-old man who was admitted to the hospital 36 hours earlier for an emergency appendectomy. The man is very agitated and is talking nonsense to the nurse, who is unable to calm him down. His blood pressure is 200/100 and his pulse is 95. He does not know the date and thinks that he is in a hotel. Review of the chart shows that he was fully oriented and had stable vitals at the time of admission. You suspect alcohol withdrawal. How long after this patient's last drink would you expect to see these significant withdrawal symptoms develop?

(A) 6 hours
(B) 12 hours
(C) 1 day
(D) 3 days
(E) 7 days

123. A 33-year-old man with a history of bipolar I disorder is admitted to the inpatient unit with acute mania. Because he has failed previous trials of lithium, valproic acid, and olanzapine, he is started on oxcarbazepine. Three days later, he complains of nausea and weakness; he appears confused about why he is in the hospital. Which of the following laboratory studies should be ordered first?

(A) BUN and creatinine

(B) CBC

C

(C) electrolytes

(D) liver function tests

(E) oxcarbazepine level

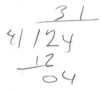

Answers and Explanations

1. **(C)** Phenelzine is a monoamine oxidase inhibitor, used for the treatment of severe depression. Phenelzine, tranylcypromine, and isocarboxazid are irreversible blockers of MAO-A (monoamine oxidase-A) and MAO-B activity; selegiline, given orally or in the form of a skin patch, is an MAO-B inhibitor that was developed for the treatment of Parkinson disease; at higher doses, it is a nonselective MAO inhibitor and is used in the treatment of depression. These medications are extremely dangerous in overdose and, after a brief asymptomatic period of 12 to 24 hours, may produce hyperpyrexia and autonomic excitability sufficient enough to cause rhabdomyolysis. Supportive care should be instituted. If delirium develops, small doses of IV benzodiazepines should be used. Lorazepam is preferred because of its short elimination half-life. Neuroleptics, especially short-acting agents such as chlorpromazine, should be avoided because of their tendency to contribute to hypotension. If ventricular arrhythmias develop, they can be treated with lidocaine. Cyproheptadine is a 5-HT$_{2a}$ antagonist that is sometimes used in the treatment of the most severe cases of serotonin syndrome. Meperidine should be avoided because it may contribute to the adrenergic crisis. Phenytoin may be used if seizures develop. Other medications that are contraindicated with MAOIs include stimulants, decongestants, amine precursors such as L-dopa and L-tryptophan, and the antihypertensives methyldopa, guanethidine, and reserpine.

2. **(E)** Blocking reuptake of catecholamines and indolamines in patients already using an MAOI can result in a potentially life-threatening drug interaction known as serotonin syndrome. Medications that block such reuptake include the SSRIs, TCAs, buspirone, and other antidepressants such as venlafaxine. Features of mild serotonin syndrome include a triad of mental status changes, autonomic hyperactivity, and neuromuscular abnormalities. Symptoms include tachycardia, flushing, fever, hypertension, ocular oscillations, and myoclonic jerks. Severe serotonin syndrome may result in serious hyperthermia, coma, autonomic instability, convulsions, and death; therefore, one must wait at least 14 days after discontinuing an MAOI before starting a serotonergic agent. Acute dystonia (including opisthotonos) occurs with the use of antipsychotic medication, not MAOIs. Akathisia, or the inner feeling of restlessness, is another extrapyramidal side effect of neuroleptic drugs. Neuroleptic malignant syndrome is an idiosyncratic reaction to neuroleptic drugs resembling malignant hyperthermia.

3. **(C)** This patient is likely suffering from a major depressive episode. Because of her weight gain, hypersomnia, and mood reactivity, her depression has atypical features. Although atypical features respond best to MAOIs such as phenelzine, these medications are rarely used because of the potential risk of a fatal hypertensive crisis when eating certain tyramine-containing foods. SSRIs such as fluoxetine and sertraline are also beneficial even though response rates to SSRIs may not match those of the MAOIs. Because of their favorable safety profile, SSRIs have become a first-line treatment in major depression. Tricyclic antidepressants such as nortriptyline are less

effective than MAOIs for atypical depression. Trazodone is an extremely sedating antidepressant that is generally used for adjunctive treatment of insomnia.

4. **(C)** Approximately 60% of patients who are going to have a response to an antidepressant do so within the first 6 weeks. However, it can take up to 12 weeks to achieve a full response. Only 30% of people with major depressive disorder achieve full remission from their first antidepressant trial.

5. **(E)** Alcohol withdrawal should be strongly considered in this patient. Benzodiazepines are the drug of choice for control of alcohol withdrawal symptoms as well as for prophylaxis against withdrawal seizures and the potentially life-threatening delirium tremens. Long-acting benzodiazepines such as chlordiazepoxide and diazepam are appropriate; however, both are extensively metabolized by the liver. Because this patient has elevated transaminases, oxazepam or lorazepam, which only undergo glucuronidation (and are therefore not dependent on liver functioning) prior to elimination, are preferable. The mnemonic "LOT" (Lorazepam, Oxazepam, Temazepam) can be helpful in remembering which benzodiazepines are metabolized in this way. A high-potency antipsychotic agent such as haloperidol may be necessary to help control this patient's agitation; however, an antipsychotic will not prevent alcohol withdrawal, and low-potency antipsychotics, such as chlorpromazine, should be avoided because they may actually lower the seizure threshold. Disulfiram is used to treat alcohol dependence, not acute alcohol withdrawal.

6. **(E)** This patient has delirium tremens, which is a medical emergency. He should be transferred to an intensive care setting where IV benzodiazepines can be administered with greater safety. The IV route is preferred in this situation to ensure adequate and rapid absorption. Haloperidol can be used for its sedative effect but it should not take the place of a benzodiazepine. Similarly, IV labetalol may be useful in the intensive care unit but it will not manage the underlying withdrawal and should not replace a benzodiazepine.

7. **(B)** This patient is suffering from major depression with psychotic features. Best practice recommends a combination of an antidepressant and an antipsychotic medication, such as fluoxetine and risperidone. Electroconvulsive therapy, not listed among the answer choices, is another effective treatment for psychotic depression. Of note, a recent Cochrane Review demonstrated that antidepressant monotherapy *may* be just as effective, but this is not yet standard practice. Antipsychotic monotherapy is also not nearly as effective. Clozapine, a second-generation antipsychotic, is reserved for the treatment of patients with schizophrenia who have failed two or more antipsychotic trials. Clonazepam, a benzodiazepine, may provide some relief from anxiety, but will not treat the underlying condition.

8. **(D)** This patient is experiencing symptoms of lithium toxicity, the severity of which is determined by checking a lithium level. A therapeutic lithium level is 0.8 to 1.2. At levels around 1.2, patients experience tremor, nausea, diarrhea, and ataxia; this is followed by seizures at levels 1.5 to 2.0, then acute renal failure (requiring dialysis) at levels greater than 2.0, with subsequent coma and death at levels above 2.5. Because lithium has such a narrow therapeutic index, dehydration can lead to toxicity. While carbamazepine and depakote are both used to treat bipolar disorder, they have much wider therapeutic indexes. A head CT is not indicated in this case, given that the most likely cause of the patient's symptoms is lithium toxicity. Similarly, there is nothing in the vignette to suggest substance intoxication as a cause of her symptoms.

9. **(D)** Akathisia, a movement disorder that is a frequent side effect of antipsychotic medication, can be difficult to distinguish from anxiety in a psychotic individual; however, new-onset restlessness in a patient recently started on antipsychotic medication suggests this diagnosis. Although more common with first-generation antipsychotics, it can be seen with second-generation antipsychotics as well at rates as high as 20%. Onset usually begins between 5 and 60 days after initiation of treatment

but can occur after just one dose. First, the neuroleptic dose should be reduced as much as possible. If symptoms of akathisia continue, in the absence of other extrapyramidal side effects, many clinicians would then start treatment with a beta-blocker such as propranolol. In general, anticholinergic agents such as benztropine are used to treat extrapyramidal symptoms such as dystonia or parkinsonism. Diphenhydramine is helpful in acute dystonias but not in akathisia. Lorazepam, a benzodiazepine, is an appropriate second-line treatment for akathisia if symptoms are still not managed or the patient cannot tolerate a beta-blocker. Given the patient's improvement of his psychotic symptoms, it is preferable to continue treatment with aripiprazole plus the above adjunctive medications rather than switching to another antipsychotic.

10. **(C)** This patient is suffering from bipolar II depression, with a history characterized by a current major depressive episode and a history of hypomania. The treatment of bipolar depression is controversial. Most treatment guidelines recommend lithium, lamotrigine, or quetiapine as first-line options. Valproic acid may be a reasonable second-line choice. Monotherapy with antidepressants (eg, bupropion, fluoxetine, venlafaxine) is not recommended due to the risk of inducing mania, and the use of antidepressants in conjunction with mood stabilizers remains debatable.

11. **(E)** This patient is experiencing neuroleptic malignant syndrome (NMS), a rare but serious side effect of antipsychotic medications. Rhabdomyolysis is the most common dangerous complication of NMS, occurring in up to 25% of patients in one series. Dialysis may be required to protect patients from renal failure. The white blood cell count and creatinine phosphokinase are often elevated in NMS but there are no specific laboratory findings. All of the other listed complications have been reported in NMS but with less frequency.

12. **(D)** Retinal pigmentation is known to occur when thioridazine is used in high doses (>1000 mg/d). It may not remit when thioridazine is discontinued and can eventually lead to blindness. The other choices can occur with all neuroleptics and are not specific to thioridazine.

13. **(C)** This patient is suffering from panic disorder with agoraphobia. There are many medications that have demonstrated efficacy in this condition, including TCAs, SSRIs, MAOIs, and high-potency benzodiazepines. Of the agents listed, only fluoxetine, an SSRI, is one of them. Bupropion, an antidepressant with dopamine activity, and buspirone, a partial 5-HT$_{1a}$ antagonist with antianxiety activity, are not effective in panic disorder. Propranolol, a beta-adrenergic blocker, may help to alleviate the physical symptoms of panic such as tachycardia, but it does not prevent the attacks. Trazodone, an antidepressant with mixed serotonergic effects, has also shown conflicting results.

14. **(C)** Clonazepam is the most potent benzodiazepine listed. Using 1 mg of lorazepam for the equivalent dose in milligrams, the potency relationship of some common benzodiazepines is as follows: clonazepam 0.25 mg, alprazolam 0.5 mg, diazepam 5 mg, oxazepam 15 mg, and chlordiazepoxide 25 mg.

15. **(E)** Because lithium is a Group IA monovalent ion, the kidney handles it much as it does sodium. Ninety-five percent of lithium is excreted unchanged through the kidneys. Therefore electrolytes, creatinine, and BUN are required to check baseline kidney function. Thyroid studies are also required because lithium inhibits the synthesis of thyroid hormone and its release from the thyroid. A CBC is optional, although lithium may cause a benign elevation in the WBC. Fasting glucose and lipids should be checked prior to initiating treatment with antipsychotic agents. Liver function tests should be performed prior to initiating treatment with divalproex sodium; rare cases of fatal hepatotoxicity have been reported with divalproex sodium. In addition, divalproex sodium may also elevate serum ammonia levels, but this is also rare.

16. **(E)** In some individuals, nonsteroidal anti-inflammatory agents (NSAIDs) cause an

increase in lithium levels. Therefore, these agents should be used with caution in patients taking lithium, and avoided if possible. Aspirin and sulindac, however, do not affect lithium levels and are therefore safe for use with lithium. Given his bipolar disorder, the patient's mood stabilizer should not be discontinued, and the other choices are not appropriate in this case.

17. **(C)** Difficulty falling asleep and decreased appetite are the two most common side effects of methylphenidate. Stimulants have been reported to slow growth; however, it is believed to be less common with methylphenidate and dose related. When drug holidays are given, a growth rebound is seen. Methylphenidate may also cause an increase in systolic blood pressure.

18. **(E)** Stimulants have been frequently reported to exacerbate the tics associated with Tourette disorder, and some studies have warned that they should not be given to children with tics or a family history of Tourette. However, this is complicated by the fact that some studies have identified frequent comorbidity of attention-deficit hyperactivity disorder (ADHD) and Tourette disorder. The other symptoms are not associated with stimulant use.

19. **(D)** This patient is suffering from Tourette disorder. Pharmacologic treatment is strictly symptomatic and not curative. Dopamine (D_2) receptor antagonism with antipsychotic medication such as haloperidol provides the greatest symptom relief in children suffering from Tourette disorder. Clonidine, an alpha-2-agonist, is preferable in the treatment of mild Tourette's as it does not have the same long-term side effects as antipsychotics. The other medications listed are not used for Tourette.

20. **(C)** Only 30% of patients achieve remission from depression after treatment with an SSRI. Best practice would be to change to another SSRI (citalopram) or an SNRI (venlafaxine); however, because of his history of hypertension, venlafaxine, which carries with it a 5% to 7% rate of hypertension, is not the best choice. Nortriptyline, a tricyclic antidepressant, is a potentially dangerous choice in a patient with a history of myocardial infarction. Augmentation with lithium and thyroid hormone are reasonable choices for a patient with a *partial* response, but are not appropriate when a patient has no response to treatment.

21. **(E)** The most likely syndrome is tardive dyskinesia (TD), a movement disorder that may occur after long-term treatment with antipsychotic medications (especially first generation) such as haloperidol. In patients on first-generation antipsychotics, TD occurs at an average rate of about 5% per year, with about 20% developing TD within 5 years, and 40% developing it within 20 years. TD consists of a number of abnormal and involuntary movements such as lip smacking, facial grimacing, and choreoathetoid-like movements of the limbs and trunk. Anticholinergic toxicity, which usually presents as delirium, is not present. In Huntington disease, an autosomal dominant genetic disorder, the involuntary movements are accompanied by a progressive dementia. Meige syndrome is an oral facial dystonia involving blinking and chin thrusting, sometimes lip pursing or tongue movements, and occasionally shoulder movement. Sydenham chorea, associated with rheumatic fever, occurs in children.

22. **(B)** It was once believed that if patients developed signs of tardive dyskinesia, they would eventually progress to severe dyskinesias. Recent evidence, however, indicates that most patients stabilize and some may actually improve, even if they continue taking the antipsychotic. However, the only medication that may improve these symptoms is clozapine, a second-/third-line antipsychotic that requires regular white blood cell count monitoring.

23. **(E)** This patient likely has generalized anxiety disorder (GAD). Benzodiazepines are the most effective medications for quickly reducing symptoms of GAD. All benzodiazepines are effective and the choice should be based on potency, half-life, and side effects. Bupropion is an antidepressant with dopaminergic and noradrenergic properties, but is not useful in the treatment of GAD.

Buspirone is effective for reducing symptoms of GAD but requires several weeks for significant improvement. The tricyclic agent clomipramine and SSRIs such as fluoxetine have anxiolytic properties but also do not work as quickly as benzodiazepines.

24. **(B)** This patient likely has the Axis II diagnosis of borderline personality disorder (BPD) with comorbid depression. Borderline personality disorder is primarily treated by psychotherapy, particularly dialectical behavioral therapy. However, medication can provide useful adjunctive treatment. Given her comorbid depressive symptoms, fluoxetine would be the most appropriate treatment. However, a recent meta-analysis of pharmacotherapy of BPD showed that mood stabilizers (eg, valproic acid, lamotrigine, topiramate, carbamazepine) and second-generation antipsychotics (aripiprazole, olanzapine, ziprasidone) may be the most effective medications for this condition in the absence of comorbid depression.

25. **(E)** Decisions about whether to continue antidepressants during pregnancy are highly individualized, based on weighing risks and benefits for each individual woman. In one study of pregnant women with histories of major depression, 68% of those who discontinued medication relapsed, versus 26% of those who continued medication. One of the most serious potential risks of SSRI exposure during pregnancy is persistent pulmonary hypertension of the newborn (PPHN), a rare condition (1-2 per 1000 live births) in which newborns develop respiratory failure due to postnatal persistence of elevated pulmonary vascular resistance. In one case-control study, infants exposed to SSRI antidepressants after 20 weeks gestation had six times the rate of PPHN as control infants; however, the absolute numbers were extremely small. Epstein anomaly, a malformation of the tricuspid valve, is seen with lithium exposure. Gestational diabetes is not associated with antidepressant use. Infant developmental delay can be seen with exposure to valproic acid. Neural tube defects are seen with exposure to mood stabilizers such as carbamazepine and valproic acid.

26. **(C)** Unless there is a comorbid psychiatric disorder such as depression or obsessive compulsive disorder, pharmacotherapy generally has a limited role in the treatment of anorexia nervosa. Reports on the usefulness of cyproheptadine to stimulate appetite have been mixed. Generally, these patients already have a good appetite, but work hard not to give in to their own hunger. Fluoxetine, an SSRI, and topiramate, an anticonvulsant, have both shown to be effective in the treatment of bulimia nervosa, but not in the treatment of anorexia. The second-generation antipsychotic olanzapine can induce weight gain, but because of this, most patients with anorexia will not agree to take it.

27. **(A)** This patient likely has SSRI discontinuation syndrome, which may occur within 1 to 3 days of abruptly stopping an SSRI. The most common physical symptoms are dizziness, nausea and vomiting, fatigue, lethargy, and flu-like symptoms. Psychological symptoms of anxiety, irritability, and crying spells are also not unusual. Paroxetine may be more likely to cause this because of its short half-life and lack of an active metabolite. Fluoxetine has a long half-life (2-4 days) as well as an active metabolite with a very long half-life (7-15 days), and therefore, does not require tapering. The discontinuation syndrome is not known to be lethal; however, restarting the paroxetine and then tapering it is a reasonable choice. Acetaminophen is unlikely to significantly help. Bupropion is an antidepressant without sexual side effects, and would be a reasonable choice for the treatment of depression, although would not help with the discontinuation symptoms. Depakote is a treatment for bipolar disorder, which this patient does not have. Venlafaxine is a serotonin-norepinephrine reuptake inhibitor with similar withdrawal side effects.

28. **(A)** Concurrent use of lamotrigine and oral contraceptives can affect levels of both medications. The clearance of lamotrigine is significantly greater in women exposed to oral contraceptives; lower levels of the medication would account for the patient's lack of improvement. Additionally, lamotrigine may induce the

metabolism of oral contraceptives, potentially rendering them less effective. Ibuprofen, lithium, and ziprasidone do not affect lamotrigine metabolism. Valproic acid *decreases* the clearance of lamotrigine, necessitating lower lamotrigine doses with concurrent use.

29. **(E)** Trazodone is an antidepressant medication which affects the serotonin system by weak reuptake inhibition and antagonist activity at 5-HT_{1a}, 5-HT_{1c}, and 5-HT_2 receptors. It has a sedative effect, produced by alpha-adrenergic blockade and modest histamine blockade. It is extremely sedating at antidepressant doses (300-500 mg), but is often used at smaller doses (50-200 mg) as an adjunct to other antidepressants to help with sleep. Both diazepam (a benzodiazepine) and diphenhydramine (an antihistamine) are used as sedatives, but neither is an antidepressant, and both can cause delirium in the elderly. Both fluoxetine and bupropion are activating antidepressants and may initially worsen insomnia.

30. **(E)** Priapism, a painful, prolonged erection, is a rare side effect of trazodone. The manufacturer has reported the incidence of any abnormal erectile function to be about 1 in 6000 men. This side effect usually occurs within the first month of treatment but can occur at any time. Any abnormal erectile function should prompt immediate discontinuation of the medication. The other symptoms are not common or dangerous enough to warrant informing the patient.

31. **(E)** Lithium causes ECG changes in about 30% of patients, most commonly T-wave depression or inversion, but the changes are usually not clinically significant. First-degree AV block and sinus node dysfunction are rare. Lithium toxicity can rarely cause sinoatrial block, AV block, AV dissociation, bradyarrhythmias, ventricular tachycardia, and ventricular fibrillation, but these are usually due to underlying cardiac disease.

32. **(C)** Thiazide diuretics such as hydrochlorothiazide can increase lithium levels owing to decreased lithium clearance. Other medications that can increase lithium levels are the diuretics

ethacrynic acid, spironolactone, and triamterene; NSAIDs (except aspirin and sulindac); and the antibiotics metronidazole and tetracycline. Nitroglycerin and propranolol do not interfere with lithium clearance.

33. **(A)** Clomipramine, a mixed serotonin and norepinephrine reuptake inhibitor (but classified as a tricyclic antidepressant) was approved for the treatment of obsessive-compulsive disorder (OCD) in the United States in 1989. Trials comparing SSRIs to clomipramine report equal effectiveness; however, the side effect profile favors the SSRIs, which are the most common first-line treatment in clinical practice. Other tricyclic agents (such as nortriptyline) are not as effective as clomipramine because they are not as serotonergic. Clonazepam may be helpful for the anxiety associated with OCD, but it is not effective in treating the underlying disorder (ie, obsessions or compulsions). Olanzapine is a second-generation antipsychotic which may be used for augmentation of antidepressants in severe OCD, but it is not recommended as monotherapy. Phenelzine is a monoamine oxidase inhibitor (MAOI), used infrequently for depression but not used in OCD.

34. **(C)** Just like in the treatment of refractory depression, treatment of refractory OCD is largely based on case reports and clinical preferences. There are very few controlled blinded trials in refractory OCD. Practice guidelines recommend augmenting SSRIs with a second-generation antipsychotic (such as risperidone) for patients with a moderate response to the SSRI. For patients with no response, one should consider switching to a different SSRI or to clomipramine. In all cases, psychotherapy— in particular, exposure therapy with response prevention—should be recommended. Buspirone and lithium may have some utility as augmenting agents, but their evidence base is less than for antipsychotics. Antipsychotics are not generally used as monotherapy in OCD. Cingulotomy, a surgical procedure, should be reserved for severe, refractory cases.

35. **(B)** This patient is suffering from command auditory hallucinations, which have not sufficiently

responded to adequate trials of one first-generation antipsychotic medication (haloperidol) or two second-generation antipsychotics (quetiapine and olanzapine). Therefore, a trial of clozapine is warranted. Clozapine was the first second-generation antipsychotic and has been found to be superior to other antipsychotics in reducing both positive and negative symptoms. It may also improve cognitive deficits in patients with schizophrenia. It is not used as first-line treatment because of a 1% risk of agranulocytosis. Aripiprazole, risperidone, and ziprasidone are all second-generation antipsychotics that are not as effective as clozapine for treatment-refractory schizophrenia. Perphenazine is a first-generation antipsychotic like haloperidol.

36. **(C)** Clozapine acts at many receptors, including D_1, D_2, and D_4; histamine-1; muscarinic; alpha 1-adrenergic; and serotonin types 5-HT$_2$, 5-HT$_{2c}$, and 5-HT$_3$. Efforts to identify the exact mechanism of the antipsychotic action of clozapine have revealed at least two possibilities. Unlike first-generation antipsychotics, clozapine has much more potent antagonism at the D_4 receptor compared to the D_2 receptor, especially in the limbic system. This has led to speculation that the D_4 receptor may mediate psychotic symptoms. Clozapine also has activity at the 5-HT$_2$ receptor, activity that first-generation antipsychotics lack.

37. **(C)** Tricyclic antidepressants, including imipramine and nortriptyline, block various receptors, including muscarinic, alpha-1- and alpha-2-adrenergic, dopaminergic, and histaminergic, to varying degrees. As a class, their blockade of alpha1-receptors is generally believed to be responsible for any orthostatic hypotension that may occur, especially in the elderly. Imipramine is a tertiary amine which blocks multiple receptors and therefore has many side effects; nortriptyline, a secondary amine, has relatively less alpha1-blocking potency and tends to be better tolerated in general. Bupropion, fluoxetine, and mirtazapine are not associated with orthostatic hypotension.

38. **(E)** This patient is presenting with mania. First-line treatment for mania includes valproic acid or lithium, with or without a concurrent antipsychotic agent. Antidepressants such as citalopram should not be used in the setting of acute mania, as they may worsen the condition. Lamotrigine is an anticonvulsant, used for bipolar depression and maintenance; it is not an effective anti-manic agent. Olanzapine is a reasonable alternative to valproic acid, but due to the risk of weight gain, may not be the optimal choice for this patient. Topiramate is an anticonvulsant used in the treatment of bulimia nervosa. While it may be useful for adjunctive treatment, it is not considered effective as monotherapy for treatment of bipolar disorder.

39. **(D)** All of the commonly used mood-stabilizing medications carry some risk of fetal malformations or a potential deleterious effect on later cognitive development. Use of lithium during the first trimester increases the risk of Ebstein's anomaly, a malformation of the tricuspid valve, from 1:20,000 to 1-2:1000 patients. If a fetus has been exposed to lithium, a fetal echocardiogram should be done between weeks 16 and 18 of pregnancy. Lithium may be used in the second and third trimesters with careful attention to adequate hydration. Carbamazepine can cause craniofacial defects, fingernail hypoplasia, neural tube defects, and developmental delay (20%). Divalproex sodium is associated with neural tube defect rates of 5% to 9%, and may cause intrauterine growth retardation. Benzodiazepines such as diazepam may be associated with cleft lip and palate, although this remains controversial.

40. **(E)** It is not unusual for delirious patients to become hostile or combative, posing a risk to themselves or to hospital staff. Low-dose atypical antipsychotics, such as risperidone, are very effective in reducing agitation in delirious patients. Diphenhydramine should be avoided as the anticholinergic effects may worsen the delirium and confusion. Donepezil is an anticholinesterase inhibitor used for dementias. Although benzodiazepines like lorazepam can be used for agitation in delirium, they should be avoided in elderly patients due to the risk of worsening delirium and potential disinhibition. Orientation to surroundings is often

additionally helpful in delirium, but it will not immediately calm the patient.

41. **(C)** Mirtazapine is an antidepressant whose pharmacologic profile is different from other available agents. It is a central alpha-2-adrenergic antagonist and an antagonist of 5-HT$_2$ and 5-HT$_3$ receptors, as well as H$_1$ receptors. Blockade of alpha-2-receptor leads to enhanced serotonin release; however blockade of 5-HT$_2$ and 5-HT$_3$ leads to relative enhancement of 5-HT$_1$ activity giving mirtazapine a different side effect profile than SSRIs. For example, mirtazapine tends to increase appetite and cause weight gain compared to placebo. In addition, its H$_1$ antagonism causes sedation. However, at higher doses, alpha-2-adrenergic blockade also leads to increased norepinephrine release, which may counteract the H$_1$-mediated sedation. In this patient, use of mirtazapine (to exploit its potential increased appetite and sedation side effects) should be considered. Bupropion is an antidepressant whose side effect profile includes insomnia and weight loss, neither of which would be beneficial in this patient. Fluoxetine and sertraline are SSRI antidepressants which, while effective, may initially cause activation. Nortriptyline is a tricyclic antidepressant that is lethal in overdose and whose anticholinergic properties can lead to delirium in the elderly.

42. **(C)** Tricyclic antidepressants (TCAs) produce several cardiovascular side effects, the most significant being a quinidine-like effect slowing cardiac conduction. Some clinicians avoid TCAs if there are any ECG changes. Certainly, if there are changes in conduction, such as a prolonged QT interval, widening of the QRS complex, or AV conduction abnormalities, TCAs should be avoided. In overdose, they can widen the QRS complex, cause a bundle branch block, and cause tachyarrhythmias; however, even at therapeutic concentrations, they may have adverse effects on cardiac conduction. Estrogen replacement therapy and amlodipine are not contraindications. TCAs can be used in patients with prior cerebral infarctions. While TCAs may exacerbate urinary retention from their anticholinergic effects, this is not a contraindication to their use.

43. **(B)** This patient is likely delirious and prompt identification and treatment of the underlying cause is indicated. To help control the agitation that may accompany delirium, low-dose haloperidol is frequently used. Haloperidol does not treat the delirium, however. It is used most frequently because it is the most potent of the typical antipsychotics, therefore requiring lower doses, with fewer anticholinergic or orthostatic side effects. Low-potency agents (such as chlorpromazine or thioridazine) are not only associated with orthostatic hypotension and anticholinergic side effects, but also with prolongation of the QT interval. Lorazepam may help sedate the patient but it will not help his psychosis and could cause disinhibition and a worsening of his delirium. Risperidone is not available in a parenteral form, and is therefore not as useful in an agitated patient who requires IV or IM medication.

44. **(A)** Of the first-generation antipsychotics listed (haloperidol, perphenazine, and thioridazine), haloperidol is the most potent and has the least activity at alpha1-receptors. Therefore, it is the least likely to cause orthostatic hypotension. The second-generation agents listed (risperidone and quetiapine) have activity at alpha-1-receptors and are both associated with orthostatic hypotension.

45. **(B)** The metabolism of ethyl alcohol involves a two-step enzymatic process. The first enzyme, alcohol dehydrogenase, metabolizes ethanol to acetaldehyde, which is quickly metabolized by aldehyde dehydrogenase. Disulfiram inhibits aldehyde dehydrogenase, resulting in an accumulation of acetaldehyde. Acetaldehyde causes facial flushing, tachycardia, hypotension, nausea and vomiting, and physical discomfort. Therefore, a patient on disulfiram has an incentive to remain abstinent. Obviously, disulfiram works only if patients continue to take it. Acamprosate, a GABA-ergic agonist, and naltrexone, an opioid antagonist, are both used to reduce cravings for alcohol. Flumazenil is a benzodiazepine antagonist used in benzodiazepine overdose. Naloxone is an opioid antagonist used in emergency management of opiate intoxication and overdose.

46. **(E)** Multiple neurotransmitter systems have been investigated in attempts to control alcohol cravings. One system that likely plays a role in the reward pathway is the opioid system. Naltrexone is an opioid antagonist that has been shown to decrease the number of days a person with alcohol dependence drinks and to increase the time before relapse of heavy drinking. Treatment of depression with an agent such as bupropion may help control drinking if a comorbid depression exists, but use of antidepressants in the absence of a mood disorder has not been effective in reducing cravings. Disulfiram is an alcohol-sensitizing agent which deters patients from drinking. Flumazenil is a benzodiazepine antagonist used in benzodiazepine overdose. Naloxone is an opiate antagonist that is used to acutely reverse the effects of opiate intoxication.

47. **(C)** This patient is likely suffering from post-traumatic stress disorder (PTSD). First-line pharmacologic treatment for PTSD is the selective serotonin reuptake inhibitors (eg, fluoxetine, paroxetine, sertraline), which several randomized controlled trials have shown are useful in reducing the core symptoms of PTSD (reexperiencing, numbing, and hyperarousal). Benzodiazepines such as alprazolam are not beneficial in treating these symptoms. Anticonvulsants are not routinely used; open-label studies of divalproex, carbamazepine, and topiramate have showed mixed results. Naltrexone, an opioid antagonist, has not been extensively studied in PTSD. Antipsychotics such as thioridazine have generally not been useful, although the second-generation antipsychotics may be useful as adjunctive medications, especially if the patient has comorbid psychotic symptoms.

48. **(E)** Prazosin is an alpha-1-adrenergic receptor blocker, traditionally used to treat hypertension and benign prostatic hypertrophy, which has demonstrated efficacy in treating nightmares and other symptoms in patients with PTSD. Sedative-hypnotic agents, such as lorazepam, may be helpful in the short-term but have larger potential for dependence.

Naltrexone has not been extensively studied in PTSD. Olanzapine, a second-generation antipsychotic, and perphenazine, a first-generation antipsychotic, may be useful in severe PTSD with psychotic symptoms, but they carry a risk of weight gain and metabolic side effects, as well as tardive dyskinesia over the long term.

49. **(E)** This patient is likely experiencing delirium, as evidenced by his acute change in mental status, with confusion, disorientation, and agitation. Elderly patients can be particularly sensitive to the adverse effects of benzodiazepines. This patient is taking 8 mg/d of lorazepam, which is a large dose. Slowly tapering the lorazepam, while investigating other potential causes of delirium, is a reasonable first step. Hydrochlorothiazide levels are not measured, and the other choices will not address or help to manage his delirium or the likely underlying cause.

50. **(B)** This patient is likely suffering from Alzheimer dementia. He has clear cognitive decline, and, although reversible causes of cognitive impairment should be investigated, there is no indication that any reversible cause is present. There are five medications currently available to treat Alzheimer disease: the anticholinesterase inhibitors donepezil, galantamine, rivastigmine and tacrine, and the N-methyl-D-aspartate (NMDA) receptor antagonist, memantine. Of these medications, tacrine is rarely used due to the risk of hepatic failure. Aspirin or trazodone will not improve cognitive ability. There does not appear to be an indication for fluoxetine in this patient (such as a depressive disorder). Pemoline is a stimulant that does not appear to be indicated in this case.

51. **(C)** Trazodone is a serotonergic agent frequently used in patients to help with sleep, and in this patient may help with his wandering behavior. It can cause orthostatic hypotension and should therefore be used with caution in those with risk factors for falls. Quetiapine and haloperidol are antipsychotic medications that should both be used carefully in the elderly. Haloperidol is a high-potency first-generation

antipsychotic that is sometimes used to manage severe agitation, but it may cause extrapyramidal symptoms. Quetiapine is a second-generation antipsychotic; however, given the black box warning about the risk of sudden death in elderly patients with dementia-related psychosis, second-generation antipsychotics should be used sparingly in the geriatric population. Benzodiazepines such as lorazepam and triazolam should also be used with caution in the elderly. They may actually worsen the behavior and cause delirium. If necessary, starting doses should be much lower than standard dosing and slowly tapered up.

52. **(E)** Patients who present with severely altered levels of consciousness need to be medically evaluated and quickly treated for several reversible causes. These include hypoglycemia, opioid overdose, and alcohol intoxication. Airway protection and monitoring of air exchange and cardiovascular status are required. Several treatments that should be immediately considered include IV dextrose, usually D_{50}, to treat hypoglycemia; thiamine to guard against the development of Wernicke encephalopathy in an alcoholic patient with thiamine deficiency; and naloxone, an opioid antagonist, to reverse the effects of opioid intoxication. Flumazenil is a benzodiazepine antagonist that should not be used before obtaining further history because it may acutely lower the seizure threshold.

53. **(A)** Buprenorphine is one of the most effective medications for opioid detoxification. Given in sublingual form, it is a mixed opioid agonist-antagonist which suppresses opioid withdrawal and blocks the effects of other opioids. Benzodiazepines such as chlordiazepoxide may be helpful as adjuncts to control anxiety, but they are not sufficient for opiate withdrawal. Clonidine, a central alpha-2-agonist, suppresses the sympathetic response to the heroin withdrawal and helps to control agitation and autonomic instability, such as elevated blood pressure and heart rate; however, it will not address the heroin craving and is less effective in managing withdrawal than buprenorphine. Naloxone would not be appropriate beyond

the initial resuscitation efforts. Propranolol is not used for heroin detoxification.

54. **(A)** Bupropion (marketed as Zyban) is an antidepressant that has also been shown to be effective as part of a smoking cessation program. The mechanism of action is unclear, but it is believed to have an effect on dopaminergic transmission. Giving up cigarettes may be extremely difficult for a patient who is also suffering from major depression; however, starting bupropion during the depression may help her quit smoking in the future. The other antidepressants listed have no impact on smoking cessation.

55. **(E)** Duloxetine is a serotonin-norepinephrine reuptake inhibitor (SNRI) that is used in the treatment of both major depression and pain, including neuropathic pain and fibromyalgia. Alprazolam and bupropion will not help with the treatment of pain. Several tricyclic antidepressants, including amitriptyline and nortriptyline, are also used to treat chronic pain. However, tricyclic antidepressants are more lethal in overdose than newer medications like selective serotonin reuptake inhibitors (SSRIs) and SNRIs, and they generally have more side effects, particularly anticholinergic and cardiovascular ones. SSRIs such as citalopram may play a role in chronic pain management, but the data are not as robust as with duloxetine.

56. **(B)** Carbamazepine is an anticonvulsant that is used to treat both bipolar mania and trigeminal neuralgia. Amitriptyline and fluoxetine are both antidepressants, which are not appropriate in his patient who is in the middle of a manic episode. Gabapentin is an anticonvulsant that has demonstrated efficacy in the treatment of trigeminal neuralgia; however, it is not considered effective as an antimanic agent. Lithium should not be restarted due to concerns about its prior effect on her thyroid functioning.

57. **(E)** Weight gain is a side effect of most antipsychotic medications, both first and second generation; however, it is particularly concerning with olanzapine. In a seminal study of

antipsychotic use in people with schizophrenia, 30% of patients on olanzapine gained more than 7% of their body weight within an 18-month period; olanzapine induces more weight gain than other antipsychotic agents. Agranulocytosis is a rare but potentially fatal side effect of clozapine. Olanzapine is not associated with the development of cataracts or increased excitability. Olanzapine is likely to cause sedation and is usually administered in the evening. As an antipsychotic with mood-stabilizing properties, it is useful for both psychotic disorders and bipolar disorder. Elevated prolactin and potential galactorrhea are side effects of first-generation antipsychotics and risperidone, but less common with olanzapine.

58. **(E)** Given that the patient tolerates and responds to oral risperidone but suffers exacerbations due to poor compliance, he is a good candidate for a long-acting medication. Risperidone (Risperdal Consta) is a long-acting form of risperidone given in bimonthly injections. Continuing his current regimen or switching to another oral medication such as olanzapine will likely only lead to a continuation of the vicious cycle of poor compliance and relapse. Clozapine is appropriate for patients who have failed two or more antipsychotic medications, which is not the case in this patient, and the regular blood monitoring also requires a compliant patient. While haloperidol is also available in a depot form, it is not as good a choice for this patient, given his prior response to risperidone.

59. **(D)** Risperidone is an atypical or second-generation antipsychotic agent that has potent 5-HT$_{2a}$ antagonist properties as well as blocking at D$_2$ and alpha-1-receptors. Because of the alpha1-blocking activity, it may cause orthostatic hypotension. Agranulocytosis is a concern with clozapine, not risperidone. Risperidone may cause weight gain rather than weight loss, and it does not cause appreciable anticholinergic effects. A benign leukocytosis can occur with lithium use, but not with risperidone.

60. **(C)** Second-generation antipsychotic agents, like clozapine and risperidone, are considered atypical because of their decreased propensity

for causing extrapyramidal side effects (EPS) and presumably a reduced (but not zero) risk of tardive dyskinesia. Unfortunately, only clozapine appears to truly obey this "rule." The other second-generation antipsychotic agents all appear to have some degree of EPS, with risperidone as the leading culprit; at doses higher than 6 mg/d, risperidone causes EPS at rates comparable to haloperidol. Agranulocytosis is a concern with clozapine, not risperidone. Risperidone may cause weight gain rather than weight loss, and it does not cause appreciable anticholinergic effects. A benign leukocytosis can occur with lithium use, but not with risperidone.

61. **(E)** Antipsychotic agents block dopamine receptors in several pathways in the brain. Blockade of dopamine receptors in the tuberoinfundibular tract results in increased prolactin release (dopamine acts as an inhibitor of prolactin release), which may cause infertility, amenorrhea, galactorrhea, and gynecomastia. Risperidone causes more prolactin increase than other antipsychotic medications–in fact, it may raise prolactin levels up to 100-fold. Dopamine antagonism in the mesocortical and mesolimbic tracts is responsible (in part) for the antipsychotic effect. Blocking dopamine receptors in the nigrostriatal system causes the extrapyramidal symptoms. The locus ceruleus, located in the brain stem, is the most important noradrenergic nucleus in the brain.

62. **(B)** This patient is suffering from bulimia nervosa. First-line pharmacologic treatment is an SSRI such as fluoxetine, which decreases symptoms of bingeing and purging independent of any mood disorder. Bupropion is contraindicated in patients with eating disorders due to an increased risk of seizure. Lamotrigine is an anticonvulsant used in the treatment of bipolar depression and maintenance. Lithium is also used to treat bipolar disorder. Mirtazapine is an antidepressant which frequently causes weight gain, and is therefore a poor choice for a patient with body-image issues.

63. **(D)** Topiramate is an anticonvulsant used in the treatment of bulimia and binge eating

disorder. In several controlled trials, topiramate decreased the frequency of binge episodes and led to weight loss. Lithium and valproic acid are both used to treat bipolar disorder. Bupropion is an antidepressant but is contraindicated in patients with eating disorders due to an increased risk of seizure. Paroxetine is an SSRI that can be used in the treatment of bulimia; however, this patient has already failed two SSRI trials, and is unlikely to benefit from a third.

64. **(E)** Zolpidem, a non-benzodiazepine hypnotic, exhibits affinity for benzodiazepine alpha-1-receptors and is cross-reactive with the benzodiazepines. However, unlike the benzodiazepines, it lacks significant anxiolytic, muscle relaxant, or anticonvulsant effects, and is therefore extremely useful for the short-term treatment of insomnia. Diphenhydramine is used for insomnia but can leave patients feeling drowsy the next day. Amitriptyline and quetiapine are sedating but have serious side effects and should not be used for primary insomnia. Short-acting benzodiazepines such as temazepam can be useful in the treatment of insomnia; however, these medications carry with them a risk of dependence and rebound insomnia.

65. **(E)** This patient likely has panic disorder. Sertraline is a selective serotonin reuptake inhibitor approved for the treatment of panic disorder. Although other medications are effective, SSRIs are the safest in overdose and have fewer side effects. Bupropion, an antidepressant with a dopaminergic mechanism, is not effective in the treatment of panic disorder. Imipramine is a tricyclic antidepressant and phenelzine is a monoamine oxidase inhibitor. Quetiapine is an antipsychotic medication that would not be appropriate for this patient.

66. **(A)** The tricyclic antidepressants, such as amitriptyline, have been shown to increase mortality in cardiac patients because of their quinidine-like effects and tendency to both increase heart rate and decrease blood pressure. Bupropion is an antidepressant that is safe in cardiac patients. As a class, amphetamines, such as methylphenidate, have been found to be safe in patients with cardiac disease.

As there may be minor changes in blood pressure and pulse, patients should be monitored closely. Sertraline is also safe for patients with cardiac disease and possesses few drug–drug interactions. Venlafaxine can increase the blood pressure an average of 8 to 10 mm Hg but this effect is dose related. At doses less than 150 mg/d, clinically significant changes are relatively rare.

67. **(D)** The symptoms the patient is experiencing are common effects of elevated prolactin levels. Haloperidol's mechanism of action is dopamine receptor blockade (D_2). Dopamine normally inhibits prolactin secretion in the tuberoinfundibular pathway, but because haloperidol blocks dopamine, prolactin secretion is unopposed. Haloperidol does not significantly increase ACTH, dopamine, norepinephrine, or serotonin.

68. **(B)** This patient most likely has akathisia, which is a neuroleptic-induced side effect. Patients generally experience subjective feelings of restlessness and can be seen swinging their legs, rocking back and forth while sitting, pacing, and rapidly alternating between sitting and standing. Acute dystonias are characterized by painful contraction of muscles resulting in abnormal movements or postures, such as spasms of the jaw, abnormal positioning of the head, or difficulty swallowing. The onset of acute dystonia usually develops within the first week of initiating or increasing a neuroleptic medication. Akathisia can sometimes be mistaken for anxiety or mania, but in this case there are no other signs (such as delusions of grandeur, decreased need for sleep, increased energy, or hypersexuality) to indicate a manic episode. Neuroleptic malignant syndrome is a life-threatening complication involving muscle rigidity and dystonia as well as autonomic symptoms such as elevated temperature, increased heart rate, and increased blood pressure. Tardive dyskinesia is a long-term consequence of antipsychotic use, and it is characterized by involuntary, choreoathetoid movements of the body, especially in the extremities. It is not painful, although may be somewhat disabling, and is often irreversible.

69. **(A)** Transcranial magnetic stimulation is a new treatment for depression, approved in 2008 by the FDA for treatment of major depression that has failed at least one antidepressant trial. The treatment involves applying a series of electromagnetic pulses to the left orbital prefrontal cortex; a full treatment consists of roughly 20 daily sessions, each lasting about 40 minutes. Unlike electroconvulsive therapy (ECT), which requires general anesthesia, rTMS can be performed in the office, without any anesthesia. The most common side effect is headache at the site of the application. The treatment is very loud and patients are asked to wear earplugs; however, hearing loss has not been reported. Also, unlike with ECT, there is no memory loss associated with the procedure. Seizures and tooth pain are rare complications.

70. **(D)** Decisions about medications during pregnancy are highly individualized, based on weighing risks and benefits for a particular individual. ECT has been used in pregnancy for more than 50 years and its safety and efficacy is well documented. Valproic acid and lithium (in addition to second-generation antipsychotics) are indicated as first-line agents for the treatment of manic episodes, with carbamazepine as a good alternative; however, all three are all associated with an increased risk of congenital abnormalities when taken during the first trimester. Benzodiazepines such as diazepam are not first-line treatment for mania, and may be associated with an increased risk of oral clefts with first-trimester exposure.

71. **(D)** Cessation or a reduction in sedative, hypnotic, or anxiolytic medications that have been used heavily or for a prolonged period of time may result in a withdrawal syndrome characterized by symptoms that develop within hours to a few days after cessation or reduction. Autonomic hyperactivity, orthostatic hypotension, muscle weakness, tremor, insomnia, nausea, vomiting, auditory/visual/tactile hallucinations, agitation, or anxiety may occur. By far, the most serious sequelae are grand mal seizures or delirium. As many as 75% of patients may experience grand mal seizures on the second or third day of withdrawal, and

two-thirds of these patients have more than one seizure. Delirium may develop between the third and eighth day of withdrawal. Minor symptoms may persist for up to 2 weeks. Withdrawal from the other medications listed is unpleasant, but is not life-threatening.

72. **(B)** Chronic alcoholics often take in calories from little else besides alcohol and are thus at risk for thiamine deficiency. If a thiamine-deficient patient is given food (glucose), he or she can develop Wernicke encephalopathy (a delirium) from the body's attempts to metabolize glucose in the absence of thiamine pyrophosphate. Although the other choices are important concerns, none are of the same acuity as thiamine deficiency.

73. **(D)** This man will probably suffer from alcohol withdrawal. Benzodiazepines and alcohol have near identical modes of action in their modulation of GABA receptors in the brain. This similarity makes a benzodiazepine such as lorazepam a sensible and popular choice for treatment of alcohol withdrawal. Acamprosate, disulfiram, and naltrexone are all used for relapse prevention in patients with alcohol dependence, but not for managing alcohol withdrawal. Clonidine, an alpha-2-agonist that modulates autonomic instability, is used to manage symptoms of opiate withdrawal, and actually may block (mask) the autonomic warning signs of alcohol withdrawal.

74–81. [74 (H), 75 (B), 76 (F), 77 (C), 78 (B), 79 (F), 80 (E), 81 (B)] Psychiatric drugs can have serious side effects, some of which are the subjects of "black box" warnings on prescribing information packets. Pimozide, a first-generation antipsychotic, interacts with a number of medications, including citalopram; the combination of these two medications can prolong the QTc. Although clozapine, haloperidol, perphenazine, pimozide, and ziprasidone are all antipsychotics used to treat schizophrenia, clozapine is the most likely to cause hyperglycemia and lead to the development of diabetes. After a controversial set of hearings on the subject of children and antidepressants in the United Kingdom and United States in 2003 and 2004, regulators decided there was enough evidence to show that some of the SSRIs, including paroxetine, may increase the risk of suicidal thoughts in children. This warning is now extended to young adults, up to age 24. Although carbamazepine, divalproex sodium, and lithium are all used to treat bipolar disorder, only valproic acid carries a warning of an increased risk of pancreatitis. Although carbamazepine and clozapine can both cause agranulocytosis, clozapine is more likely to be used (and is FDA approved) for treatment of refractory schizophrenia.

Paroxetine is the only antidepressant listed and has a very short half-life such that it produces a significant withdrawal syndrome after just 2 days. While carbamazepine, divalproex sodium, and lithium (as well as antipsychotics) may all be used to treat bipolar disorder, only lithium causes both polyuria (a benign side effect) and nephrogenic diabetes insipidus, resulting in frequent urination. While all antipsychotics have the risk of increasing cholesterol, of those listed, clozapine has the most significant effect.

82. **(I)** Haloperidol, clozapine, and risperidone are all useful in the treatment of schizophrenia, but only haloperidol and risperidone are available in a depot injection. Risperidone would be preferable because it is a second-generation medication with a better side effect profile.

83. **(K)** Trazodone, a serotonergic antidepressant, is an effective sleeping aid that is not habit forming. While benzodiazepines such as alprazolam may help with insomnia, it is wise to avoid prescribing them in a patient with a history of alcoholism because of the cross-reactivity with alcohol.

84. **(D)** The recommended length of treatment of a first episode of unipolar depression is at least 6 months and usually on the scale of 8 to 12 months, and possibly longer, depending on patient factors such as family history of mood disorder, severity and duration of the depressive episode, and comorbid psychiatric symptoms such as anxiety and substance abuse.

Discontinuation within the first 16 weeks of treatment is associated with a high risk of relapse.

85. **(A)** Bupropion is the one antidepressant listed that does not cause sexual dysfunction, and is sometimes added to SSRIs in order to help with sexual dysfunction. Citalopram, fluoxetine, and fluvoxamine are all SSRIs that have been reported to cause varying degrees of sexual dysfunction. Clomipramine is a tricyclic antidepressant that has a greater incidence of sexual dysfunction than other TCAs, possibly due to its potent serotonin reuptake inhibiting properties.

86. **(C)** Sialorrhea is a common side effect of treatment with clozapine (up to 30% of patients). It can be extremely bothersome to the patient and others but does not usually require discontinuation of treatment. Often, behavioral measures are sufficient, such as the use of lozenges or placing a towel on the patient's pillow at night. Anticholinergic agents such as propylthiouracil often help to reduce the volume of saliva. Amantadine may be helpful in the treatment of parkinsonian symptoms and propranolol is useful in the treatment of akathisia.

87. **(D)** Patients on clozapine often develop a persistent sinus tachycardia that does not require cessation of treatment. Often, the tachycardia resolves without necessitating further intervention; however, should it persist, it may be treated with the beta-antagonist propranolol. Benztropine is an anticholinergic agent that will not help the tachycardia, and may, in fact, worsen it. Clozapine has significant alpha-receptor blockade, which often causes orthostatic hypotension, requiring a gradual titration of the dose. Because of this, labetalol would not be appropriate as it may exacerbate this side effect. Lorazepam is a benzodiazepine that may calm the patient, but will not directly affect heart rate.

88. **(C)** This patient presents with signs and symptoms suggestive of a first manic episode. Lithium and divalproex sodium remain the mainstay of initial and maintenance treatment

of bipolar I disorder. Antipsychotics, such as haloperidol and olanzapine may be used in conjunction with lithium or divalproex sodium initially; however, due to their side effects and risk of tardive dyskinesia, they are not routinely used as maintenance treatment. Lamotrigine is an anticonvulsant that is used for treatment of bipolar depression and maintenance treatment; it is not useful during an acute manic episode. Lorazepam can be used initially for sedation and sleep, but it is not effective for treating or maintaining patients with bipolar disorder.

89. **(E)** The neurovegetative symptoms (changes in appetite, poor concentration, anergia, and sleep disturbances) tend to respond first with antidepressant treatment, prior to significant mood changes or reduction in suicidality. This is why it is a common wisdom in psychiatry that the person who begins to recover from depression may be at greater risk for suicide than when he is at the height of his depression. As he starts to function better physiologically (with improved sleep, energy, and motivation), he may be more capable of carrying out a suicidal impulse.

90. **(E)** In cases of suspected liver impairment, it is advisable to use a benzodiazepine minimally metabolized by the liver (eg, lorazepam and oxazepam). These benzodiazepines do not go through oxidation, but rather only through glucuronidation. The other benzodiazepines listed are metabolized mostly by the liver and could quickly build to toxic levels in a cirrhotic patient.

91. **(A)** The patient has likely developed tardive dyskinesia (TD). All of the second-generation antipsychotics listed have lower rates of TD when compared to the first-generation antipsychotics. Although they all have warnings regarding the increased risk of diabetes and hyperlipidemia (metabolic syndrome), they are believed to cause it at different rates, so this is often a factor in choosing a particular antipsychotic medication. The least likely to cause metabolic syndrome are aripiprazole and ziprasidone, followed by risperidone and quetiapine.

Clozapine and olanzapine have the highest rates of weight gain, hyperlipidemia, and insulin resistance.

92. **(D)** The need for increasing amounts of a drug to achieve the same effect or a diminishing effect with the same amount of a drug describes tolerance, a sign of physiological dependence. Withdrawal, another characteristic of dependence, is a syndrome of behavioral, emotional, and physiologic signs and symptoms that occur in a setting of the discontinuation of a drug. Abuse is defined by a maladaptive pattern of use leading to significant impairment or distress, manifested by occupational, legal, or social problems, or using in situations that are physically hazardous. As mentioned, dependence requires either tolerance or withdrawal, or a persistent desire to stop or cut down, spending a lot of time using or recovering from the substance, or continuing to use despite an ongoing medical problem complicated by use. There is not enough history given to clearly determine whether the patient is suffering from abuse or dependence. Addiction is more of a lay term for substance dependence.

93. **(D)** All of the medications listed are sleep aids; however, only zaleplon, a non-benzodiazepine hypnotic with a half-life of only 4 hours, is appropriate for middle insomnia (falling asleep but frequently awakening during the night). All of the alternatives listed are more useful for people who have initial insomnia (difficulty falling asleep) and require a medication at bedtime. Amitriptyline and trazodone are both sedating antidepressants. Ramelteon is a melatonin-receptor agonist. Zolpidem is another non-benzodiazepine hypnotic with a longer half-life than zaleplon.

94. **(E)** ECT has relatively few contraindications and in some cases is preferred for its rapid onset of action. However, because of the cardiovascular effects of ECT, a history of a recent myocardial infarction (within the past 6 months) is a relative contraindication. Another relative contraindication is the presence of a clinically significant intracranial space-occupying lesion due to the risk of brain stem herniation.

ECT may be performed in patients with degenerative disc disease or hypertension, and during pregnancy. ECT is a safe and effective treatment for psychotic depression. The most common complaints patients have following ECT are impairments in both anterograde and retrograde memory. Although most memory problems resolve, some may persist indefinitely.

95. **(D)** This patient has delirium, a common complication in the ICU. Low-dose antipsychotics such as olanzapine can be very helpful if used judiciously. Haloperidol is often used in clinical practice; however, IV haloperidol can lengthen the QTc and therefore should not be used for this particular patient. Benzodiazepines such as diazepam and lorazepam can worsen delirium in the elderly and should be avoided. Risperidone (Risperdal Consta) is the long-acting form of risperidone, and would not be appropriate in this setting.

96. **(E)** The patient likely suffers from performance anxiety, a form of social phobia. Propranolol, a beta-blocker, is extremely helpful in managing performance anxiety. Taken immediately before the feared event, it decreases heart rate, blood pressure, and tremor, and consequently decreases anxiety. Buspirone is an anxiolytic agent that is helpful in the treatment of generalized anxiety disorder. Fluoxetine and fluvoxamine are antidepressants used in the treatment of generalized anxiety disorder and panic disorder. Lorazepam is a benzodiazepine that can be helpful in managing acute anxiety, but its accompanying sedation may be problematic in a performance context.

97. **(B)** A subjective feeling of restlessness and a need to constantly move about and pace is known as akathisia, a common side effect of antipsychotic medication that can occur soon after such medications are started. The other choices listed are also antipsychotic side effects, seen most often with first-generation medications. Dystonias are uncontrolled, painful, muscle contractions, seen early in treatment. Neuroleptic malignant syndrome is a rare, idiosyncratic, but serious side effect of antipsychotics, manifested by fever, muscle rigidity, delirium, and autonomic instability. Parkinsonism refers to symptoms evoked by neuroleptics that are commonly seen in Parkinson disease, such as tremor (a 3-6-cycle/sec motion), akinesia (or bradykinesia), and rigidity. Tardive dyskinesia is a rhythmic, involuntary movement of the tongue, jaw, trunk, or extremities appearing months to years after the initiation of antipsychotic therapy.

98. **(D)** Although there are various side effects of lamotrigine, the most dangerous is that of a severe rash, which can develop into Stevens-Johnson syndrome, a potentially life-threatening complication. Beginning at a low dose and slowly increasing reduces the risk significantly. Acute dystonia and akathisia are both side effects of antipsychotic medications. Aplastic anemia is a rare side effect of carbamazepine. Renal failure can occur with lithium.

99. **(C)** All of these are types of dystonic reactions that are induced by the use of neuroleptics. Opisthotonos, also known as *arc de cercle*, is a spasm of the neck and back that causes the patient to arch forward. The most alarming of these dystonias is laryngospasm, which is the spasm of the muscles controlling the tongue and the throat; this can lead to respiratory distress. Oculogyric crisis is spasm of the extraocular muscles, often resulting in the patient looking up and unable to look down. Pleurothotonos, also known as Pisa syndrome, is a leaning posture induced by the spasm of the torso muscles. Torticollis is a spasm of the neck muscles that usually brings the neck to one side or another but may also pull forward or backward.

100. **(B)** Although any of the listed antidepressants will treat her depression adequately, only duloxetine, a combined serotonin-norepinephrine reuptake inhibitor, has been approved in the treatment of both depression and neuropathic pain. Given her likely major depressive disorder, reassurance would not be appropriate or efficacious.

101. **(A)** With the exception of mirtazapine, bupropion, and nefazodone (now off the market due to risk of hepatic failure), all antidepressants can cause significant sexual dysfunction, including decreased libido, erectile dysfunction, and anorgasmia. Given the recurrent nature of his

illness, leaving him without medication would likely lead to a relapse of his major depression. Restarting sertraline would be likely to cause the same problems and lead to nonadherence.

102. **(D)** This patient has symptoms of generalized anxiety disorder. All of the medications listed, except clonazepam, a benzodiazepine, can interact negatively with warfarin. Bupropion is also likely to worsen anxiety. Buspirone and citalopram are reasonable choices for his anxiety, but his PT/PTT and INR would have to be monitored carefully. Venlafaxine may also elevate blood pressure.

103. **(D)** Priapism, a painful, prolonged erection, is a rare but serious side effect of trazodone. Nymphomania is insatiable sexual desire in a woman while satyriasis is its counterpart in men. A parapraxis, or slip of the tongue, is also known as a "Freudian slip." Erectile dysfunction refers to difficulty obtaining or maintaining an erection, a common side effect of SSRIs.

104. **(A)** Sexual dysfunction (eg, decreased libido, erectile dysfunction, anorgasmia) is not uncommonly seen with SSRIs and other antidepressants (such as those listed). Bupropion is one of the few antidepressants which causes little to no sexual dysfunction, and, in fact, may reverse the side effect when added to treatment. In addition, many other psychotropic medications including lithium and antipsychotics can also cause sexual dysfunction.

105. **(D)** Topiramate is an anticonvulsant used in the treatment of bulimia and binge eating disorder. It carries with it a 1.5% risk of renal stones. Topiramate often causes cognitive impairment, particularly word-finding difficulty, short-term memory problems, and problems with attention. Pancreatitis is a rare side effect of valproic acid, and polyuria is seen with lithium use. Topiramate causes weight loss, not weight gain.

106–109. **[106 (E), 107 (B), 108 (F), 109 (I)]** Formication is the feeling of bugs crawling on the skin, usually associated with alcohol withdrawal, but also with intoxication, such as with cocaine. Amotivational syndrome is a lack of drive or motivation usually associated with chronic drug use, especially marijuana. Inhalants, including gasoline, are volatile substances that have rapid-onset intoxicating effects. Tolerance is the need for higher doses of a drug in order to achieve the same effect. Abuse is substance recurrent use in spite of adverse consequences related to the substance. Marijuana is classified as cannabis. Dependence is a physical or psychological need to continue taking a drug. Intoxication is represented by behavioral, cognitive, or perceptual changes taken in relationship to drug ingestion. Posthallucinogen perception disorder is also known as a flashback. It is characterized by a distressing return of perceptual changes without the ingestion of hallucinogens. Withdrawal is a set of signs and symptoms, physical and psychological, that are associated with drug cessation.

110. **(E)** Antipsychotic agents, in addition to blocking dopamine receptors in the nigrostriatal pathway (causing extrapyramidal symptoms) and the mesolimbic pathway (decreasing hallucinations), also block dopamine in the tuberoinfundibular system. Dopamine normally inhibits prolactin release in this pathway, and therefore dopamine blockade increases prolactin levels, causing sexual dysfunction, gynecomastia in men, and galactorrhea in women. This effect is seen with first-generation antipsychotics and with risperidone.

111–121. **[111 (N), 112 (M), 113 (A), 114 (L), 115 (O), 116 (G), 117 (E), 118 (K), 119 (B), 120 (H), 121 (J)]** Antipsychotics, also known as neuroleptics, can cause a wide variety of side effects. These side effects can be broken down into some of the following categories for an easier approach. The dopaminergic side effects include those that are due to the blockade of the natural dopamine inhibition of prolactin release from the anterior pituitary causing galactorrhea **(E)** and gynecomastia **(F)**. The side effects that arise from dopamine blockade in the basal ganglia cause various dystonias, including blepharospasm (spasm of the eyelids) **(C)**, opisthotonos (spasm of the neck and back causing an arched posture) **(I)**, and torticollis (spasm of the sternocleidomastoid) **(P)**. The blockade of D_2 receptors in the nigrostriatal pathway can also cause other extrapyramidal syndromes such as akathisia (subjective feeling of restlessness) **(B)**, pseudoparkinsonism **(L)** which resembles Parkinson disease, characterized by muscle rigidity and a short festinating gait, rabbit syndrome **(M)** (a rare side effect of long-term antipsychotic use characterized by involuntary, fine, rhythmic motions of the mouth and lips), and tardive dyskinesia **(O)**, a disorder of abnormal involuntary movements caused by prolonged use of neuroleptics. An idiosyncratic but rare complication of neuroleptics is neuroleptic malignant syndrome **(G)**. This is characterized by hyperthermia, change in mental status, and increased muscle tone. It can lead to a rise in muscle breakdown products (creatine kinase levels are typically elevated), renal failure following dehydration, pulmonary complications, and death. Clozapine can cause agranulocytosis **(A)**, a dangerous side effect that sometimes can present with sore throat and fever; if this occurs, the drug must be stopped immediately. Constipation **(D)** is a complicating side effect of some antipsychotics, particularly those with anticholinergic effects. This can often be relieved with use of a laxative. Obstructive jaundice **(H)** is rare and occurs mainly with chlorpromazine. Symptoms include fever, nausea, malaise, and pruritus. Orthostatic hypotension **(J)**, a sudden drop in blood pressure upon standing, is due to alpha-1-adrenergic blockade. It is especially troublesome with chlorpromazine and clozapine and

best handled by raising doses slowly. Pigmented retinopathy **(K)** is observed with high doses of thioridazine and best detected with a good ophthalmologic examination. An additional side effect of some antipsychotic medications that may decrease compliance is retrograde ejaculation **(N)**; orgasm may be achieved but ejaculation is abnormal, with retrograde propulsion of the semen, resulting in a cloudy appearance of the urine.

122. **(D)** Alcohol withdrawal can take the form of minor withdrawal symptoms such as sweating, flushing, and tremulousness, or more serious consequences including withdrawal seizures or withdrawal delirium, formerly known as delirium tremens. Minor withdrawal symptoms can last for several days. Withdrawal seizures are rarely focal and usually occur within 48 hours after alcohol consumption ceases. Delirium tremens most often occurs within 72 hours of cessation of drinking, although may peak for several days further.

123. **(C)** This patient is exhibiting symptoms of hyponatremia, a relatively common side effect of oxcarbazepine (2.5%), so obtaining serum electrolytes would be critical. The other tests would not help in diagnosing hyponatremia, and oxcarbazepine levels are not routinely checked (unlike levels of carbamazepine).

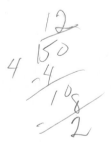

CHAPTER 4

Psychological Treatment and Management
Questions

DIRECTIONS (Questions 1 through 42): For each of the multiple choice questions in this section, select the lettered answer that is the one *best* response in each case.

Questions 1 and 2

A 38-year-old male thinks that he is a "failure and will never find a partner" whenever he feels rejected. He often finds himself getting depressed and isolating himself when he thinks like this. His therapist thinks that it would be a good idea for him to make a log of the situations, his immediate thoughts, his immediate feelings, alternate responses to those thoughts and feelings, and re-rate his feelings after completing the exercise so they can examine them during their sessions.

1. Which of the following types of therapeutic approaches is the therapist using?

   (A) cognitive behavioral
   (B) expressive
   (C) hypnotherapy
   (D) psychoanalysis
   (E) psychodynamic

2. Which of the following terms refer to the immediate thoughts that the patient experiences and records in this type of therapy?

   (A) automatic thoughts
   (B) core beliefs

   (C) ego strengths
   (D) premonitions
   (E) unconscious thoughts

3. A 43-year-old man is chastised at work. When he comes home, his friend asks him how his day went. He responds angrily saying that a "real friend wouldn't be so nosy." Which of the following defense mechanisms characterizes this reaction?

   (A) denial
   (B) displacement
   (C) humor
   (D) intellectualization
   (E) isolation of affect

4. A 20-year-old woman diagnosed with borderline personality disorder thinks of her therapist as "the best person I've ever known." The next week, the therapist announces that he will be going on vacation. The patient becomes enraged and states that he is "the cruelest doctor in the world!" Which of the following defense mechanisms characterizes this reaction?

   (A) devaluation
   (B) idealization
   (C) intellectualization
   (D) repression
   (E) splitting

5. A 16-year-old boy has just lost his mother and father in a car accident. In your office, he talks philosophically about death and its implications. When asked how he feels about his parents' death, he responds by saying that "it is the nature of things to pass away." Which of the following defense mechanisms best demonstrates this patient's inability to talk directly about his emotional experience concerning personal loss?

(A) denial
(B) intellectualization
(C) lying
(D) projection
(E) suppression

Questions 6 and 7

A 44-year-old woman with schizophrenia is struggling with paranoia, auditory hallucinations, and delusions. She lives with her mother but has a poor relationship with her. She tells you that everyone wants her to spend a lot of money and buy drugs.

6. Which of the following responses would be the most useful?

(A) "Well, deciding for yourself is best."
(B) "If you buy drugs, I'll call the police."
(C) "Perhaps we should look at what your mother would think about that."
(D) "Why do you think everyone wants you to do that?"
(E) "No, they don't."

7. You decide that supportive therapy would be helpful to this patient. Which of the following would be the most appropriate goal of supportive therapy for this patient?

(A) correcting faulty ideas
(B) exploring the feeling of meaninglessness in life
(C) investigating the freedom of individuals
(D) personality change
(E) strengthening of defenses

8. A 32-year-old psychiatry resident is in psychoanalysis 4 days per week. He is encouraged to lie on the couch and say "whatever comes to mind." Which of the following analytic techniques does this represent?

(A) free association
(B) hypnosis
(C) repression
(D) thought records
(E) transference

9. A psychotherapist has been meeting regularly with a 10-year-old boy for 18 months. During one of the therapy sessions, she finds herself feeling very angry at the patient after he reports "beating up" his little brother. Which of the following phenomena is the psychotherapist most likely exhibiting?

(A) countertransference
(B) extinction
(C) interpretation
(D) resistance
(E) transference

10. In an acute inpatient psychiatric unit, the resident psychiatrist is in charge of leading a group consisting of patients newly admitted to the ward. During group she asks two participants to act out a scenario, describe their feelings about the situation, and then explore the individual conflicts which arose. Which of the following techniques of psychotherapy does this most represent?

(A) feedback
(B) free association
(C) go-around
(D) psychodrama
(E) resistance

Questions 11 and 12

A 28-year-old female patient who is addicted to opiate analgesics states that she has been upset with family for not continuing to support her financially and allow her to stay with them. She has been unemployed for many years since leaving college. Since they informed her that she should start working and find a place of her own 1 year ago, she has felt that they are abandoning her and "kicking her out on the street," although they have continued to support her.

Her therapist believes that she is very dependent, but tells the patient that she should continue to be upset with her family, and also blame them for her inability to be independent and not continuing to support her.

11. Which of the following therapeutic techniques best describes the therapist's response?

(A) countertransference
(B) empathy
(C) interpretation
(D) paradoxical intervention
(E) working through

12. The patient's family members and close friends work with the therapist and join the patient in a session. During the meeting, they tell her about her maladaptive behaviors and how they have affected her and her family negatively. They then give her an ultimatum whereby if she does not get treatment for her addiction they will not continue to support her. Which of the following techniques best describes this scenario?

(A) behavioral therapy
(B) family therapy
(C) group therapy
(D) intervention
(E) relapse prevention

13. A 24-year-old female patient who has been diagnosed with post-traumatic stress disorder and borderline personality disorder is referred for medication management. During the beginning of her first visit she initially praises the psychiatrist and how understanding he is of her problems. However, after her request for a certain medication is denied, she becomes very upset and begins to berate the psychiatrist, telling him that he is the "worst psychiatrist" she has met, that he is uncaring and does "not understand human needs." Which of the following concepts best describes this behavior?

(A) abreaction
(B) dependency

(C) projection
(D) reaction formation
(E) splitting

14. A 34-year-old male is referred by his job because of ongoing interpersonal conflicts. During the interview, he appears very focused on his health, his attractiveness to others, and his success at work. When confronted with his difficulties, he becomes defensive, blaming others and accusing them of being "jealous of me." He describes himself as "better" than his friends and colleagues and admits to taking advantage of others in order to "get what I deserve." Which of the following treatment modalities would be the most appropriate for this patient?

(A) anger management
(B) combined individual and group therapy
(C) psychoanalysis
(D) psychopharmacotherapy
(E) social skills training

15. A 29-year-old woman has been depressed for 2 months prior to seeking medical attention. She believes that nobody likes her even though she is always cordial, and that there is nothing she can do to change the way other people perceive her. The patient consistently thinks that she is a failure and she will never be successful; this in turn worsens her depression. She adamantly refuses to take antidepressants. You believe that cognitive therapy is indicated for this patient. Which of the following thoughts would most likely be the focus of your therapy?

(A) genetically determined thoughts
(B) thoughts at the edge of conscious awareness that regularly precede unpleasant feelings
(C) thoughts that cannot be changed
(D) thoughts that impede free association
(E) thoughts that occur while sleeping

16. After several weeks, a 40-year-old female patient who is in psychodynamic psychotherapy begins to show up late and miss appointments; each time this happens she has a reason for doing so. However, the therapist begins to feel that her behavior is interfering with her treatment. The therapist is not sure if the patient understands her behavior is inappropriate and potentially damaging to her therapy. Which of the following topics would be the most important to review with the patient before making an interpretation of her behavior?

    (A) boundaries and rules defining the way in which therapy is conducted
    (B) focus on the therapeutic goals
    (C) method used to change the patient's maladaptive thoughts
    (D) patient's need for attention
    (E) reasons the patient is late to the appointments

17. A 45-year-old man presents to your outpatient clinic handicapped by a fear of parking lots and fields. The fear started 4 months prior to this visit. At the beginning of cognitive therapy, he tells you that his behavior is constantly being scrutinized and criticized by other people. He claims that he cannot change his behavior, because if he does others will think he is a fool. Which of the following would be the most appropriate response?

    (A) "That's silly. People will not think you are a fool."
    (B) "Yes, I can see that."
    (C) "What makes you think that others are constantly scrutinizing your behavior?"
    (D) "How can you possibly think other people care enough about you to constantly scrutinize your behavior?"
    (E) "Well, maybe you are a fool. Have you ever thought of that?"

18. A 32-year-old female in therapy describes how she feels that she should have a life partner; the fact that she is not currently dating means that she is unlikely to ever get married and is therefore unlovable. Her therapist points out to her that she has had a few meaningful long-term relationships in the past and that she has dated as recently as a couple of months ago. The therapist also explains that many people may not date, but this does not mean they are unlovable or will never get married. Which of the following terms best describes the therapeutic intervention described above?

    (A) clarification
    (B) confrontation
    (C) empathy
    (D) interpretation
    (E) reframing

Questions 19 and 20

An 18-year-old, single man presents to your office complaining that he cannot pass a movie theater without stopping, going inside, and buying candy. This behavior is troublesome to him and interferes with his daily activities causing him to be constantly late to other appointments. You decide to help the patient with behavior therapy.

19. Which of the following would be the most appropriate focus of the therapy?

    (A) analyzing the patient's relationships
    (B) decreasing the maladaptive behavior of stopping by movie theaters
    (C) examining the patient's negative eating habits
    (D) exploring the patient's childhood traumas
    (E) working on resolving the patient's unconscious conflicts

20. Which of the following behavioral interventions would be the most helpful in this case?

    (A) aversion therapy
    (B) environmental modification
    (C) exposure and response training
    (D) modeling
    (E) relaxation training

21. A 39-year-old man presents to your office complaining of chronic "stress," anxiety, and poor sleep. He also admits to intermittent headaches, which you diagnose as tension headaches. You recommend behavioral therapy for reduction

of his headaches. Which of the following behavioral techniques would be most appropriate for this patient?

(A) aversive stimuli
(B) biofeedback
(C) negative reinforcement
(D) stimulus control
(E) systematic desensitization

Questions 22 and 23

A 32-year-old male complains of ongoing depression for the past month which he attributes to the break-up with his fiancée. He has been having insomnia, decreased appetite, and low energy, although he denies anhedonia or problems concentrating. He also denies any suicidal ideation. He has just started to date someone else within the last week. After discussion with the patient, it is decided to utilize both medication and interpersonal psychotherapy for his depression.

22. Which of the following goals would be the most likely focus of his psychotherapy?

   (A) character change
   (B) clarifying communication patterns
   (C) hypnosis
   (D) interpreting transference
   (E) pointing out resistance

23. Which of the following techniques would be most likely utilized during this patient's therapy?

   (A) dream interpretation
   (B) defense analysis
   (C) free association
   (D) regression
   (E) role playing

Questions 24 and 25

A 22-year-old college student presents complaining of having "no goals" in his life, not doing as well as he could in school, and desiring but having no serious long-term romantic relationships. He has not chosen a major and states that his indecision is paralyzing him from "moving on with the rest of my life." After discussing various forms of psychotherapy with the

patient, you recommend psychoanalysis four times per week.

24. Which of the following is the most important reason for the frequency of psychoanalysis?

   (A) Allow the patient to get enough support during the course of their treatment.
   (B) Allow transference to build between patient and therapist.
   (C) Complete homework frequently to better learn about their issues.
   (D) Prevent conflicts from arising between the therapist and patient.
   (E) Require more intensive treatment due to severity of mental illness.

25. Which of the following would be the most important tool in his psychoanalysis?

   (A) altering cognitive distortions
   (B) altering maladaptive behaviors
   (C) interpretation of transference
   (D) interpreting dreams
   (E) solving interpersonal problems

26. A male therapist has been working with a female patient for over 3 years, enabling her to improve her self-esteem and confidence, and to eventually divorce her emotionally-abusive husband 1 year ago. The patient continually thanks the therapist and explains that she is sexually attracted to the therapist. He is initially taken aback and then somewhat flattered by her sexual interest. However, he also notes that he also feels a strong attraction to her and feels the need to care for her. Which of the following would be the most appropriate next step for the therapist to take?

   (A) Act cold, show less empathy, and set more rigid boundaries during sessions.
   (B) Explore the patient's feeling in order to increase her erotic transference.
   (C) Ignore the patient's disclosure of her sexual attraction.
   (D) Seek supervision with a mentor or colleague.
   (E) Terminate or fire the patient from his care.

Questions 27 and 28

You are seeing a 25-year-old man in cognitive-behavioral therapy who suffers from generalized anxiety disorder, as well as epilepsy. He often talks about the many dreams he has while in his sessions, and he is having a hard time with the restructuring of maladaptive thoughts. You decide that hypnosis may be helpful as an adjunctive therapy for this patient, as he has been hypnotized before with good results and you have a skillful hypnotist in your clinic. The patient is hopeful that hypnosis will be beneficial for him again.

27. Which of the following characteristics is the best predictor of response to hypnosis in this patient?

    (A) Patient has a lot of dreams.
    (B) Patient is responsive to suggestion.
    (C) Patient's diagnosis.
    (D) Patient with low seizure threshold.
    (E) Trained hypnotist will be doing his treatment.

28. The patient is started in hypnosis, but there is a concern as to whether he is in a trance during the sessions. Which of the following indicators would be most likely increased in a trance state?

    (A) amnesia
    (B) pain perception
    (C) pulse
    (D) reflexes
    (D) respirations

29. You are treating an 11-year-old boy for oppositional defiant disorder and have heard from the parents that his disorder has had an impact on the family. They have two older children who often feel left out and feel distanced from the family unit. You recommend a trial of family therapy. In this case, which of the following would be the most appropriate focus of the family therapy?

    (A) assigning roles in a household
    (B) early childhood experiences
    (C) impulsive behavior
    (D) relationship patterns
    (E) unconscious conflicts

30. A 32-year-old man presents for psychotherapy. He denies pervasive depression or anxiety symptoms, but he has had a string of failed relationships. He blames the problem on "his sabotaging things" when the women "start to get serious." He is clearly ambivalent about his desire to "settle down" with someone. According to Erik Erikson, which of the following stages of development is the patient most likely in?

    (A) trust versus mistrust
    (B) autonomy versus shame
    (C) initiative versus guilt
    (D) intimacy versus isolation
    (E) identity versus role confusion

31. A 9-year-old boy with attention-deficit hyperactivity disorder (ADHD), predominantly hyperactive type, presents to your office accompanied by his mother. He is currently on methylphenidate (Ritalin) and they both wonder if there is something else that can be done to help the patient. Despite some benefit and tolerability, the child continues to have difficulty in school, not remembering his homework assignments and not paying attention in class. He has also recently gotten into a minor physical fight with a peer. Therapy is recommended for the child. Which of the following aims best illustrates how behavioral therapy would help this patient?

    (A) focusing on maladaptive communication in the family
    (B) focusing on the patient's interpersonal relationships
    (C) interpreting a transference
    (D) positively reframing a negative experience
    (E) reinforcing attention to necessary tasks and ignoring disruptive behaviors

32. A 14-year-old boy with attention-deficit hyperactivity disorder (ADHD) is frequently late for school and forgets to do his chores around the house due to his disorganization. His parents are fed up with him and ask you what they can do to help change his behavior. Which of the following represents the most helpful behavioral tool for patients with ADHD?

(A) a report card of behaviors to be rewarded by parents

(B) aversion

(C) a well-timed interpretation of maladaptive behaviors

(D) positively reframing a negative experience

(E) punishment

Questions 33 and 34

A 25-year-old unmarried man in his fourth year of medical school presents to your office complaining of not being able to remain in a relationship with a girlfriend for longer than 3 months. He says that he would like an insight-oriented therapy, and you agree that this form of therapy would help him. You decide to treat this patient with brief psychodynamic psychotherapy.

33. Which of the following factors would best predict a positive outcome with brief psychodynamic psychotherapy in this particular patient?

(A) age

(B) gender

(C) marital status

(D) motivation for change

(E) socioeconomic status

34. Which of the following aspects best distinguishes his specific type of psychotherapy from other forms of therapy?

(A) correcting cognitive errors

(B) identification of a focal conflict

(C) interpreting dreams

(D) interpreting resistance

(E) modifying maladaptive behaviors

35. A 20-year-old man is currently in college and has completed the first semester of his sophomore year. Halfway into the second semester, his grades drop from As to Fs over a 3-month period. He becomes increasingly isolated and

paranoid, believing that the government is after him because he has solved "all theological problems" through direct communication with God. He is started on olanzapine (Zyprexa) 10 mg by mouth (PO) daily and is tentatively diagnosed with schizophreniform disorder. He recovers after 4 months but has another relapse 6 months later in the absence of elevated, irritable, or depressed mood. He is then given a diagnosis of schizophrenia. Which of the following types of psychotherapy would most likely worsen his condition?

(A) behavioral therapy

(B) family therapy

(C) group psychotherapy

(D) psychoanalysis

(E) supportive psychotherapy

36. A 50-year-old man is in psychoanalysis because he feels stagnant in his personal life. He notes he is not having any problems with his work or relationship with his wife, although he feels that he has never had more than a platonic relationship with her. He notes that he feels capable and confident in most spheres of his life and most of his relationships. He feels like he is at a "road block" in therapy and does not know how to proceed. He has, however, mentioned a reoccurring dream about his wife turning into his mother and taking care of him. The therapist thinks that interpreting his dream may be a good tool to use in therapy. Which of the following uses of his dream would be the most appropriate in this case?

(A) Interpreted by the analyst to subliminally influence the mind of the patient.

(B) Provide information about psychic conflicts.

(C) Represent the conscious framework for behavior.

(D) Used to alter cognitive errors.

(E) Used to change behavior.

37. You have been assigned to lead various groups that help patients who suffer from personality disorders. To accomplish this task, you need to know which disorders are appropriate for group psychotherapy and which benefit from combined individual and group psychotherapy. Which of the following personality disorders is best treated with combined individual and group psychotherapy?

    (A) antisocial personality disorder
    (B) avoidant personality disorder
    (C) borderline personality disorder
    (D) schizoid personality disorder
    (E) schizotypal personality disorder

Questions 38 and 39

A 33-year-old woman presents to the emergency department saying that she wants to kill herself. She has felt increasingly depressed for many months, with terminal insomnia, poor appetite, weight loss, distractibility, and fatigue. She currently feels hopeless and helpless, and has a plan to overdose of pills that she has stockpiled at home.

38. Other than her feelings of helplessness and hopelessness, which of the following cognitive difficulties would she most likely also exhibit?

    (A) begging the question
    (B) circular reasoning
    (C) personalization
    (D) rigid, black-or-white thinking
    (E) selective abstraction

39. Which of the following forms of psychotherapy would be most appropriate to help minimize this patient's suicidality?

    (A) behavioral therapy
    (B) cognitive therapy
    (C) hypnosis
    (D) interpersonal psychotherapy
    (E) paradoxical therapy

40. In the context of a women's group, one member begins crying as she relates her story of her abusive partner. As she is telling her story, three other members begin crying and are upset because they have been through similar situations. Which of the following terms best describes this phenomenon?

    (A) competition
    (B) contagion
    (C) corrective experience
    (D) differentiation
    (E) imitation

41. A 38-year-old lawyer is referred for behavioral therapy because of extreme social anxiety which is interfering in his ability to litigate. In his early therapy sessions, he is told to make a hierarchy of situations that make him anxious. The therapist then begins working with him by first exposing him to the least anxiety-provoking items on the list and then gradually increasing the severity. Which of the following therapeutic techniques is the therapist most likely utilizing?

    (A) aversion
    (B) flooding
    (C) modeling
    (D) suggestion
    (E) systematic desensitization

42. A 47-year-old, divorced male has been attending psychotherapy for 8 months due to ongoing "stress" and conflicts at work. During most of his therapy sessions, the psychiatrist responds to his comments with empathic responses. Which type of psychotherapy is the psychiatrist most likely utilizing in this case?

    (A) behavioral
    (B) cognitive
    (C) dynamic
    (D) existential
    (E) supportive

DIRECTIONS (Questions 43 through 50): The following group of questions is preceded by a list of lettered options. For each patient scenario, select the one lettered option that is *most* closely associated with it. Each lettered option may be used once, multiple times, or not at all.

(A) anxiety
(B) biofeedback
(C) countertransference
(D) flooding
(E) hypnosis
(F) negative reinforcement
(G) positive reinforcement
(H) posttraumatic stress disorder
(I) projection
(J) projective identification
(K) punishment
(L) real relationship
(M) schema
(N) splitting
(O) therapeutic alliance
(P) transference
(Q) undoing

43. You are seeing a 26-year-old woman who complains of migraines. She is otherwise healthy. You explain to her that you would like to try a technique in which you give her information on muscle tension and temperature.

44. You are seeing a 45-year-old man in psychoanalysis four times per week. After about 6 months, the patient tells you that you are the "center of his universe" and that "no one could be a better psychiatrist."

45. A patient who is afraid of clowns is taken to the circus in the beginning of her therapy in order to get over her fear.

46. To train a 4-year-old boy to say "thank you," his mother gives him a sweet whenever he does.

47. To train a 4-year-old boy not to bite his classmates, his mother puts soap in his mouth whenever he does.

Questions 48 through 50: The following group of questions is preceded by a list of lettered options. For each question, select the one lettered option that is *most* closely associated with it.

(A) Josef Breuer
(B) Jean-Martin Charcot
(C) Erik Erikson
(D) Sigmund Freud
(E) Heinz Kohut
(F) Franz Anton Mesmer

48. Made many contributions to psychiatry and neurology with a special interest in describing hysteria.

49. Known as the inventor of the "cathartic" treatment or talking therapy.

50. Known as the developer of self-psychology.

Answers and Explanations

1. **(A)** Cognitive-behavioral therapy refers to a variety of techniques that concentrate on the construction and reconstruction of people's cognitions, emotions, and behaviors. Cognitive-behavioral therapists use a range of modalities to help patients assess, recognize, and deal with problematic and dysfunctional ways of thinking, emoting, and behaving. In this case, a thought record is being used to examine their feeling and beliefs. Expressive therapy uses different forms of expression (ie, art, movement, music, or writing) to have a patient express their feelings and work through them. Hypnotherapy uses hypnosis to uncover underlying conflicts and hypnotic suggestion to change behaviors. Psychoanalysis encourages a patient to verbalize all their thoughts, including free associations, fantasies, and dreams, and the analyst formulates the unconscious conflicts causing the patients symptoms or character problems. Psychodynamic therapy tries to find out the unconscious content of a client's psyche and then work on the issues in therapy; it has its root in psychoanalysis.

2. **(A)** Automatic thoughts are the immediate thoughts that come to mind in any situation that are based on underlying core beliefs; these are deeply held ideas regarding the world and oneself that drive a patient's emotional responses and behavior. Ego strength is the ability of the ego to cope with competing conflicts between the id, ego, and superego which help one manage stress and maintain stability. Premonitions are thoughts predicting the future. Unconscious thoughts are instinctual thoughts, drives, and needs out of one's awareness, arising from the unconscious mind.

3. **(B)** Displacement is a defense that transfers a feeling about, or a response to, one object (person) onto another object (person). Denial is a defense that keeps out of conscious awareness an aspect of external reality or subjective distress that is too uncomfortable for the person to accept. Humor is considered a mature defense mechanism that emphasizes the amusing or ironic aspects of the stressor. Intellectualization is a defense in which the individual favors abstract thinking over dealing with the disturbing feelings of an idea or experience. Isolation of affect involves detachment of feelings from a particular idea or experience.

4. **(E)** Splitting occurs when an individual is unable to see others moderately, with positive and negative qualities (ie, people's actions are either all good or all bad). Devaluation is a defense that attributes excessive negative qualities to another. Idealization attributes excessive positive qualities to another. Intellectualization is a defense that utilizes excessive abstract thinking or generalizations to manage threatening emotions. Repression expels disturbing wishes, thoughts, or experiences from conscious awareness. The feeling component may remain but be divorced from the idea.

5. **(B)** This is an example of intellectualization, a defense that utilizes excessive abstract thinking or generalizations to manage threatening emotions. Denial is a defense that keeps out of conscious awareness an aspect of external reality or subjective distress that is too uncomfortable for the person to accept. Lying is not considered a defense mechanism. Projection is a defense whereby a thought, feeling, or idea

that is unacceptable to the person is falsely attributed to another. Suppression is where one intentionally avoids thinking of distressing thoughts, feelings, ideas, or experiences.

6. **(D)** The best strategy in any communication is to try to gain clarity. Asking this patient why she believes what she does may lead nowhere but it may help to understand the patient's concerns. Choice A may be helpful in some situations and certainly has a positive ring to it. However, this patient's comment is an implicit question. She is asking for help and genuinely does not know what to do. Hiding behind pithy maxims is not usually helpful. Choices B and C are coercive and block communication. Giving supportive guidance is appropriate in this situation, but coercion is never appropriate in a therapeutic relationship. Choice E is not coercive but also blocks communication. While the patient may require reality testing, the response may sacrifice a more insightful, empowering reply.

7. **(E)** The goal of supportive therapy is the strengthening of current defense mechanisms. Through supportive care, the patient can learn to cope with difficult problems using already established abilities. Correcting faulty ideas is the expressed goal of cognitive therapy. Exploring the feeling of meaninglessness in life and investigating the freedom of individuals are goals of existential psychotherapy. Personality change is a goal of psychodynamic psychotherapy, where defenses are examined gradually in order to achieve a more optimal level of functioning.

8. **(A)** This is an example of free association. Freud believed that all mental activity is causally related, meaning that free associations are not truly random. They follow logically, but the missing connection is being held down or repressed unconsciously by defenses. Hypnosis is where a patient is placed in a trance and their unconscious is explored. Repression is a defense mechanism that expels disturbing wishes, thoughts, or experiences from conscious awareness. Thought records is when a patient records a situation, feeling, automatics thoughts, and

alternative responses then re-rates the initial feelings; this technique is commonly used in cognitive-behavioral therapy. Transference, in strict terms, is the reexperiencing of past experiences with the analyst in the setting of psychoanalytic psychotherapy. Countertransference is the analyst's response to this. However, these terms have come to mean the transferring of emotions and feelings that one has from one's past to the physician or care provider in the case of transference and the physician toward the patient in countertransference.

9. **(A)** Countertransference is the conscious or unconscious emotional reaction of the therapist to the patient. Transference is the conscious or unconscious emotional reaction of the patient to the therapist based on a past relationship the patient had with a significant other person (eg, a parent). Extinction is a term frequently used in learning theory, which refers to the reduction in frequency of a learned response as a result of the cessation of reinforcement. Interpretation is insight offered by the therapist regarding patterns of thought or behavior. Resistance is the patient's unconscious opposition to full disclosure of feelings or ideas.

10. **(D)** Psychodrama is a technique in which group members are used as the audience and the cast in reenactments of scenarios and conflict. The content of the drama is used to explore individual problems in a group setting. Feedback, a cardinal feature of group psychotherapy, comes from peers as well as from the leader. Feedback from peers in the group can be a powerful stimulus for insight and change. Free association is used in psychoanalytically oriented groups. These groups are largely outpatient groups whose members can tolerate and effectively use this technique. Members are encouraged to be spontaneous with their thoughts and feelings, and the therapist assists in pointing out common themes and possible connections. Go-around is a common technique where each group member is asked to introduce themselves, state how they are feeling, or otherwise specifically respond; this gives each individual a chance to participate. Resistance is the unconscious opposition to full disclosure of thoughts or feelings.

11. **(D)** Paradoxical intervention is a therapeutic technique where a therapist instructs a patient to hold onto a symptom in order to get the patient to understand that the symptom is not helpful (in this case her dependency). Countertransference is when the therapist's feelings and emotions are directed toward a patient. Empathy is when a therapist identifies and understands a patient's situation or feelings. Using hypotheses to explain the psychological meaning of a behavior or symptom is called interpretation. Working through refers to thinking about and discussing a problem in order to lessen its intensity or impact.

12. **(D)** Intervention is an orchestrated attempt by one or many to get an individual to accept professional help or treatment, usually for an addiction or crisis. Behavioral therapy concentrates on changing a patient's maladaptive behaviors or actions, and its purpose is not to try to get a patient to commit to treatment. Family therapy involves an entire family in therapy together working to change the dynamics, development, and systems of interaction; family therapy does not usually focus on the problems of one member. Group therapy is when a group of individuals work on issues in conjunction with each other; it can be helpful because the different backgrounds and problems can be looked at together in order to help each person with their own difficulties. Relapse prevention is used in addictions treatment, where individuals are taught self-control and how to maintain changes in behavior, as well as how to anticipate and cope with relapse.

13. **(E)** This patient is demonstrating the concept of splitting, a defense mechanism where one views themselves or others (in this case the doctor) as "all good" or "all bad." It is commonly seen in patients with borderline personality disorder. Abreaction is when a patient relives an emotional or traumatic experience to get rid of or purge negative emotions and move forward. Dependency is where one needs another person or addictive substance in order to maintain their level of emotional or physical functioning. Projection is a primitive defense consisting of attributing one's own undesirable thoughts, desires, or emotions onto someone or something else. Reaction formation is when unacceptable or anxiety-provoking emotions are dealt with by acting in the opposite manner, for example, unconsciously wishing for someone to die and then repeatedly saving them from danger.

14. **(B)** This individual has features of narcissistic personality disorder. Although patients with narcissistic personality disorder have difficulty with confrontation, it is necessary to help them work toward change; therefore, group therapy is a good setting for this to take place. In addition, in individual therapy patients can process these situations and examine how possible insults to the ego can be dealt with, as well as addressing the other individual issues. Anger management as well as social skills training can be helpful, but are not enough to examine the deep underlying issues and defenses that patients with narcissistic personality disorder have. Similarly, psychoanalysis alone would not be enough to help patients in which many of their relationships and social interactions are affected by their personality disorder. Pharmacotherapy is often not helpful with personality disorders unless severe impulsivity or psychosis is present, or unless a patient has a comorbid axis I disorder (eg, major depressive disorder).

15. **(B)** One of the goals of cognitive-behavioral therapy is to identify and modify automatic thoughts so that individuals do not constantly view themselves or their environment in a negative light. Automatic thoughts are constant ways of perceiving situations and oneself in relation to the environment; they can be thought of as a set way of evaluating oneself and events. Automatic thoughts are not genetically determined. They have not always been present and can be changed. There is no moral imperative from automatic thoughts and they do not impede free association. They are not thoughts that occur during sleep.

16. **(A)** In this case, it would be important for the therapist to review the "frame" for therapy. In psychodynamic psychotherapy the "frame" refers to the boundaries and rules defining the

way the therapist and patient interact (eg, the meeting time, place, length, other details down to where the therapist and patient usually sit, how fees for service are collected, what happens when a patient starts missing appointments). The frame is important as it gives psychotherapy a structure and sets up a specific dynamic between the patient and therapist. Therefore, if boundaries or rules are challenged the therapist can use this to better understand the reasons as well as determine any transference issues at play. In this case the therapist suspects the patient may not understand the frame used for her therapy sessions and why it is important. Reviewing the goals of and the type of therapy provided may both be reasonable topics for the therapist to discuss; however, it would not address her reasons for being late and not showing up for appointments. Interpreting the patient's behavior as a need for attention may not only be incorrect, but it may be experienced by the patient as an attack or hurtful, particularly if she does not understand the therapeutic frame correctly. Similarly, looking at the individual reasons why she is late avoids the subject of why this pattern of behavior is present.

17. **(C)** One reason this is the best response is that it is a question. Patients with cognitive distortions often take their view of the world as a given. They do not question their perspectives. Asking a question invites patients to examine their perspectives and thereby become open to the possibility that their thoughts may be inaccurate. Choices **(D)** and **(E)** are also questions but are authoritarian and punitive, not to mention insulting; to have the best outcome in any form of therapy, there must be a good relationship or alliance between the patient and therapist. Choice **(A)** may also be harmful as a patient should not be called "silly." Choice **(B)** is ambiguous—to which part of the question are you responding? The patient may believe that you are insulting him rather than attempting to be supportive.

18. **(E)** Reframing is a technique commonly used in cognitive-behavioral therapy. First, a therapist will examine how patient's thoughts or beliefs

about themselves or the world may be skewed. Then the thoughts or beliefs are reframed by comparing them to a more normalized perspective. Clarification is when a therapist asks for further details about a patient's experience or situation they are describing. Confrontation is when a therapist directly asks patients about their maladaptive behaviors or symptoms. Empathy is when a therapist shows understanding or agrees with patients, showing them that they are able to "put themselves in the patient's shoes" or see their perspective. Interpretation is when a therapist tells a patient a hypothesis regarding the reason(s) (often unconscious) a patient has certain behaviors or symptoms.

19. **(B)** Behavior therapy is focused on behaviors, not on possible underlying factors that cause the behaviors. In this case, addressing the negative or maladaptive behavior (eg, stopping by movie theaters to buy candy) would be addressed. Behavior therapy is a here-and-now approach to maladaptive behaviors. It may utilize information surrounding the emergence of a particular maladaptive behavior to construct a behavior modification plan. Although behavior therapy can and does change neurobiology, this is not its expressed goal. It does not focus on the patient's relationships or seeking the sources for the patient's negative eating habits. This is also why childhood issues such as trauma are not addressed in behavioral therapy. Changing underlying conflicts in an attempt to change behavior is a description of the goals of psychodynamic psychotherapy or psychoanalysis.

20. **(C)** In this case, exposure and response training would be the most helpful in decreasing the patient's maladaptive behavior of stopping at movie theaters. It would teach more adaptive behaviors through exposing him to situations where he could stop by movie theaters and practice healthier ways of coping. Aversion therapy is when a negative (painful) stimulus is paired with a maladaptive behavior in order to extinguish the behavior; it is not commonly used and often the behavior returns over time. In this case, environmental modification would

be less helpful as the patient will likely encounter situations where he may pass movie theaters in the future; in addition, changing the environment does not address the behavior. Modeling is where adaptive behaviors are taught by demonstration, which would be difficult to teach in this particular case. Relaxation training is used to help a patient to handle anxiety-provoking situations, not change an unhealthy behavior.

21. **(B)** Biofeedback and stress reduction are used to reduce the frequency and severity of headaches. They are equally effective in accomplishing this goal. Substance withdrawal syndromes are examples of aversive stimuli, and the resultant negative reinforcement theoretically leads to a decrease in substance use. Stimulus control is used in the treatment of insomnia: The negative association between multiple failed attempts at falling asleep and the specific environment where they occurred is eliminated by reducing distractions and creating an environment more conducive to sleep (eg, taking televisions and computers out of the bedroom), as well as teaching good sleep hygiene. Systematic desensitization is a behavioral technique which can be used in asthma, where the patient becomes relaxed and visualizes typical situations that precipitate asthma attacks.

22. **(B)** The major focus of interpersonal psychotherapy is communication analysis. Indirect, unclear interpersonal communication patterns are identified in the course of therapy. These communication patterns are then altered, for instance, by role playing or asking the patient to try out different forms of communication during the session. Character change, interpreting transference, and pointing out resistance are more the focus of psychodynamically-oriented psychotherapy. Hypnosis is a sleep-like state induced by a therapist, which has been of some use in behavioral modification such as stopping smoking. It is not a goal or component of interpersonal psychotherapy.

23. **(E)** Interpersonal psychotherapy focuses on the patient's role and communication style within important relationships and how their position

may be causing or complicating the illness (eg, depression). If one or two specific ways of communicating can be altered so that a relationship improves, the depressive illness also improves. This therapy also has the added benefit of durability; once a communication pattern is improved and the patient better understands how his or her role in a relationship may create distress, the depressive illness is not as likely to recur. Various techniques used in interpersonal psychotherapy are role playing, supportive listening, clarification, and communication analysis. Analyzing dreams and psychic defenses are used in more psychodynamically-based therapies, such as psychoanalysis; regression often occurs in these therapies, but is to be avoided in interpersonal therapy due to the short-term nature.

24. **(B)** Psychoanalysis tends to be among the longest of therapies and involves the process of free association in which the patient lies on a couch, facing away from the therapist, and says whatever comes to mind. It takes four to five sessions a week to successfully complete an analysis because it is difficult for patients to build, sustain, and work through their transference and defensive structure; less frequent sessions decrease the formation of a "transference neurosis" and increase defenses. Psychoanalysis is based on an expressive or exploratory model of therapy, as opposed to a supportive model aimed at stabilizing crisis and reestablishing a baseline level of function. Homework is a method used on cognitive-behavioral therapy and not psychoanalysis. In psychoanalysis conflicts between therapist and patient are analyzed and discussed as they often represent a recreation of childhood conflicts and relationships. There is no correlation between severity of mental illness and length of therapy. Patients who are in psychoanalysis are not more likely to be severely ill and will need a certain level of insight and competence to gain the benefits of psychoanalysis without encountering severe problems.

25. **(C)** The major tool of psychoanalysis is the careful interpretations of the transference neurosis. Altering cognitive distortions is the main

ODD

goal of cognitive therapy. While psychoanalysis may accomplish many tasks, including changing maladaptive thoughts and behaviors and "solving" interpersonal problems, these are the consequences of analysis, not the instruments of change. Although interpreting dreams can lead to insights into a patient's unconscious thoughts and feelings, it is an adjunctive tool.

26. **(D)** In this case, the therapist is having an inappropriate attraction to his patient and should seek supervision in order to understand the reasons for his (and the patient's) sexual feelings. In addition, a supervisor can help to make sure that the transference or countertransference is not significantly interfering in the therapy. Not addressing the situation, or acting less empathetic or cold would be evasive and confusing to the patient, making it difficult for the patient to move forward in therapy. The therapist should not try to elicit more behaviors or continue to deepen any erotic transference that could lead to power differential or more seductive behavior which could put the relationship in jeopardy or cross boundaries inappropriately. Although the therapist can fire or terminate the patient, the situation may not be serious enough to warrant such severe actions; it may also send the message to the patient that her sexual feelings are dangerous and that the therapy was not a safe place to discuss them.

27. **(B)** While a skilled hypnotist is very important, far and away the most important factor in hypnosis is a patient who is highly responsive to suggestion, as indicated by the patient's prior positive experience with hypnosis and belief that it will be helpful. Some individuals are able to alter their subjective experience in response to suggestion more than others; some patients can be taught self-hypnosis. None of the other characteristics is as important in the success of hypnosis.

28. **(A)** There are numerous indicators of a trance state, such as amnesia, anesthesia, and reduced pulse, reflexes, and respiration. Other changes include changed voice quality, eye closure, lack of body movement, pupillary changes, reduced blinking, and time distortion.

29. **(D)** Family therapy concentrates on the relationships between members and how to make them more adaptive to the situations. In this case, family therapy will help the parents and children understand why there are conflicts between them and work with the family as a unit; the purpose is neither to blame nor change the brother's behavior. Family therapy does not give attention to assigning roles to each member. Unlike psychoanalysis or psychodynamic therapy, family therapy does not focus on any individual's early childhood experiences or trauma, unconscious conflicts, or impulses that lead to the family members' pathology.

30. **(D)** This patient is in the Erikson stage of intimacy versus isolation which occurs in young adults from the approximate age of 20 to 40 years. This is the period when adults are struggling with becoming emotionally close and physically intimate with another versus feelings of loneliness. Trust versus mistrust occurs from birth to 1 year when infants learn whether or not primary caregivers can satisfy basic needs. The autonomy versus shame/doubt stage occurs in toddlers from ages 1 to 3 years when children attempt to master tasks on their own (as well as their own impulses), and, if supported (as opposed to punished), they will grow confident and secure in their ability to survive. Initiative versus guilt occurs from age 3 to 5 years where preschool children gain a sense of well-being from displaying initiative without feeling guilty. The identity versus role confusion stage occurs during adolescence from ages 11 to 19 years when teenagers attempt to determine who they are and what they wish to accomplish in life.

31. **(E)** Behavioral therapy helps patients who suffer from ADHD to derive satisfaction and positive reinforcement from learning, but to negatively reinforce disruptive behaviors. The other choices can also be very helpful, but they are not aims of behavioral therapy.

32. **(A)** A behavioral tool that is used quite effectively is a report card. This tool can function as a bridge between school and home. In addition, a report card can serve as a positive incentive to "good" behavior when the report is

positive and is then rewarded. The rewards can be adjusted for the degree of positive behavior obtained. Neither aversion therapy nor punishment is helpful in teaching patient with ADHD new, more constructive behaviors to help cope with their symptoms. Interpretive strategies such as a well-timed interpretation of maladaptive behaviors or positively reframing a negative experience are not behavioral tools.

33. **(D)** Motivation for change goes beyond a desire for removal of symptoms and includes a willingness to tolerate discomfort and to take risks in a search for understanding. The other demographics do not play as significant a role.

34. **(B)** In brief psychodynamic therapy a single, focal area of conflict is identified, and during the therapy the time is spent actively interpreting transferences as they pertain to this identified focal conflict. Many types of therapy correct cognitive errors and modify maladaptive behaviors, although cognitive therapy and behavioral therapy, respectively, are specifically concerned with these outcomes. Interpretations of dreams and resistance may certainly take place in brief psychodynamic therapy; however, they are only interpreted in so far as they relate to the identified focal conflict.

35. **(D)** Psychoanalysis is usually not indicated in patients who have difficulty with reality testing, such as those with schizophrenia. The inevitable regression, introspection, and self-examination required in psychoanalysis are usually overwhelming to psychotic patients and actually may cause more harm than good, with a worsening of psychosis. All of the other types of psychotherapies can be helpful in the treatment of schizophrenia or other psychotic disorders.

36. **(B)** Dreams provide information about psychic conflicts. In this case, dream interpretation may help the patient learn more about his current unhappiness and conflict in his married life. Dreams are used to uncover psychic conflicts, which, when interpreted appropriately and consciously (not subliminally), can lead to a productive change in behavior. According to

psychoanalytic theory, dreams represent the unconscious workings of the mind, not the conscious ones, and may be symbolic in content. Interpreting dreams may eventually lead to an alteration in a patient's conduct, but reducing cognitive errors or changing behavior is not its primary purpose.

37. **(C)** Patients with borderline personality disorder develop intense transferences in individual treatment. This can impede the work of psychotherapy. Transference is usually diluted in group psychotherapy because of the number of other peers. The group can offer stability and moderation to the extreme ways of viewing others that distort borderline perceptions. The combined modes of treatment, individual and group, offer the patient with borderline personality disorder a higher probability for personality change. Borderline patients are known for their intense personal relationships, self-destructive behaviors, anger management difficulties, and poor sense of self-image. Antisocial patients demonstrate a pervasive pattern of disregard for and violation of the rights of others. They respond poorly to group or individual therapy due to their deceitfulness, impulsivity, aggressiveness, and irresponsibility. The other personality disorders do not necessarily benefit more from combined psychotherapies as do borderline personality disordered patients. Patients with avoidant personality disorder long for relationships yet are extremely shy and fear them. Schizoid personality disorder is marked by significant isolation, emotional coldness, and indifference to praise or criticism. Schizotypal patients display odd beliefs, suspiciousness, eccentric behavior, and magical thinking.

38. **(D)** Patients who are suicidal characteristically have severe hopelessness and think about events in rigid, black-and-white ways. They see very few options and become overwhelmed with their feelings of hopelessness which are exacerbated by seeing "no way out." Personalization is one's tendency to relate events to oneself without any reason for doing so. Begging the question and circular reasoning are both logical fallacies. They

occur when an idea is "proven" to be true when assumed implicitly or explicitly in the premise (eg, only weak people put themselves in my position, therefore I am a weak person). Selective abstraction is term from cognitive therapy where details of a scenario are taken out of context and believed while everything else contrary about the scenario is ignored.

39. **(B)** Cognitive therapy is the psychotherapy that would be most appropriate to help this particular patient solve problems more productively. Behavioral therapy is focused on behaviors, not on the possible underlying factors that cause behaviors. Hypnosis is a sleep-like state induced by a therapist, which has been of some use in uncovering psychodynamic processes and in behavioral modification such as stopping smoking. Interpersonal therapy is aimed at understanding communication patterns and roles in relationships. In paradoxical therapy, developed by Bateson, the therapist suggests that the patient engage in the behavior with negative connotations (eg, a phobia or compulsion).

40. **(B)** Contagion is when expression of emotion elicits emotional response in other members of the group. A corrective experience is when the group recreates a family of origin or the original dynamics of a conflict which helps a patient work through their original conflict. Competition is when members compete for time or attention of the other members (in this case their emotion is from having shared experience and is more empathetic in nature). Differentiation is when group members test norms and compete with each other to establish autonomy. Imitation is when one group member models their behavior after another group member's behavior.

41. **(E)** Systematic desensitization is the process of exposing a patient to feared objects or situations and teaching them to decrease their anxiety and fear in order to overcome them. Systematic desensitization is sometimes called graduated exposure therapy and can be used with many types of anxiety, including social and specific phobias. Aversion therapy is when a stimulus is paired with something negative or discomforting in order to get a patient to avoid or stop a certain maladaptive behavior. Flooding is when a patient is exposed to the most feared situations all at once. Modeling is when observed behaviors are imitated. Suggestion is when an idea or change is consciously suggested to a patient in order to change the behavior.

42. **(E)** Supportive psychotherapy attempts to fortify psychological defenses by providing empathic reassurance as opposed to probing into a patient's psychological conflicts. Behavioral therapies utilize operant conditioning, relaxation training, and exposure techniques (among others) in order to change dysfunctional behavior, mostly for anxiety disorders. Cognitive therapy is often combined with behavioral therapy; it was developed by Aaron Beck and is used for depressive and anxiety disorders. It is based on the belief that the way that patients think and act are due to cognitive schemas which derive from childhood experiences and temperamental factors. Dynamic psychotherapy delves into current and past conflicts in order to bring unconscious material into consciousness. Existential psychotherapy is based on existential philosophy and emphasizes personal feeling and experience over rational thinking.

43. **(B)** Biofeedback is the process whereby a patient receives information on physiologic variables in order to alter those variables and ultimately the corresponding behavior. For example, patients with migraine headaches obtain information on muscle tension or temperature. They will then use this information to decrease the intensity of the headaches by directly trying to relax and alter the known parameters.

44. **(P)** Transference (and transference neurosis) can be understood as a general phenomenon in which the patient displaces onto others (including the therapist) the feelings, thoughts, and conflicts from the patient's past (particularly the earliest years of life).

45. **(D)** Flooding is a technique used in behavior therapy where a patient is exposed to a feared or anxiety-provoking stimuli all at once to

help them overcome the fear or anxiety. It is used most frequently in specific phobias as in this case.

46. **(G)** Positive reinforcement is a behavioral technique where a reward (a sweet) is given after a specific behavior (saying "thank you") in order to increase the frequency of that behavior.

47. **(K)** Punishment is presenting an aversive stimulus (soap in the mouth) after a behavior (biting) in order to decrease that behavior. Anxiety **(A)** is a state of uneasiness or fear, triggered by environmental or intrapsychic processes. Countertransference **(C)** is the compilation of a therapist's feelings toward a patient. Hypnosis **(E)** is a sleep-like state induced by a therapist, which has been of some use in uncovering unconscious processes and in behavioral modification such as stopping smoking. Negative reinforcement **(F)** is an operant conditioning technique where an aversive stimulus is removed in order to increase a desired behavior. Posttraumatic stress disorder **(H)** is an anxiety disorder seen after life-threatening traumas, characterized by reexperiencing symptoms, avoidance, irritability, and hyperarousal. Projection **(I)** is an unconscious defense where unwanted feelings, attitudes, and thoughts are attributed to others. Projective identification **(J)** is similar to projection, but where the other individual is induced to behave in such a way as to confirm the projections. The real relationship **(L)** is considered to be the relationship between a psychoanalyst and patient which is not influenced by transference. A schema **(M)** refers to an organized pattern of thoughts or behaviors relating to oneself, others, and the environment around. Splitting **(N)** is another defense mechanism characterized by viewing feelings, others, and situations in "all good or all bad" terms. Therapeutic alliance **(O)** refers to the healthy relationship between a caregiver and patient. Undoing **(Q)** is a defense mechanism where a patient attempts to "undo" an unwanted thought (eg, an obsession) by engaging in contrary behavior (eg, a compulsion).

48. **(B)** Jean Martin Charcot is known for his contributions to neurology including the description of many medical diseases including Charcot-Marie tooth disease amyotrophic lateral sclerosis (ALS), Charcot joint, Charcot aneurysms, and Charcot triad. He was also known for his descriptive work on hysteria and other neuroses.

49. **(A)** Josef Breuer is known for his use of cathartic treatment or talking therapy in the famous case of Anna O, which was subsequently followed closely by Sigmund Freud.

50. **(E)** Heinz Kohut is most well known for his development of self-psychology. It was a very influential school of thought within psychoanalysis and helped direct modern approaches to therapy, particularly concerning the treatment of narcissism. Erik Erikson **(C)** was a psychoanalyst who posited eight stages of development, from infancy to old age. Sigmund Freud **(D)** was the founder of psychoanalysis, best known for his theories of the unconscious mind. Franz Anton Mesmer **(F)** is considered the father of modern hypnosis; the word mesmerism is derived from his name.

CHAPTER 5

Legal and Ethical Issues in Psychiatry and Medicine
Questions

DIRECTIONS (Questions 1 through 51): For each of the multiple choice questions in this section, select the lettered answer that is the one *best* response in each case.

Questions 1 and 2

The case manager for an 18-year-old man that you are treating notifies you that your patient has been acting strangely lately. You learn from the case manager that the patient makes provocative sexual comments toward her on a daily basis. During your session, the patient expresses concern that his case manager is somehow conspiring against him and he plans to do something about it. On further questioning, he becomes increasingly anxious and abruptly storms out of your office. You hear him in the hallway, exclaiming, "That woman, I'm going to stab her and she won't bother me anymore."

1. Your first course of action should be which of the following?

   (A) Respect the patient's confidentiality and wait until your next scheduled appointment with him to discuss his feelings.

   (B) Contact the patient's family and let them know about his threats toward the case manager.

   (C) Inform the police of the content of your previous sessions and his recent threat toward the case manager.

   (D) Notify the case manager of the potential danger.

   (E) Attempt to contact the patient over the next several hours to discuss the intent of his parting comments.

2. The legal precedent that guides the appropriate course of action in this case is which of the following?

   (A) *Rogers v Commissioner of the Department of Mental Health*

   (B) *Tarasoff v Regents of University of California*

   (C) *Durham v United States*

   (D) *Zinerman v Burch*

   (E) *Kansas v Hendricks*

Questions 3 through 5

Two years ago, you were the anesthesiologist involved in a cesarean delivery of a baby born with cerebral palsy. You had heard from your obstetrical colleague that the family was planning to sue, and today a process server delivers papers notifying you that the family has brought an action against the physicians involved in the surgery, including you.

3. In medical malpractice cases, the plaintiff must establish which of the following?

   (A) burden of proof beyond a reasonable doubt

   (B) clear and convincing evidence of wrongdoing

   (C) harm or damage

   (D) criminal intent

   (E) criminal mischief

4. Which of the following best protects a physician against a malpractice suit?

(A) seeing the patient in clinic on a weekly basis

(B) maintaining a good therapeutic alliance with the patient

(C) hiring a malpractice attorney to examine the physician's treatment practices

(D) having the patient sign a "no harm" contract

(E) refusing to prescribe medications that may have adverse effects

5. When determining medical malpractice, the term "standard of care" refers to the use of medical and psychiatric treatments that are

(A) the most current treatments available

(B) evidence based

(C) used by average, reasonable practitioners in similar circumstances

(D) safe and free from any potential negative side effects

(E) endorsed by the American Medical Association

Questions 6 and 7

An 80-year-old widow with a history significant for schizophrenia was recently diagnosed with end-stage hepatic cancer. She is concerned about the disposition of her estate and does not want her family to receive any of her money; she plans to donate her entire estate to the local humane society.

6. Which of the following is most important in establishing a legally valid will?

(A) mens rea

(B) informed consent

(C) lack of mental illness

(D) testamentary capacity

(E) conservatorship of estate

7. The patient's family hires an attorney to challenge the integrity of her will. Which of the following items, if present, would undermine this patient's competence to make a will?

(A) paranoid delusions regarding the patient's family

(B) the presence of a diagnosable Axis I disorder

(C) the patient's non-delusional explanation of why she wants to donate her estate to the local humane society

(D) inability to read and write

(E) refusal to undergo treatment with chemotherapy

Questions 8 and 9

A 23-year-old man with no prior psychiatric history is charged with murdering his next-door neighbor. His friends note that he became increasingly isolative and suspicious of others in the weeks prior to the crime. The examining psychiatrist found him to be having paranoid delusions regarding his neighbor and noted that his thought processes were too disorganized to complete the examination.

8. Which of the following legal standards is the current basis for establishing an insanity defense?

(A) M'Naghten rule

(B) American Law Institute test (Model Penal Code)

(C) Durham rule

(D) Extreme emotional disturbance

(E) Irresistible impulse rule

9. Criminal responsibility requires demonstration of the criminal act along with which of the following elements?

(A) diminished mental capacity

(B) mens rea

(C) modus operandi

(D) product test

(E) "wild beast" test

Questions 10 and 11

An obese 54-year-old woman presents to the emergency department by ambulance complaining of severe substernal chest pain lasting 40 minutes, profuse sweating, and nausea. Her vital signs are blood pressure 195/96 mm Hg, heart rate 63 beats/min, respiratory rate 18 breaths/min, temperature 98.8°F. An electrocardiogram reveals 3-mm ST-segment elevations in leads V_4, V_5, and V_6. Cardiac enzymes and laboratory workup are pending. You suspect a lateral wall myocardial infarction and recommend immediate thrombolytic therapy. The patient states, "You're crazy if you think I'm gonna let some intern care for me...my family will drive me across town to the private hospital." The patient then jumps from the gurney and begins walking toward the exit.

10. Which of the following is the most appropriate next step?

   (A) Sedate the patient and begin thrombolytic therapy.

   (B) Allow the patient to leave against medical advice.

   (C) Admit the patient to the cardiology service on a physician emergency certificate.

   (D) Detain the patient until the results of the cardiac enzymes are available.

   (E) Detain the patient until you can assess her ability to provide informed consent.

11. On further evaluation, the patient demonstrates a thorough understanding of the information you have given to her and appreciates the consequences of not being treated immediately. The appropriate next step is which of the following?

   (A) Sedate the patient and begin thrombolytic therapy.

   (B) Allow the patient to leave against medical advice.

   (C) Admit the patient to the cardiology service on a physician emergency certificate.

   (D) Detain the patient until the results of the cardiac enzymes are available.

   (E) Detain the patient so that her family may make decisions on her behalf.

12. A 19-year-old man with a history significant for bipolar I disorder is charged with assaulting a police officer. This is the man's fifth arrest in the past 4 months for aggression toward an authority figure. The assigned attorney has informed the forensic psychiatrist involved in the case that the patient has been noncooperative and belligerent while attempting to prepare for his defense. The attorney also questions whether the patient has an understanding of the severity of his crime given his acute mental state and lack of formal education. Which of the following items would be consistent with the assertion that the patient is incompetent to stand trial?

   (A) failure to comprehend the criminal charges

   (B) inability to read and write

   (C) presence of a diagnosable mental illness

   (D) inability to provide informed consent

   (E) history of prior assault charges

13. A 35-year-old man is brought to the emergency room by his family for threatening to shoot his mother in the chest. Urine toxicology is negative for cocaine, phencyclidine (PCP), or opioids, and his blood alcohol level is 0.04. You learn from the patient's family that he has been threatening to assault his mother for several days and has even written notes about executing his plan. On mental status examination (MSE), the patient's speech is loud, pressured, and very threatening toward the emergency department staff. Family history is significant for bipolar disorder. The patient states that he has not done anything wrong and wants to be released immediately. Which of the following next steps would be the most appropriate?

   (A) Notify the police about the patient's homicidal threats.

   (B) Warn the patient's mother about the threats.

   (C) Arrange for a police hold given the patient's potential for violence.

   (D) Involuntarily admit the patient to a locked psychiatric ward.

   (E) Medicate the patient with a mood stabilizer and arrange for outpatient follow-up.

Questions 14 and 15

You are the psychiatrist on duty when a man, arrested by police for stabbing his lover, is brought into the emergency room for evaluation. The man's behavior is wild and unpredictable. At one point he starts to pick up a chair and look menacingly at a nurse before being subdued by police officers. Detectives tell you that the man's only chance of staying out of a jail cell that night is to be admitted to the locked unit, but the man makes it clear that he does not want to stay in the hospital.

14. Which of the following should justify the physician's decision to involuntarily admit the patient?

    (A) medication noncompliance
    (B) imminent threat to others
    (C) history of prior psychiatric hospitalization
    (D) presence of a diagnosable mental disorder
    (E) refusal to follow-up with psychiatric outpatient services

After being admitted to the psychiatric unit, the patient becomes increasingly aggressive toward staff. He adamantly refuses all medications offered to help calm his agitated behaviors. The patient at one point accuses a male staff member of having an affair with his lover and attempts to punch him. You place a stat order for a haldol 5 mg intramuscular (IM) injection to sedate the patient and prevent further escalation of his combative behaviors.

15. Administering the haldol without his consent directly challenges which of the following ethical principles?

    (A) autonomy
    (B) beneficence
    (C) confidentiality
    (D) justice
    (E) nonmaleficence

16. A 36-year-old woman with delusional disorder is brought to the emergency room by police after she was found trespassing on the governor's private estate. She claims she has been having an affair with the governor and demanded that he acknowledge that he is the father of her 5-year-old son. This is the third time the patient has been caught stalking the governor. The patient is subsequently admitted to the inpatient unit and discharged several days later to her parents with whom she lives. The governor ultimately decides to pursue charges against the woman. A forensic psychiatrist is asked by the woman's attorney to evaluate the woman and render an opinion about her mental status at the time of the crime. Which of the following statements regarding her incarceration is most accurate if found not guilty by reason of insanity?

    (A) She will serve her original criminal sentence once she is deemed sane.
    (B) She will not serve any time and will be released with close psychiatric follow-up.
    (C) She will serve less time than if found guilty.
    (D) She will serve more time in a locked psychiatric unit than she would in prison if she were found guilty.
    (E) She will serve half her criminal sentence incarcerated and the other half in a locked psychiatric facility.

Questions 17 and 18

A 9-year-old girl is brought to the pediatric emergency department by her parents for evaluation of a persistent cough. She is withdrawn and complains of a "scratchy throat." Vital signs are stable and the patient is afebrile. On examination, the lungs are clear to auscultation bilaterally and the posterior oropharynx is clear. There are multiple bruises on her buttocks and back. A chest x-ray demonstrates several rib fractures in different stages of healing. Her parents report that their daughter is quite active with her younger siblings and often gets into fights with them. The patient agrees with her parents.

17. Which of the following is the most likely diagnosis?
    (A) age-appropriate "rough play"
    (B) major depressive disorder (MDD)
    (C) physical abuse
    (D) sexual abuse
    (E) somatization disorder

18. Which of the following is the most appropriate next step?

(A) Discharge the patient with follow-up in 1 week to reevaluate her bruises.

(B) Refer for family therapy to address the issue of rough play.

(C) Treat the patient with intramuscularly (IM) penicillin.

(D) Notify Child Protective Services.

(E) Confront the siblings about their behavior.

Questions 19 and 20

A 17-year-old girl presents to your office complaining of a burning vaginal discharge. She informs you that she has been involved in a consensual sexual relationship with her boyfriend and is worried that she has contracted a sexually transmitted disease (STD). You start the patient on antibiotics. Three days later, you discover that the culture of her vaginal discharge grew *Neisseria gonorrhoea*.

19. A few days later, you receive a call from the patient's parents demanding to know why their daughter was seen in your office. Which of the following is the most appropriate next step?

(A) Explain to the parents that their daughter has contracted an STD and requires immediate antibiotic treatment.

(B) Maintain confidentiality by disclosing no information, but encourage the patient to discuss this issue with her parents.

(C) Ask the parents about their daughter's sexual history.

(D) Alert the parents that their daughter is at risk for human immunodeficiency virus (HIV) and should be tested.

(E) Find out the boyfriend's name and telephone number to confirm the history.

20. At the patient's next follow-up visit, she requests to be tested for HIV. She reports that her boyfriend recently tested negative, but given her promiscuity, she wonders if she has contracted HIV. Which of the following should be done prior to administering the HIV test?

(A) Notify her parents about the patient's request for an HIV test.

(B) Directly inform the patient's boyfriend that he is at risk for HIV.

(C) Inform the department of public health of your intent to administer an HIV test.

(D) Explain to the patient how the test is performed and interpreted, along with information on confidentiality and how you will proceed if the result is positive.

(E) Perform a pregnancy test.

21. A 44-year-old man with insulin-dependent diabetes mellitus and end-stage renal failure has been on dialysis several years while awaiting a kidney transplant. He feels as though he has "waited long enough" and does not want to continue "living tied to a machine." After several family meetings and consultations with other physicians, he informs you that he no longer wishes to be dialyzed. You obtain a psychiatric consult that concludes no evidence of mood or thought disorder. The family is upset with the patient's decision and demands that you continue to administer dialysis until a transplant is available. Which of the following is the most appropriate next step?

(A) Respect the patient's wishes and discontinue dialysis.

(B) Coerce the patient into continuing treatment.

(C) Continue dialysis until you convince the ethics committee to support the family's decision.

(D) Tell the patient you're sure a transplant will arrive soon and encourage him to remain in treatment.

(E) Place the patient on a physician's emergency certificate because he is a danger to himself.

22. A 40-year-old surgical attending is admitted to the medical unit after developing severe right flank pain. Further workup confirms a diagnosis of nephrolithiasis. One of the surgical residents asks you about the attending's diagnosis so that coverage can be arranged. Which of the following is the most appropriate next step?

   (A) Reveal only the estimated length of stay.
   (B) Inform the chief surgical resident of the attending's condition and length of stay.
   (C) Tell the surgical resident that you will not say anything, but she could take a look in the attending's chart.
   (D) Tell the resident to address the questions directly to the attending.
   (E) Arrange a conference between your medical attending and the surgical house staff.

23. A 43-year-old man is referred for continued treatment of depression after release from jail. The court mandated psychiatric treatment while he is on probation. The patient's probation officer calls you for information regarding his condition, progress, and treatment compliance. You should do which of the following?

   (A) Discuss the case with the probation officer because the treatment is court mandated.
   (B) Limit your discussion with the probation officer to only treatment compliance because the rest of the information is confidential.
   (C) Obtain a confidentiality waiver from the patient before speaking to the probation officer.
   (D) Ignore the request altogether because psychiatric treatment bears no relation to law enforcement.
   (E) Correspond with the probation officer only through written documents.

24. A 23-year-old woman with a known history of heroin use is admitted for intravenous (IV) antibiotic treatment for infective endocarditis. The nurse informs you that the patient was accidentally given the wrong antibiotic but has suffered no adverse reaction. Which of the following is the most appropriate next step?

   (A) Enforce the "no harm, no disclosure" rule.
   (B) Inform the patient that she was given the wrong medication.
   (C) First report the mistake to the hospital advisory committee.
   (D) Notify the patient's family of the mistake.
   (E) Encourage the patient to seek legal action because a critical mistake has occurred.

25. A 38-year-old woman is admitted to the oncology unit with severe aplastic anemia. She appears pale and weak. Vital signs indicate a blood pressure of 110/75 mm Hg and a pulse of 110/min. Hematocrit is 18%. On MSE, cognition is intact and there is no evidence of a mood or psychotic disturbance. The patient states that she is a Jehovah's Witness. She refuses any blood transfusion on the basis of her religious beliefs. Which of the following best applies to your next step in the treatment of this patient?

   (A) administering packed red blood cells
   (B) persuading the patient that she must accept the transfusion
   (C) explaining the implications of no treatment but respecting the patient's refusal for treatment
   (D) utilizing a "confrontation method" to secure lifesaving treatment
   (E) referring the patient for involuntary psychiatric treatment based on her life-threatening decision

26. The parents of a newborn with Down syndrome find their daughter to be lethargic and minimally responsive. Medical evaluation is significant for the following cerebrospinal fluid findings: opening pressure of 100 mm Hg, white blood cell count of 5000/μL (predominantly neutrophils), protein more than 40 mg/dL, glucose content more than 40 mg/dL, and Gram stain positive for bacteria. You suspect group B streptococcal meningitis and recommend IV antibiotic therapy. The parents feel as though their child will ultimately have a poor quality of life and request that treatment be withheld. Which of the following is the most appropriate next step?

(A) Respect the parents' wishes because they are the primary decision makers.

(B) Refer the case to the ethics committee for review at their next scheduled meeting.

(C) Inform the parents that after reviewing the laboratory data you realize the patient has viral meningitis and care will be mostly supportive.

(D) Start intravenous ampicillin against the parents' wishes.

(E) Repeat the lumbar puncture to verify the diagnosis.

27. You are a psychiatrist who hosts a morning radio show dedicated to educating the general public about mental illness. During a question and answer segment, a caller phones in to ask about your opinion regarding a prominent politician whose recent erratic behaviors have gained significant media attention. The caller asks you directly whether you believe the politician has a bipolar illness. Which of the following best applies?

(A) Stating your opinion publicly is legitimate as long as the politician is not your private patient.

(B) Offering a psychiatric diagnosis in such instances is unethical.

(C) Comment in written form only.

(D) Provide an "off-the-record" or anonymous opinion.

(E) State your diagnosis but indicate that other problems may account for the symptoms.

28. An 84-year-old widowed man with severe dementia, for whom you have been the primary care physician for years, is diagnosed with hepatocellular carcinoma. The patient does not have an advance directive and never designated a power of attorney. Psychiatric consultation concludes that the patient is unable to make an informed decision regarding treatment options, and you turn to his family for guidance. The patient's oldest son is adamant that his father receive chemotherapy, while the two younger daughters feel that he should not suffer the adverse effects of chemotherapy "especially because he's so

demented." Which of the following is the next appropriate step?

(A) Ask the patient which family member he would like to designate power of attorney.

(B) Let the patient decide whether or not to proceed with treatment.

(C) Abide by the son's wishes because he is the oldest.

(D) Abide by the daughters' wishes because the patient's quality of life is already poor.

(E) Consult the hospital's ethics committee.

29. A 27-year-old woman who is 3 months postpartum is brought to the emergency room by her husband and mother with concerns that the patient "is not acting like herself." The husband informs the consulting psychiatrist that for the past few weeks the patient has been increasingly irritable, withdrawn, and crying almost daily. He doesn't understand why the patient is behaving like this given that the pregnancy was planned and the patient was looking forward to having a family. The patient tearfully admits that this is her first child and that she is overwhelmed with the responsibilities of being a new mother. On further questioning, she hesitantly confesses to intrusive thoughts of suffocating her child and sometimes worries about being alone with the baby. She denies suicidal ideation. The patient is willing to seek outpatient treatment but adamantly refuses voluntary admission. Her mother states that the patient is "just exhausted" and that "everything will be fine after she gets some rest." Which of the following is the most appropriate next step?

(A) Admit the patient involuntarily.

(B) Call Child Protective Services because the infant is at risk of harm.

(C) Give the patient a 2-week supply of fluoxetine to treat her depression and then arrange outpatient follow-up.

(D) Administer a stat dose of lorazepam 2 mg IM and reevaluate when the patient is calmer.

(E) Discharge the patient and inform the husband and mother to bring the patient back to the hospital if her symptoms do not improve in the next few weeks.

30. A physician is at a community fair with her spouse when a patient approaches the psychiatrist to say hello. The spouse does not recognize the patient. The patient does not introduce himself to the spouse, nor does the physician acquaint the two. After a brief conversation, the patient politely excuses himself and leaves. On the way home, the spouse asks, "Who was that man you were talking to earlier?" The physician should do which of the following?

(A) Answer the spouse's question truthfully.

(B) Lie to the spouse to protect the identity of the patient.

(C) Inform the spouse that revealing such information would compromise confidentiality.

(D) Ask the spouse to guess the identity of the person.

(E) Inform the spouse that he must first promise not to reveal the identity of the patient before answering the question.

Questions 31 and 32

You have been treating a female patient who has been seeing you for psychodynamic psychotherapy for approximately 6 months. Near the end of the suggested course of treatment, the patient reports that she feels markedly better about her progress and attributes her improvement to your expertise. Prior to the last session, she confesses that she has always found you attractive and that she would like begin an intimate relationship with you. You feel flattered by the patient's sexual interest and are surprised by your own interest in the patient.

31. Which of the following is the most appropriate course of action?

(A) Decline participation in the relationship because sex with a former psychiatric patient is unethical.

(B) Engage in sexual relations because there is no established professional code of ethics regarding sex with psychiatric patients.

(C) Engage in sexual relations because sex with a current or former psychiatric patient is ethical.

(D) Engage in sexual relations because sex with a former psychiatric patient is permissible only if you do not exploit your past position of authority.

(E) Inform the patient that the professional code of ethics requires that you wait 1 year after termination before you can ethically engage in sexual relations.

32. Which of the following would be the most appropriate course of action if the above patient were your medical or surgical patient?

(A) Decline participation in the relationship because sex with a current patient is unethical.

(B) Engage in sexual relations because there is no established professional code of ethics regarding sex with nonpsychiatric patients.

(C) Engage in sexual relations because sex with a current nonpsychiatric patient is ethical.

(D) Engage in sexual relations because sex with a current nonpsychiatric patient is permissible only if you do not exploit your past position of authority.

(E) Inform the patient that the professional code of ethics requires that you wait 1 year after termination before you can ethically engage in sexual relations.

33. A 52-year-old man, for whom you have been the primary care physician for the last 20 years, was recently diagnosed with amyotrophic lateral sclerosis. The disease has rapidly progressed and he has experienced multiple respiratory complications that likely will require a tracheotomy. Severe muscle weakness and atrophy are apparent in all limbs. The patient states that there is no meaning in continuing without his physical capacities. He asks for your help in ending his life in a humane and dignified manner. MSE is at baseline and there is no evidence of any psychiatric disorder. You discuss the patient's request with his family and they unanimously support his desire to "end the suffering." The most appropriate course of action would be which of the following?

(A) Respect the patient's wishes by helping him end his life in a painless and respectful manner.

(B) Refuse to participate in assisting the patient with suicide and focus on responding to the patient's end-of-life issues.

(C) Provide the patient with plenty of medication refills to provide a lethal dose.

(D) Provide the patient with information regarding how to effectively end his life.

(E) Ignore the patient's request.

34. You are an inpatient psychiatrist treating a patient with bipolar I disorder. The patient has a long history of medication noncompliance resulting in severe, persecutory delusions during his manic episodes. After 1 week of treatment, you receive a phone call from hospital administration informing that the patient's insurance will not cover the cost of additional inpatient stay. You are encouraged to discharge the patient so that the hospital will not have to incur these costs. You feel, however, that the patient requires more time on the inpatient unit because of safety concerns. You should take which of the following actions?

(A) Contact the insurance company without the patient's permission and request coverage for additional days.

(B) Keep the patient on the unit as long as it is medically necessary.

(C) Establish follow-up at the patient's outpatient community mental health facility prior to discharge

(D) Ensure that the patient is established with a caseworker to supervise the patient in the community before discharge.

(E) Speak with the inpatient social worker to determine whether the patient is eligible for a loan.

Questions 35 and 36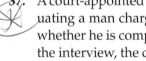

You receive a subpoena from an attorney representing a party that has filed a lawsuit against one of your patients. The subpoena pertains to releasing the medical records of your patient.

35. Which of the following is the appropriate next step?

(A) Contact the attorney who obtained the subpoena to discuss the process of releasing the medical information.

(B) Release the medical records upon receiving the subpoena.

(C) Sign a release of information form and turn over the records.

(D) Do not release the information and contact your patient regarding the subpoena.

(E) Release the medical records directly to the presiding judge.

36. A court hearing has been organized by your patient's attorney to quash the subpoena you have been issued. At the hearing, the judge rules that you should release the medical record even though your patient has not consented to the release of information. Which of the following would be the most appropriate next step?

(A) Appeal to the state's Supreme Court to block the release of the medical record.

(B) Refuse to disclose the patient's medical record regardless of the court orders.

(C) Release only information that will not incriminate your patient.

(D) Release the complete medical record to the judge.

(E) Work out a plan of legal action with your patient.

37. A court-appointed forensic psychiatrist is evaluating a man charged with theft to determine whether he is competent to stand trial. During the interview, the defendant confesses to murdering a woman 3 years ago and hiding her body in an undisclosed area. The psychiatrist should do which of the following?

(A) Immediately notify authorities of the defendant's confession.

(B) Encourage the defendant to speak with his attorney about the murder.

(C) Include this detail in the final report.

(D) Withdraw from the case.

(E) Avoid details of the defendant's prior criminal history in the report.

38. A 28-year-old woman with dysthymic disorder has been seeing you in weekly psychotherapy and has failed to pay her bill for 2 months. Which of the following is the most appropriate next step?

    (A) Contract with a billing collector to demand immediate payment.
    (B) Terminate the treatment.
    (C) Contact the patient's family to determine if the patient is financially stable.
    (D) Inquire as to the reasons she has been avoiding payment at the patient's next visit.
    (E) Inform the patient that you will not see her if she doesn't pay for her treatment.

39. A wealthy 46-year-old male banker is in psychotherapy with you for treatment of a single episode of depression. After significant improvement in his symptoms, he offers you the opportunity to take part in one of his financial ventures. The investment appears to be sound. Which of the following is most appropriate comment to make to the banker?

    (A) "Thanks for thinking about me...I'd be honored to invest with you."
    (B) "Because your depression is improved, it would be appropriate for us to be business partners."
    (C) "I can invest with you only when our treatment is nearing its end."
    (D) "It is probably a bad idea; I'm already committed in other investments."
    (E) "I have to decline; it potentially may interfere with our treatment relationship."

Questions 40 and 41

A 23-year-old Caucasian Catholic woman with a history of schizophrenia and multiple medical illnesses presents to your office after arguing with her husband. She is unemployed and has been staying at home taking care of their children. She notes feeling sad recently and reports thoughts of killing herself. She has a past history of an overdose attempt with aspirin.

40. Which of the following is her strongest risk factor for suicide?

    (A) age
    (B) gender
    (C) marital status
    (D) past history of suicide attempt
    (E) terminal medical illness

41. Which one of the following, if documented, may legally protect a physician in the event of a patient suicide?

    (A) a written "no self-harm" contract signed by the patient
    (B) the patient's refusal to consider pharmacological treatments
    (C) the patient's verbal promise to seek medical attention if feeling suicidal
    (D) an assessment of suicide risk and protective factors
    (E) the patient's missed appointments

42. A 36-year-old man with a history of bipolar I disorder is brought to the emergency department by police after stabbing a patron in a bar room brawl. His blood alcohol level was 0.320 upon arrival, and the patient required intramuscular (IM) haldol for agitation. The patient has no recollection of the event, and the victim died 2 hours later. The patient has a history of assault while psychotic and is currently in weekly psychotherapy. His lawyer has chosen to assert an insanity plea in defense of the patient. Which of the following factors is most likely to undermine his assertion of the insanity defense?

    (A) inability to recall the event
    (B) mental disease or defect
    (C) prior history of assault
    (D) voluntary intoxication
    (E) violent nature of the crime

43. You are a forensic psychiatrist hired as an expert witness by the defense attorney of a mentally ill patient charged with criminal misconduct. The attorney is seeking your help in convincing the jury that the patient was mentally ill at the

time of the crime. Which of the following is your primary responsibility as an expert witness?

(A) countering evidence of criminal responsibility

(B) establishing reasonable doubt

(C) evaluation, diagnosis, and initiation of treatment of the accused

(D) obtaining a not guilty by reason of insanity verdict

(E) rendering an opinion based on reasonable medical certainty

Questions 44 and 45

A 48-year-old man is involuntarily admitted to the hospital after an acute manic episode. The patient is pressured, demanding, and increasingly talkative on the unit. He becomes intrusive, not able to be redirected, and demands immediate release. You explain to him that you feel he is gravely disabled and unable to care for himself. He respectfully disagrees with you and demands "due process."

44. On which of the following legal principles is the patient's request for a hearing based?

(A) actus reus

(B) habeas corpus

(C) mens rea

(D) parens patriae

(E) rights under the Fourth Amendment

45. The court agrees that the patient is severely disabled and in need of acute medical management. You load the patient with divalproex sodium 20 mg/kg, and 3 days later his symptoms of mania are markedly diminished. The patient requests immediate discharge and agrees to follow up with a partial hospital program. You feel that he would benefit from further inpatient treatment but is no longer gravely disabled or a threat for self-harm. Which of the following is the next appropriate step?

(A) File for another court hearing to detain the patient further.

(B) Ignore the patient's request because he has been committed by the court.

(C) Release the patient to the partial hospital program.

(D) Persuade the patient to stay for a few more days.

(E) Appease the patient by increasing smoking privileges.

Questions 46 and 47

You are consulted by the medical team to evaluate a woman on the medical unit who suffers from dementia. The internist believes that she requires a central line for fluids and medication, but is unsure if she can fully comprehend the risks and benefits of the procedure. The team is requesting help in determining her capacity to give informed consent.

46. Which of the following components is most important in obtaining informed consent in this case?

(A) absence of mental illness

(B) capacity to read and write

(C) involving family members in this discussion

(D) petitioning a court to establish the patient's competence

(E) raising alternative treatment options

47. The family is subsequently contacted about her condition, and they request a meeting with the treatment team. During the meeting, the patient's eldest son notifies you that the patient did create a living will approximately 1 year ago, but they are unsure whether it would be useful. Which of the following would you tell them best describes the purpose of a living will?

(A) absolves personal responsibility

(B) arranges for funeral services and distributing her estate

(C) establishes personal preferences regarding end-of-life issues

(D) prevents her from changing her mind about life support if she becomes terminally ill

(E) requests physician-assisted suicide if she becomes terminally ill

48. A 28-year-old man involved in a motor vehicle accident brings a lawsuit against the driver. Emergency department records do not show any physical injuries, but the patient is claiming to suffer from posttraumatic stress disorder (PTSD). You are asked to evaluate the patient's symptoms. He complains of distressing dreams of the accident, having flashbacks while awake, and avoiding the intersection where the accident occurred. His symptoms have lasted for 3 months. Past psychiatric history is significant for major depression, impulsivity, and violent behavior. He has been incarcerated numerous times, showing a blatant disregard for the law. On MSE, the patient is likable and cooperative. His mood is reported as being depressed and he currently denies any hallucinations or delusions. Which of the following items from your evaluation of the patient raises your suspicion regarding a diagnosis of malingering?

(A) duration of symptoms
(B) flashbacks while awake
(C) history of major depression
(D) lack of physical injuries
(E) prior incarcerations

49. One of your patients consistently misses appointments without giving you advance notice. After numerous failed attempts at resolving this issue with the patient, you realize that the patient's behavior is not changing and you decide to discharge the patient from your care. Which of the following most appropriately describes what you should do?

(A) Write a letter to the patient notifying her that she has been discharged due to her failure to comply with treatment.
(B) Notify your staff that the patient is not to be given further appointments.
(C) Contact the patient's family/friends to request their help in improving the patient's attendance.
(D) Write a letter to the patient stating that she will be discharged in 60 days.
(E) Notify the patient's insurance company that she is discharged from your care.

50. You are asked by the court to provide a forensic evaluation for a child custody case. The child had been living with his biological mother and stepfather since birth. Recently, the child's stepfather passed away from lung cancer leaving the unemployed mother alone to raise the child. The child's biological father, who is a renowned orthopedic surgeon in the community, is requesting full custody because he asserts that he is better able to financially support the child. The child's mother refuses to relinquish custody out of concern of how leaving her household will emotionally impact the child. She also implies that he is, in fact, not the biological father. Which of the following factors would be the most important in determining which parent should get custody?

(A) Who is the biological parent?
(B) Who can provide for the best interests of the child?
(C) Who is most financially stable?
(D) Who has the highest level of education?
(E) Who is in the best mental and physical health?

51. You are an internal medicine resident who has been assigned to rotate through the inpatient medical service for the next 2 months. Shortly after you begin, you notice that one of your colleagues consistently comes to work late and smells of alcohol. Some time later, you notice that your colleague has been making increasingly careless mistakes and missing important meetings and discussions. Occasionally, you observe that his hands shake when he is documenting his notes or holding his charts. You are concerned that he may have an alcohol dependency problem. Which of the following is the most appropriate course of action?

(A) Notify the local police.
(B) Contact the Drug Enforcement Administration to rescind his license.
(C) Do nothing so as to avoid personal liability.
(D) Admonish him for using but do not report.
(E) Notify the hospital's committee for impaired physicians.

Answers and Explanations

1. **(D)** A physician or therapist has a duty to protect identifiable victims from imminent danger. This obligation may be fulfilled by directly contacting the party at risk, notifying the police, or taking other appropriate measures to protect the victim. Contacting the patient's family fails to protect the intended victim. Although notification of the police is an acceptable intervention in this case, disclosing unrelated confidential information about the patient is inappropriate. When notifying third parties, care should be taken to release only information necessary to protect the potential victim. The remaining choices fail to protect the potential victim.

2. **(B)** *Tarasoff v Regents of University of California* is the landmark legal precedent establishing liability to third parties. It states "when a psychotherapist determines...that his patient presents a serious danger of violence to another he incurs an obligation to use reasonable care to protect the intended victim against such danger." Therefore, the physician may ethically break confidentiality in cases involving imminent harm to others. In the *Tarasoff* case, a student at the University of California (Prosenjit Poddar) expressed intentions to kill a fellow student (Tatiana Tarasoff) to his therapist. Poddar tragically followed through on his threat and murdered the young woman at her home. *Tarasoff v Regents of University of California* holds legal precedent only in the state of California; however, the case has been adopted by physicians/therapists as the standard of care and has led to nationwide legislative changes. There have been two rulings regarding the *Tarasoff* case. The original decision, *Tarasoff I* (1974), established a "duty to warn." The California Supreme Court revised its previous holding in *Tarasoff II* (1976) with a "duty to protect." In *Rogers v Commissioner of the Department of Mental Health,* the court expounded opinions regarding the treatment of involuntarily committed patients. *Durham v United States* held that an individual "is not criminally responsible if the unlawful act was the product of mental disease or mental defect." The holding of this case has become known as the "product test" for determining an insanity defense and ultimately was replaced by the American Law Institute standard. *Zinerman v Burch* and *Kansas v Hendricks* involve court decisions regarding civil commitment.

3. **(C)** The four Ds of establishing medical malpractice cases involve proving that a *d*ereliction of *d*uty *d*irectly causes *d*amage. The plaintiff must establish the presence of a fiduciary relationship (a duty), negligence (dereliction of duty), and damages directly caused by that negligence. Typically, the burden of proof in medical malpractice cases (civil cases) is by a preponderance of the evidence (greater than 50%). Proof beyond a reasonable doubt refers to criminal cases; clear and convincing evidence is reserved for special cases decided by the court. Neither criminal intent nor criminal mischief is required to prove medical malpractice.

4. **(B)** As a broad generalization, a good patient–doctor relationship is key for a physician to potentially avoid or deflect a lawsuit. It is the physician's duty as a health care provider to facilitate open communication regarding the patient's illness, treatment recommendations, risks versus benefits of such treatments, and

to acknowledge any errors that the physician may have made. Seeing the patient on a more frequent interval, hiring a malpractice attorney to monitor treatment practices, or avoiding prescribing medications with potentially adverse side effects do not decrease a physician's risk for malpractice suits. Requiring that a patient sign a "no harm" contract is not reasonable nor does it stand up as a legal document in a court of law.

5. **(C)** The standard of care for determining medical malpractice is based on how a similarly qualified practitioner would have performed under the same or similar situation. Usually the testimony of an expert witness (a physician qualified by evidence of his/her expertise, training, and special knowledge to provide an opinion about the case) is necessary to demonstrate the standard of care in medical malpractice suits. Treatments that are the most current, evidence based, free from adverse effects, or endorsed by the American Medical Association are not sufficient to establish the standard of care.

6. **(D)** Testamentary capacity refers to the level of competence required to make a legally valid will. Case law and statutes differ across states. However, the central elements of testamentary capacity include: (1) comprehension of the act of writing/signing a will, (2) knowledge of potential heirs, (3) understanding the extent of one's assets, (4) lack of undue influence, and (5) the absence of delusions compromising rational thought. Mens rea refers to criminal intent and has nothing to do with drafting a will. Informed consent is the process of obtaining permission for medical treatment. Important elements include the ability to make a voluntary decision regarding treatment, explanation of risks and benefits, and competency to make an informed decision. The presence or absence of a mental illness does not necessarily impair an individual's competency to make a will. Conservatorship of estate refers to an individual's ability to manage his or her finances.

7. **(A)** Paranoid delusions regarding the patient's family may significantly undermine this patient's assertion that she was competent to make a will. The absence of delusions, which

may compromise rational decision making, is one of several criteria required for testamentary capacity. The presence of a diagnosable Axis I disorder, the inability to read and write, and refusal to undergo treatment with chemotherapy do not automatically undermine a patient's competence to make a will as long as the criteria for testamentary capacity are met. An explanation of why the patient wants to donate her estate to the local humane society does not undermine the patient's competence to make a will unless such an explanation demonstrates that the patient is unable to meet any of the specified criteria.

8. **(B)** The American Law Institute test is the modern standard for the insanity defense. It holds that a person with a mental disease or defect should not be held criminally responsible for an act if the person (1) could not appreciate the wrongfulness of the conduct and (2) could not conform the conduct to the requirements of the law. The American Law Institute test expanded upon the 1843 M'Naghten rule, which held that an individual was not guilty by reason of insanity if, as a result of a mental defect, the person did not know the nature of what he or she was doing or did not know that what he or she was doing was wrong ("right-wrong test"). The Durham rule arose from a 1954 District of Columbia case in which the court held that "an accused is not criminally responsible if his unlawful act was the product of a mental disease or mental defect." This is also known as the "product test." Extreme emotional disturbance and the irresistible impulse rule are not modern standards for proving an insanity defense. Extreme emotional disturbance is an affirmative defense used to render the accused less culpable for the crime (ie, reduce the charge from murder to manslaughter). The irresistible impulse rule, established in England in 1922, states that an individual is not responsible for a criminal act if he was unable to resist that act due to a mental illness.

9. **(B)** Criminal responsibility requires (1) criminal intent (mens rea) and (2) a criminal act (actus reus). Diminished mental capacity can serve to avoid criminal responsibility, but it is not

required to prove criminal responsibility. Modus operandi is the pattern in which an action or crime is executed by a person. The product test and the wild beast test are antiquated standards of the insanity defense.

10. **(E)** Before discharging or transferring the patient, it is important to determine whether she can make an informed decision regarding her care. Informed consent requires that the patient (1) comprehend the issues and/or choices furnished by the physician, (2) appreciate the consequences of making a certain decision, and (3) arrive at a voluntary decision after weighing the facts. At this point in the vignette, there is not enough information to establish the patient's ability to make an informed decision regarding her care. Exceptions to informed consent include incompetence, emergency situations (eg, comatose, unresponsive patient), a competent patient's waiver of informed consent, and therapeutic privilege. The other choices are incorrect because this patient's ability to make an informed decision has not been assessed.

11. **(B)** A competent patient has the right to refuse treatment, even if the consequences are life threatening. In the extension of this vignette, the patient has adequately demonstrated the elements of an informed decision. The other choices are incorrect because they would prevent a competent patient from making an informed decision in her treatment.

12. **(A)** In *Dusky v United States* (1960), the Supreme Court ruled that competency to stand trial requires the ability to (1) rationally consult with one's attorney and (2) understand the proceedings in both factual and rational terms. A history of prior assault charges or illiteracy does not constitute grounds for incompetency. A person can suffer from a mental illness and be competent to stand trial. Informed consent is important in making decisions related to medical treatments but has little bearing on one's competency to stand trial.

13. **(D)** Involuntary commitment is used when a physician believes that an individual is an imminent threat to themselves, or others, or is otherwise gravely disabled. Medicating the patient and arranging for outpatient treatment when the patient is actively homicidal is an improper course of action. Notification of the police or warning the patient's mother is not immediately necessary because this patient is well-contained in a locked unit. Arranging a police hold is incorrect as police holds are issued when an individual who is arrested requires a psychiatric evaluation. If the arrested individual does not require inpatient psychiatric care, he is released back into the custody of the police.

14. **(B)** Involuntary admission to the hospital is justified when the patient is judged to be (1) an imminent danger to self or others or (2) gravely disabled or unable to care for self. The criteria for involuntary commitment derive from the doctrines of police power (the state acts as protector of public safety) and parens patriae (the state acts as parent for those unable to care for themselves), respectively. State laws differ on the length of time a person can be committed to the hospital on the basis of either criterion. Permission from the conservator of person is not required for involuntary commitment. The other choices may be important factors, but are not requisite elements for involuntary hospitalization.

15. **(A)** Forcing treatment on a patient directly challenges his autonomy. In general, an adult with decisional capacity has every right to determine what may be done to his body. However, a physician may medicate a patient against his will and without a court hearing if it is done to prevent a patient from causing imminent harm to himself or others. In the vignette, the patient is grossly impaired and poses an immediate threat to others. Beneficence refers to a physician's duty to do good for the patient. Justice refers to the concept that persons who are equals should qualify for equal treatment. Confidentiality, or physician–patient privilege, is a legal concept that protects communications between a patient and his or her doctor from being disclosed to a third party. Nonmaleficence refers to a physician's intention to not harm or bring harm to the patient and others.

16. **(D)** Not guilty by reason of insanity is a verdict rendered in a criminal case which finds that the defendant was insane at the time of committing the crime. This is determined by the application of the test for insanity used in the particular jurisdiction. Contrary to popular belief, the insanity defense (1) is seldom asserted, (2) is usually unsuccessful, and (3) typically leads to a greater number of years that the defendant spends in a mental hospital. Individuals found not guilty by reason of insanity are committed to a mental facility rather than serving time incarcerated. Typically, the commitment is not for a set amount of time but rather until the individual is deemed not to be a threat to society. Releasing an individual found not guilty by reason of insanity without appropriate psychiatric treatment is unethical and fails to protect society.

17. **(C)** Typical signs of physical abuse include burns with peculiar patterns (eg, cigarette marks, geometric designs, bilateral immersion patterns), bruises in low-trauma areas (eg, buttocks, genital areas, or back), retinal hemorrhages, and multiple fractures at different stages of healing. Although there is a high rate of comorbidity between physical and sexual abuse, there is no evidence to suggest sexual abuse in this particular case. Sexual or physical abuse may predispose an individual to the development of other psychiatric disorders such as depression, PTSD, and borderline personality disorder. Although the differential in this case should include depression and somatization disorder, history and mental status do not provide sufficient evidence to diagnose either. Age-appropriate "rough play" is also not likely.

18. **(D)** Every state requires mandatory reporting of abuse or neglect to Child Protective Services. In cases in which there is a reasonable suspicion of abuse, a report should be filed even if the patient and family deny the allegations. In cases of suspected abuse, steps to ensure the safety of the minor should be taken immediately. Discharging the patient with follow-up in 1 week to reevaluate her bruises disregards her safety and potentially subjects the minor to continued abuse. Considering the extent of the physical injuries, it is unlikely that the patient's younger siblings inflicted them. Consequently, confronting the siblings about their behavior serves no purpose.

19. **(B)** Confidentiality in the treatment of minors should be maintained unless specifically prohibited by state law (eg, in cases of abortion) or when the parents' involvement is necessary to make complicated or life-threatening treatment decisions. The other choices all constitute violations of confidentiality to your patient.

20. **(D)** Informed consent for HIV testing involves a thorough explanation of the test's interpretation, information regarding confidentiality, and further evaluation needed if the test is positive. The patient should be aware of the risk of false positives and negatives, and the need for confirmatory testing if the test result is positive. Choices A and B are incorrect because they violate patient confidentiality. When a patient tests positive for HIV, state laws may require notification of the sexual partner (this is usually done without revealing the patient's identity) in addition to the department of public health. There is no reason to notify the state's health department or performing a pregnancy test before administering an HIV test.

21. **(A)** The patient's desire to stop dialysis should be respected because competent adults are able to determine which treatment they should accept or deny. The American Medical Association (AMA) Code of Ethics notes that there is no ethical distinction between withdrawing and withholding medical treatment. The remaining choices undermine the patient's right to make an informed decision.

22. **(D)** Physician–patient confidentiality should be maintained except in certain cases (ie, duty to protect others, mandatory reporting, or emergencies). The remaining choices violate physician–patient confidentiality.

23. **(C)** Confidentiality between patient and physician should be respected even in cases of court-mandated treatment. In such cases, issues around disclosure to a probation officer can be

used to explore the patient's attitudes toward probation and incarceration. Obtaining a confidentiality waiver from the patient should be done in a thoughtful manner and is essential before releasing any information to the probation officer. Ignoring the probation officer's request is inappropriate in such circumstances. The other choices are incorrect because they violate physician–patient confidentiality.

24. **(B)** The patient should immediately be informed that she was accidentally given the improper medication. The physician should also evaluate for potential adverse reactions. The fact that the patient did not suffer harm is no reason to conceal the medication error. Although many hospitals require documentation or reporting of such to the appropriate person or committee, this should not be the first course of action. Evaluating the patient for any adverse reaction and explaining the mistake is the appropriate first step. Notifying the patient's family of the mistake is a breach of confidentiality and inappropriate. Encouraging the patient to seek legal action is both alarmist and inappropriate in such a case.

25. **(C)** Explaining the implications of no treatment but respecting the patient's refusal for treatment is the most appropriate course of action. This allows the patient to make an informed decision with regard to her treatment. The elements integral to informed consent include (1) competency to make a decision; (2) an adequate explanation of the risks, benefits, rationale for treatment, and alternative treatments (including no treatment at all); and (3) a voluntary decision. In this vignette, there is no evidence that the patient suffers from a condition that might impair her competency. Further, her stated religious belief is consistent with a Jehovah's Witness's refusal of human blood products. Administering packed red blood cells infringes on the patient's right to refuse a blood transfusion and consequently is incorrect. Strongly persuading the patient to arrive at a decision for treatment or utilizing a confrontational method to secure lifesaving treatment is coercive in nature and could prevent the patient from making a voluntary decision. It is inappropriate to involuntarily hospitalize this patient if she has arrived at her decision in compliance with the elements of informed consent.

26. **(D)** According to the AMA Code of Medical Ethics, treatment decisions must be made in the best interest of the child or neonate regardless of the desires of the parents. Treatment can be withheld or withdrawn only in cases in which the risks far outweigh the benefits, there is low potential for success, or when treatment extends the child's suffering without potential for a joyful existence. The lumbar puncture results unequivocally demonstrate bacterial meningitis. In this particular case, the neonate suffers from a serious, but treatable, central nervous system infection and treatment should not be withheld. Withholding treatment until the next regularly scheduled ethics meeting would likely result in the neonate's demise.

27. **(B)** It is unethical to offer specific psychiatric diagnoses for individuals that you have not personally examined. Moreover, commenting on an individual that you have evaluated would be a breach of confidentiality.

28. **(E)** Family and/or close associates should be consulted to aid in reaching treatment decisions if there is no advance directive or designated power of attorney. Consultation with the ethics committee should be sought when the patient's prior wishes are unclear or family members are unable to agree on treatment options. Ethics committee consultations are also useful when the power of attorney's decision is unreasonable or contrary to the patient's prior wishes. It would be inappropriate to allow a severely demented patient to designate a power of attorney or make treatment decisions. Choosing sides in a family conflict would be arbitrary; consultation with the hospital ethics committee would help clarify issues in a complicated case such as this.

29. **(A)** The most appropriate course of action is to involuntarily admit the patient. Postpartum depression is a form of clinical depression that occurs in 10% to 15% of women in the general

population after childbirth. Symptoms can manifest within the first 4 weeks postpartum and can last from several months to a year. It is imperative that examining physicians inquire about the mother's thoughts toward her child when concerns for postpartum depression are present. The patient in the vignette demonstrated a significant clinical decline and acknowledged that she had thoughts of harming her infant. Discharging the patient under any circumstances is inappropriate because the infant remains at risk of harm. Child Protective Services should be notified in cases of suspected or known child abuse or neglect. Administering lorazepam and reassessing the patient does not address the issue of the baby's safety.

30. **(C)** Most physicians will someday find themselves in situations where they encounter their patients in the community. Patient–physician confidentiality does not cease once a physician leaves the hospital and must be maintained regardless of who is making the inquiry. Confidentiality can only be broken when the physician has a duty to protect others, in cases of mandatory reporting, or in medical emergencies. The remaining choices violate physician–patient confidentiality.

31. **(A)** Sexual or romantic relationships with current and former psychiatric patients (regardless of the time elapsed since treatment) are always considered unethical, making the other choices incorrect.

32. **(A)** Sexual relations with current patients are unethical and constitute sexual misconduct. The AMA Code of Medical Ethics states that sexual and/or romantic relations with former patients are unethical if the physician uses or exploits trust, knowledge, emotions, or influence derived from the previous professional relationship. At the very least, the physician has an ethical duty to terminate the physician–patient relationship prior to initiating any romantic or sexual relationships.

33. **(B)** According to the AMA Code of Medical Ethics, "physician-assisted suicide is fundamentally incompatible with the physician's role

as healer," and the physician should aggressively respond to a patient's end-of-life needs rather than assist in suicide. Physician-assisted suicide is defined as the act of facilitating a patient's death by "providing the necessary means and/or information to enable the patient to perform the life-ending act." Simply ignoring the patient's request is inappropriate because it fails to recognize and address potential end-of-life issues. End-of-life issues that should be addressed with the patient include adequate pain control, emotional/family support, comfort care, respect of patient autonomy, and appropriate multidisciplinary referrals (hospice, counseling, religious issues). The remaining choices are consistent with the definition of physician-assisted suicide and are therefore unethical.

34. **(B)** The treating physician is ultimately legally responsible for determining whether a patient is appropriate for discharge. Discharging a medically unstable or unsafe patient is considered negligence and can potentially lead to a lawsuit if there is an adverse outcome. A psychiatric patient can be considered for discharged as long as he/she does not meet the criteria for involuntary admission (ie, imminent risk to self or others, or grossly unable to care for self). The patient in the vignette is not considered safe to leave the hospital, which makes the other answer choices incorrect. Contacting the insurance company without permission violates patient confidentiality. Regardless of whether the patient has insurance or qualifies for a loan, the physician should continue to treat the patient as long as it is medically necessary.

35. **(D)** When a physician is served a subpoena to release medical information, the appropriate first step is to contact the patient to find out if he or she consents to the release. Discussing the implications of the lawsuit with your patient and clarifying whether the patient has the proper legal counsel for the lawsuit also are important. Contacting the attorney of the party requesting the subpoena and releasing the medical records without consent from the patient constitute unethical breaches of physician–patient

confidentiality. The confidentiality privilege belongs to the patient, not to the physician. Releasing the medical information directly to the judge at this stage makes no sense and would likewise be a breach of confidentiality.

36. **(D)** Turning over medical records to comply with a direct court order is ethical and legal. To defy a judge's order can potentially place a physician in contempt of court. Working out a plan of legal action or appealing to the state's Supreme Court is not the role of the physician, but rather the patient's attorney. Releasing partial records is unethical and also violates the court order.

37. **(E)** In the United States criminal justice system, a competency evaluation is an assessment of the defendant's ability to understand and rationally participate in a court process (*Dusky v United States,* 1960). The psychiatrist's goal in assessing for competency to stand trial involves evaluating whether the defendant has a rational understanding of the criminal court proceedings, the capacity to understand the different potential outcomes of the court proceedings (eg, pleading guilty vs not guilty), and have sufficient ability to communicate with and assist their attorney in their defense. The examiner should document that he or she has fully informed the defendant of the purpose and nature of the evaluation procedure and the extent of nonconfidentiality. In situations such as this where confidentiality is limited the psychiatrist must make every effort to maintain confidentiality with regard to any information that does not bear directly upon the legal purpose of the evaluation. There is no need for the examiner to withdraw from the case in the event of a criminal confession, nor is it appropriate for the examiner to persuade the defendant to act in any particular manner.

38. **(D)** Inquiring about possible reasons the patient may be avoiding payment, may help uncover important treatment issues. Such inquiry often leads to how the patient feels about the therapy and/or the therapist. These feelings can be utilized to address factors related to her symptoms. Exploring such issues

should be done in a sensitive manner to avoid alienating the patient. Requesting that the billing collector demands immediate payment and terminating treatment would be far too aggressive at this point. Contacting the patient's family violates physician–patient confidentiality. At this point, informing the patient that you will not see her if she doesn't immediately pay her bill may be perceived as confrontational and threatens the therapeutic alliance.

39. **(E)** Becoming involved in the business venture of a psychotherapy patient could have significant adverse effects on the patient's transference (feelings and memories experienced by the patient that are aroused by the therapist) as well as on the physician's countertransference (feelings aroused in the physician while working with the patient); therefore, it should be avoided. Anger, distrust, and guilt are some of the feelings that may occur if a business venture such as the one described were to fail. Further, a physician's business involvement with a patient might affect the neutral stance essential to effective psychotherapy. The central problem that involvement in a business venture might interfere with treatment should best be explained to the patient honestly.

40. **(D)** The most significant predictor of suicide is a past history of suicide attempt. Other suicide risk factors include: advancing age (>40); gender (M > F); marital status (separated or divorced > married); race (Native Americans/ Alaskan natives > Whites > Blacks/Hispanics); religion (Catholics are lowest risk); employment status (unemployed or retired > employed); support system (living alone > living with others); and health status (serious medical condition or terminal illness > good health).

41. **(D)** Suicidal behavior is among the most stressful emergencies encountered by mental health professionals. There is no algorithm or scoring tool that is able to consistently identify a patient's risk for suicide. If a malpractice claim is brought up against a psychiatrist, adequate documentation of the patient's suicide risk and

protective factors assist the courts in determining the scope and complexities of the patient's treatment. Failure to document these assessments and intervention potentially gives the courts a reason to believe they were not done. "No self-harm "contracts do not hold up as legal documents in a court of law. The remaining choices are not sufficient enough to legally protect a psychiatrist in the event of a suicide.

42. **(D)** An individual who commits a crime while voluntarily intoxicated cannot assert an insanity defense because the basis of such behavior stems from a rational decision to drink. Involuntary intoxication may be used effectively as an insanity defense if the individual had no choice in becoming intoxicated (eg, the person was drugged). A mental disease or defect or inability to recall the event might be used to enhance an insanity defense, not undermine it. Prior history of assault or the nature of the crime should have no bearing on an insanity defense. However, if prior violent behavior has been associated with mental illness and the inability to appreciate the criminality of one's conduct or conform to the law, this could be used to strengthen an insanity defense.

43. **(E)** Medical expert witnesses are called to present their professional opinions based on reasonable medical certainty. An expert witness may be called to testify in both civil and criminal trials, and is expected to perform an impartial evaluation and testify as to the findings. It is not the responsibility of the expert to ensure a particular outcome for either side. Unlike the traditional physician–patient relationship, the expert witness does not initiate treatment of patients and has limits on confidentiality.

44. **(B)** Habeas corpus refers to the US Constitution's clause that the state shall not "deprive any person of life, liberty, or property, without due process of law." Under habeas corpus, citizens have the right to petition the court when detained to decide whether they are being held lawfully. Establishing criminal responsibility requires the presence of both actus reus and mens rea. Actus reus refers to the voluntary act of committing a crime, and mens rea refers

to criminal intent. Both choices are incorrect as they have nothing to do with the patient's right to due process. Parens patriae refers to the state's function as parent for those unable to care for themselves. This is often used for justification of involuntary commitment. The Fourth Amendment protects citizens from unreasonable searches and seizures.

45. **(C)** It would be unethical to involuntarily detain a patient in treatment if he or she is no longer deemed to be gravely disabled or a threat to self or others. In this case, the patient should be promptly discharged to the partial hospital program. Ignoring the patient's request because the court has committed him is incorrect. Filing for another court hearing is appropriate only if the patient is still gravely disabled or a danger to self or others. Persuading the patient to stay a few more days even though he wishes to leave the hospital and no longer meets criteria for involuntary commitment is inappropriate. Appeasing the patient by increasing smoking privileges fails to address the key issue in this question.

46. **(E)** The key elements to informed consent include the capacity to make a decision; a voluntary choice without coercion or duress; and an adequate understanding of the rationale, risks, benefits, and alternative treatment options. The remaining choices are not required for informed consent.

47. **(C)** Living wills (or advance directives) preserve patient autonomy by establishing personal preferences regarding end-of-life issues. If patients lose their decisional capacity in the future, advance directives outline what procedures they do or do not desire without relying on physician or family member opinions. Patients are always able to change their living wills if desired. Physician-assisted suicide is not considered ethical. The remaining choices are not characteristics of a living will.

48. **(E)** Malingering is characterized by intentional feigning of symptoms for secondary gain (ie, financial remuneration, disability benefits, avoiding criminal prosecution or military

duty). A diagnosis of malingering should be suspected when there is the presence of one or more of the following factors: (1) litigation (especially when the patient is referred by a lawyer), (2) discrepancy between objective findings and the patient's complaints, (3) a diagnosis of antisocial personality disorder (which his history supports), and (4) a failure to comply with the evaluation and recommended treatments. The duration of symptoms in this case has no bearing on a diagnosis of malingering. The lack of physical injuries or the presence of flashbacks in a claim of PTSD is not sufficient to raise suspicions of malingering. PTSD occurs in individuals exposed to actual or threatened death or injury and consequently may have no physical injuries. A past history of major depression does not raise a suspicion of malingering.

49. **(D)** According to the AMA Code of Medical Ethics, physicians are obligated to provide continuity of care for their patients. When discharging a patient from your care, advance notice of the pending discharge must be given with sufficient time to obtain another physician. Contacting the patient's family breaches confidentiality and is not the appropriate procedure for discharging the patient. Notifying the insurance company fails to inform the patient of her discharge and does not provide her time to obtain a new physician. The remaining choices fail to provide the patient with sufficient notice to obtain proper medical follow-up.

50. **(B)** The prevailing concept in determining child custody is based on individual(s) who can provide for the best interests of the child. Factors that can be used to determine the best interests of the child include assessing the individual's biologic relation, financial stability, level of education, and health; however, it is the aggregate rather than any single factor which determines what is in the best interest of the child.

51. **(E)** Physicians are ethically obliged to report impaired colleagues. Reporting procedures vary from state to state. However, the AMA Code of Medical Ethics suggests initial reporting to a hospital's impaired physician program. If no such program exists, the chief of staff or clinical service director should be notified. For physicians without hospital privileges, an impaired physicians program run by a medical society or the state board licensing committee should be made aware of the impaired physician. The other choices do not meet the AMA guidelines and fail to initiate proper treatment and supervision of the impaired physician.

CHAPTER 6

Differential Diagnosis and Management
Questions

Questions 1 and 2

A 43-year-old woman presents to your office telling you that recently she has been experiencing an increase in the volume of a voice that she has been hearing for years. It constantly criticizes her behaviors regardless of her mood. She also notes that for the past month, her mood has been very low. She is no longer able to get any pleasure from watching television. Her sleep is poor and her energy is low. She also describes a 10 lb weight loss in the past month because she no longer feels the need to eat. She denies the use of any drugs or alcohol.

1. Which of the following diagnoses best accounts for this patient's symptoms?

   (A) bipolar II disorder
   (B) major depression with psychotic features
   (C) schizoaffective disorder
   (D) schizophrenia
   (E) schizoid personality disorder

2. Which of the following medication combinations could be used to best treat this patient's symptoms?

   (A) divalproex sodium and lorazepam (Ativan)
   (B) fluoxetine (Prozac) and diazepam (Valium)

   (C) haloperidol (Haldol) and perphenazine (Trilafon)
   (D) mirtazapine (Remeron) and citalopram (Celexa)
   (E) ziprasidone (Geodon) and sertraline (Zoloft)

Questions 3 and 4

A 29-year-old woman who just delivered 3 weeks ago is referred because her obstetrician noticed that she appeared to be disheveled. Upon initial interview, the patient tells you that she has been feeling down since delivering her son. She tells you that while she continues to care for her son, she is growing increasingly depressed because she does not get any pleasure from taking care of him. She is unable to sleep and has not been eating much either. She feels tired all the time. She also tells you that at times, she will hear a baby in the background crying, but when she checks on her son, he is sleeping soundly. She denies any thoughts of wanting to hurt her son or herself.

3. Which of the following diagnoses is the most likely?

   (A) adjustment disorder
   (B) brief psychotic disorder
   (C) postpartum depression with psychosis
   (D) postpartum obsessive compulsive disorder
   (E) schizoaffective disorder, depressed type

4. Which of the following is the most appropriate first step in her treatment?

(A) fluoxetine (Prozac) and haloperidol (Haldol)

(B) haloperidol (Haldol)

(C) hospitalize the patient

(D) lithium

(E) supportive therapy

Questions 5 and 6

A 64-year-old woman is brought to the emergency department by her neighbor, who says "my friend isn't acting right." The patient requires the support of a nurse while walking to an examination table. Examination reveals that she cannot correctly identify the season or the town she is in. She does not recognize her neighbor. She is inattentive and seemingly apathetic to the activity around her. She dozes off repeatedly during the interview, but each time is arousable and resumes answering questions. Her answers are illogical and inconsistent.

Vital signs are within normal limits and she is neither tremulous nor diaphoretic. Neurologic examination finds bilateral sixth nerve palsy and horizontal nystagmus. Urine toxicology screen and blood alcohol level are negative.

5. Which of the following is the most likely diagnosis?

(A) acute subdural hematoma

(B) alcohol withdrawal

(C) folic acid deficiency

(D) normal pressure hydrocephalus (NPH)

(E) Wernicke encephalopathy

6. What is the most important first step in managing this patient?

(A) administration of a benzodiazepine

(B) administration of folic acid

(C) administration of thiamine

(D) computed tomography (CT) scan of the head

(E) intravenous (IV) fluids and observation

Questions 7 and 8

A 62-year-old woman presents to your office along with her daughter. Her daughter explains to you that lately, her mother has been extremely concerned about her body odor. Despite multiple reassurances from her daughter that she does not smell, she continues to be concerned that other people find her body odor extremely offensive. The patient tells you that she knows that she smells because she can smell her own body odor all the time despite taking multiple showers throughout the day. Despite being concerned about her odor, she continues to work from home as she has done for the past 30 years and she continues to speak with friends on the telephone. She pays her monthly bills without the help of her family. Her thinking otherwise seems logical.

7. Which of the following is the most likely diagnosis?

(A) delusional disorder

(B) obsessive compulsive disorder

(C) paranoid personality disorder

(D) schizoaffective disorder

(E) schizophrenia

8. Which of the following would be the most appropriate treatment?

(A) electroconvulsive therapy (ECT)

(B) fluoxetine (Prozac)

(C) lithium (Eskalith)

(D) olanzapine (Zyprexa)

(E) carbamazepine (Tegretol)

Questions 9 and 10

A 29-year-old man with a history of chronic paranoid schizophrenia comes to the emergency department with a temperature of 102.9°F, labile blood pressure rising to 210/110 mm Hg, a pulse of 110/min, and a respiratory rate of 22 breaths/min. This patient's medications include haloperidol, benztropine (Cogentin), and clonazepam (Klonopin). He cannot correctly identify the day, date, or year, and believes himself to be in a city from which he moved 10 years ago. A family member indicates that 3 days ago he was healthy and completely oriented and that he has no significant medical or surgical history.

Physical examination reveals that he is in acute distress with hypertonicity. Laboratory examination reveals creatine phosphokinase (CPK) of 45,000 Iμ/L, white blood cell count of 14,000/μL and no left shift, sodium of 145 mEq/L, and creatinine of 2.5 mg/dL. Lumbar puncture produces clear fluid with a slightly elevated protein count.

9. Which of the following is the most likely diagnosis?

    (A) anticholinergic syndrome
    (B) central nervous system (CNS) infection
    (C) malignant hyperthermia
    (D) neuroleptic malignant syndrome (NMS)
    (E) prolonged immobilization

10. With appropriate treatment, the patient recovers completely and returns home. In a month's time, he comes to the emergency department stating that the "voices in the walls" are telling him to kill himself. He has taken no medications since he left the hospital. His vital signs are stable and a medical workup is negative. Which of the following therapies should be initiated first?

    (A) ECT
    (B) haloperidol depot injections
    (C) olanzapine
    (D) physical restraints
    (E) safety monitoring only

Questions 11 and 12

A 39-year-old woman comes to the emergency department and complains that since her boyfriend broke up with her 3 months ago, she has been sleeping and eating poorly, has lost all interest in her work, and feels guilty that she drove her boyfriend away. In the past month, she has begun to feel hopeless, helpless, and that "life may not be worth it." In the past 2 weeks, she has developed a belief that a rare disease is rotting her heart, and in the past week, a voice in her ear tells her she is no good and that she should take an overdose of a heart medication she is prescribed. At first she was able to ignore the voice, however, she is now at the point that she believes she should act on it.

11. Which of the following should be the most immediate management?

    (A) admission to a medical unit
    (B) admission to a psychiatric unit
    (C) medication and discharge to a close family member
    (D) referral to an outpatient psychiatrist
    (E) restraints and medication in the emergency department

12. Which of the following medication(s) would be the most appropriate?

    (A) benzodiazepine only
    (B) lithium and a selective serotonin reuptake inhibitor (SSRI)
    (C) lithium only
    (D) SSRI and an antipsychotic
    (E) tricyclic antidepressant (TCA) only

Questions 13 and 14

A 21-year-old man is brought to the emergency department by police after an episode in which he ransacked the office where he works looking for "evidence." He started this job 2 months ago after graduating from college. He lives with four roommates and he believes they are jealous of him because of his job and have been poisoning his food. His family reveals that once before when he began college he went through a period of "acting crazy" but got better without treatment and has done well since. In the emergency department, he is shouting that he has been up for a week writing a "classic" book about accounting and someone at the office stole it from him. He needs to be physically restrained by emergency department security. Physical examination and complete laboratory workup and toxicology screen prove to be negative.

13. Which of the following medication(s) should be initiated?

    (A) antipsychotic and benzodiazepine
    (B) buspirone (BuSpar)
    (C) carbamazepine (Tegretol)
    (D) lithium
    (E) SSRI

14. Three months later, the patient sees his doctor for follow-up. He is taking lithium and haloperidol. He is doing well, except he complains of muscle stiffness. His lithium level is 0.8 mEq/L. Which of the following would be the most appropriate next step in his management?

    (A) Decrease the haloperidol dose.
    (B) Decrease the lithium dose.
    (C) Increase the haloperidol dose.
    (D) Increase the lithium dose.
    (E) Start baclofen (Lioresal).

Questions 15 and 16

A 29-year-old woman tells her doctor that about 3 weeks ago she was caring for a child who ran into the street and was killed by a bus. Since then, she cannot get the image of the accident out of her mind. Even in sleep, she dreams about it and it prevents her from sleeping more than a few hours at night. She used to take a bus to work but she now drives because she cannot bear to be near buses as this causes her to think about the accident. In the past week, she has begun missing work because she is uncomfortable leaving her house. She feels guilty, believing the accident was her fault.

15. Which of the following is the most likely diagnosis?

    (A) acute stress disorder
    (B) adjustment disorder
    (C) major depressive disorder (MDD)
    (D) panic disorder with agoraphobia
    (E) posttraumatic stress disorder (PTSD)

16. The patient decides against any medication but follows up with psychotherapy. A year later, although she is no longer having distressful symptoms relating to the accident, she feels sad and tearful most of the time, is having trouble eating, has lost interest in gardening, and wakes up at 4 AM every morning, unable to get back to sleep. She constantly feels tired throughout the day. Which of the following is the most likely diagnosis?

    (A) acute stress disorder
    (B) adjustment disorder

    (C) MDD
    (D) panic disorder with agoraphobia
    (E) PTSD

17. A patient with a history of bipolar disorder is admitted to a psychiatric hospital in an acute manic episode. Her medications include an SSRI and a benzodiazepine, which are both discontinued on admission. A neuroleptic and a mood stabilizer are started. Two days after admission, she calls the nursing staff to her bed. She is extremely frightened and complains excitedly that she cannot stop looking up. On examination, her eyes are noted to be deviated upward bilaterally. Which of the following side effects is most consistent with her presentation?

    (A) NMS
    (B) oculogyric crisis
    (C) retrocollis
    (D) torticollis
    (E) trismus

Questions 18 and 19

A 59-year-old woman with a long history of GAD tells her primary care doctor that 2 days ago while in a crowded supermarket she felt dizzy, along with associated heart palpitations, pressure on her chest, and a frightening sense of doom. Shortly thereafter, she fell unconscious and woke up minutes later to a crowd around her. She felt somewhat better and rejected others' advice that an ambulance be called. She quickly made her way home.

18. Which of the following is the most appropriate next step?

    (A) cognitive-behavioral therapy
    (B) electrocardiogram (ECG)
    (C) reassurance that her condition is benign
    (D) short-acting benzodiazepines
    (E) SSRI

19. Which of the following diagnosis is the most important to rule out first?

    (A) acute stress disorder
    (B) cardiovascular disease

(C) GAD

(D) hypochondriasis

(E) panic attack

20. A 28-year-old male presents to your office because he wants to stop a particularly disturbing behavior. He tells you that he often goes on public trains with the intention of trying to rub his genitals on other people without their consent. He continues to have fantasies about this but he wishes to stop because he is afraid of getting into trouble. Which of the following is his most likely diagnosis?

(A) exhibitionism

(B) frotteurism

(C) masochism

(D) sadism

(E) voyeurism

Questions 21 and 22

A 53-year-old man presents to your office complaining of worsening depression. He states that he no longer enjoys spending time with his family, he is only getting a few hours of sleep at night, and his appetite is much lower than it used to be. He feels tired all day long. You decide to initiate an SSRI.

21. Which of the following side effects is he most likely to experience after 3 months of treatment?

(A) diarrhea

(B) headaches

(C) nausea

(D) sedation

(E) sexual dysfunction

22. The patient returns a few more times and during each visit, you increase the dosage of the SSRI, however, he does not report any decrease in his depressive symptoms. Because of his lack of response to an SSRI, you decide to initiate a tricyclic antidepressant. He continues to feel depressed, helpless, and hopeless, and he subsequently overdoses on his medication. His wife finds him unconscious and proceeds to call 911. Which of the following would be the most likely cause of death?

(A) cardiac arrhythmia

(B) respiratory failure

(C) seizure

(D) shock

(E) stroke

Questions 23 and 24

A 19-year-old man with no previous psychiatric history is noted by his college roommate to be acting bizarrely for the past month and a half, having conversations with people who are not there, walking around the dormitory room naked, and accusing the roommate of calling the Federal Bureau of Investigation (FBI) to have him monitored. The patient's vital signs are all within normal limits and his neurologic examination shows no deficits or abnormalities.

23. Which of the following tests would be most useful in the initial diagnosis of this patient?

(A) complete blood count (CBC)

(B) erythrocyte sedimentation rate (ESR)

(C) liver function tests

(D) noncontrast CT scan of the brain

(E) toxicology screen

24. If the above test were negative, which of the following would be the most likely diagnosis?

(A) chronic paranoid schizophrenia

(B) delusional disorder

(C) major depression with psychotic features

(D) schizophreniform disorder

(E) substance-induced psychosis

Questions 25 and 26

You have been asked by the surgery team to evaluate a 35-year-old man who had surgery to repair his fractured right wrist 24 hours ago and is now complaining of anxiety. The patient has been in the hospital for 2 days. His heart rate is 120 beats/min, and his blood pressure is 160/106 mm Hg. He is afebrile and reports that he has never suffered anything like this before. He is not in any pain and has no previous psychiatric history. His medication includes only acetaminophen for pain control. You note that he is diaphoretic and tremulous.

25. Which of the following is the most appropriate medication to treat this patient?

 (A) carbamazepine
 (B) clonidine (Catapres)
 (C) lorazepam
 (D) methadone
 (E) naltrexone (ReVia)

26. Without the above treatment, which of the following is he most at risk for developing?

 (A) abdominal pain
 (B) cirrhosis
 (C) fatty liver
 (D) muscle cramps
 (E) seizures

Questions 27 and 28

You are working in the psychiatric emergency department of a large metropolitan hospital. A 20-year-old man with unknown psychiatric history is brought in by the police after being found stumbling naked around a local college campus. He is markedly agitated, pacing, and appears to be responding to internal stimuli. On examination, you note that he is tachycardic with a heart rate in the 110s, he has tics or spasms in his face, and he has vertical nystagmus.

27. Which of the following tests would be most helpful in the diagnosis?

 (A) CBC
 (B) electroencephalogram (EEG)
 (C) magnetic resonance image (MRI) of the brain
 (D) noncontrast head CT
 (E) toxicology screen

28. Which of the following would be the most appropriate treatment for this patient?

 (A) a low-stimulus environment
 (B) benztropine
 (C) methylphenidate (Ritalin)
 (D) phenytoin (Dilantin)
 (E) propranolol (Inderal)

29. A 40-year-old divorced woman is brought in to the emergency department after being found sleeping in a pile of leaves. Initially, she is difficult to arouse and has trouble answering your questions, but she appears to be in no respiratory distress. You also notice that her pupils are pinpoint. After a few hours, she becomes more interactive and is complaining of diffuse, crampy abdominal pain and symptoms of "the flu." Her pupils are now slightly dilated, and she is yawning. Her vital signs are a temperature of 99.3°F, a heart rate of 99 beats/min, and blood pressure of 142/90 mm Hg. After the second interview, which of the following is the most likely diagnosis?

 (A) cannabis abuse
 (B) cocaine intoxication
 (C) cocaine withdrawal
 (D) opiate intoxication
 (E) opiate withdrawal

Questions 30 and 31

A 70-year-old widow is admitted for an evaluation of depression and anxiety. She tells you that for the past 15 years her family doctor has prescribed "some pills" that have helped her sleep and feel less nervous. She says that she ran out of them yesterday and since that time has felt increasingly anxious and jittery. She also notes that she's now having tremors in her hands that have not been there before.

30. Which of the following medications would be the most dangerous to suddenly discontinue?

 (A) fluphenazine (Prolixin)
 (B) imipramine (Tofranil)
 (C) nortriptyline (Pamelor)
 (D) thioridazine (Mellaril)
 (E) triazolam (Halcion)

31. Which of the following would be the most dangerous side effect of abruptly stopping the above medication?

 (A) autonomic hyperactivity
 (B) seizures
 (C) hallucinations
 (D) worsening anxiety
 (E) vomiting

Questions 32 and 33

A 73-year-old man is admitted to the hospital for community-acquired pneumonia and dehydration. On day 2 of his hospitalization, you are asked to evaluate the patient for depression; the staff has noted that he seems very withdrawn. He is not eating or sleeping well. The nursing staff reports that last night he was angry and requested to leave the hospital. You talk with the patient's family and find that the patient has no previous psychiatric history. Prior to the onset of this illness 5 days ago, he had no depressive symptoms and no difficulties with cognition. On examination, his vital signs are temperature 98.2°F, heart rate 87 beats/min, blood pressure 130/86 mm Hg, and a peripheral oxygen saturation of 95% on room air. He is drowsy and oriented only to person. His Mini-Mental State Examination (MMSE) score is 24/30.

32. Which of the following is the most likely diagnosis?

    (A) anxiety disorder
    (B) delirium
    (C) dementia
    (D) factitious disorder
    (E) MDD

33. The medical team asks for medication recommendations if the patient becomes agitated. Which of the following would be the most appropriate medication to recommend?

    (A) benztropine
    (B) diphenhydramine
    (C) lorazepam
    (D) haloperidol
    (E) thioridazine

Questions 34 and 35

A 34-year-old female presents to your office as she has been feeling depressed and angry for the past couple of days because she thinks her boyfriend is going to leave her. As a result, she has been calling him every hour just to confirm that he is not leaving her. She tells you that she has had many relationships in the past which have always been very rocky, causing her emotions to constantly go up and down.

When many of these relationships ended, she purposely cut on her arms superficially to "relieve stress." At this time, she tells you that she does have some thoughts of wanting to cut herself, but no thoughts of wanting to end her life.

34. Which of the following is the most likely diagnosis?

    (A) bipolar disorder
    (B) borderline personality disorder
    (C) histrionic personality disorder
    (D) major depressive disorder
    (E) narcissistic personality disorder

35. Which of the following is the most appropriate treatment for this diagnosis?

    (A) dialectical behavioral therapy
    (B) initiate aripiprazole (Abilify)
    (C) initiate citalopram (Celexa)
    (D) initiate lithium
    (E) psychoanalysis

Questions 36 and 37

A 65-year-old woman with a past medical history of non-insulin-dependent diabetes mellitus and depression is admitted with increasingly depressed mood over the last month. She is unable to complete her crossword puzzles because of difficulty concentrating. She has trouble falling asleep and also wakes up in the middle of the night. She denies suicidal ideation, but does feel guilty that she is depressed. Prior to this episode, she was doing well and was actively engaged in community volunteer groups. In the last month, she has lost 13 lb due to poor intake. When asked why she is not eating, she states she is worried that she will become infected with bacteria. She has been to her primary physician for an evaluation, but she claims everything was normal. Her husband confirms that the patient has been very worried about "getting a disease" to the point where she will eat only food in sealed containers. He also confides in you that she has been worried that she might have cancer and despite reassurances from her primary care physician, she continues to voice her concerns to her husband that "my intestines are not working."

36. Which of the following is the most likely diagnosis?

(A) dysthymia

(B) MDD without psychotic features

(C) MDD with psychotic features

(D) OCD

(E) somatization disorder

37. Which of the following medication(s) is the treatment of choice for this patient?

(A) divalproex sodium

(B) lithium and sertraline

(C) nortriptyline and lorazepam

(D) sertraline

(E) sertraline and risperidone

Questions 38 and 39

An 18-year-old man is brought to the psychiatric emergency department by his parents for evaluation of his behavior. Three months ago, the patient started classes at the state university located in a different city, although he would come home each weekend to visit. His parents have noticed that over the past 3 weeks he has become increasingly withdrawn and does not seem to be taking care of himself. The parents were recently called by the patient's roommate who informed them that the patient has not been going to classes for the last week, has not been eating or bathing, and has been speaking about how people in his classes are trying to kill him. The patient denies any drug use and is not on any medication. On examination, the patient's vital signs are all within normal parameters. His physical and neurologic exams are unremarkable. He is pacing and appears to be responding to internal stimuli. His mood is "OK" and his affect is flat. He is fully oriented. He says that he hears a number of people talking to him, "maybe in my head," saying bad things about him. He looks frightened and asks, "What is happening to me?"

38. Which of the following diagnoses is most likely?

(A) brief psychotic disorder

(B) chronic undifferentiated schizophrenia

(C) delusional disorder

(D) schizophreniform disorder

(E) substance-induced psychotic disorder

39. Which of the following laboratory tests or procedures would be the most helpful in narrowing the above differential?

(A) CBC

(B) EEG

(C) electrolytes

(D) noncontrast head CT

(E) toxicology screen

Questions 40 and 41

A 35-year-old woman with no previous personal or family psychiatric history is brought to the emergency department by her husband, who reports that his wife was attempting to kill herself by cutting her wrists. Her husband tells you that 6 months ago the patient's grandmother died. Since that time, her husband believes that the patient has been becoming more depressed. She has difficulty falling asleep and has lost 15 lb in 2 months. She was recently fired from her job as a paralegal because she was unable to concentrate and made frequent mistakes. She feels guilty that she is unable to feel better, and she endorses feelings of hopelessness and worthlessness. She believes that her "only way out of this" is to kill herself.

40. Which of the following would be the most appropriate treatment?

(A) flumazenil (Romazicon)

(B) fluoxetine

(C) fluphenazine

(D) phenelzine (Nardil)

(E) triazolam

41. After being begun on the appropriate medication, which of the following side effects may mimic a worsening symptom of her illness?

(A) akathisia

(B) constipation

(C) diarrea

(D) insomnia

(E) nausea

Questions 42 and 43

A 46-year-old man with no previous psychiatric history presents with complaints of feeling depressed since his wife died 1 month ago from pancreatic cancer. He shares that although he knows she is dead, he sometimes hears her calling his name. This has occurred several times and usually happens more often at night when he is falling asleep. He denies any visual hallucinations, paranoia, or delusional beliefs. He expresses guilt about not spending more time with his wife when she was alive but denies any thoughts of wanting to end his life. He is now sleeping only about 3 to 4 hours at night and has had a 5 lb weight loss over the past month. He is still able to work on a daily basis.

42. Which of the following is the most likely diagnosis?

   (A) adjustment disorder
   (B) bereavement
   (C) dysthymic disorder
   (D) major depressive episode
   (E) schizophrenia

43. Which of the following would be the most appropriate treatment for this patient?

   (A) amitriptyline (Elavil)
   (B) fluoxetine (Prozac)
   (C) haloperidol (Haldol)
   (D) lithium
   (E) no intervention at this time

Questions 44 and 45

You are asked to see an 18-year-old woman with no previous psychiatric or medical history because the dean of her college is concerned about her and worried that she may be depressed. The patient tells you that despite being far away from her home for the first time, she was enjoying school and her new friends until 2 months ago, when she learned that her parents were getting divorced. Since that time, her grades have gone from As and Bs to Bs and Cs because she is concerned about her parents and her sister at home. She feels "bummed out" most of the time, and her friends note that she seems unhappy and occasionally becomes tearful when talking about her family. She denies difficulty sleeping or changes in appetite or weight, and she continues to enjoy daily trips to the gym to exercise.

44. Which of the following is the most likely diagnosis?

   (A) acute stress disorder
   (B) adjustment disorder with depressed mood
   (C) bereavement
   (D) GAD
   (E) MDD

45. Which of the following treatments would be most appropriate?

   (A) alprazolam
   (B) fluoxetine
   (C) nortriptyline
   (D) psychotherapy
   (E) risperidone (Risperdal)

Questions 46 and 47

A 26-year-old woman with no previous psychiatric history is referred to you by her primary care physician for evaluation of "anxiety attacks." She tells you that approximately 2 months ago she began having periods lasting 10 or 15 minutes during which, she says, "I feel like I'm going to die." During these episodes, her heart races, she feels as though she cannot catch her breath, she is dizzy and afraid she may pass out, and she has tingling and tremors in her hands. She is concerned because she is now having difficulty leaving her house due to worry that these episodes will occur, making it impossible for her to get home. She is unable to identify any triggers leading to the episodes. She is not on any medication and has no medical problems.

46. Which of the following is her most likely diagnosis?

   (A) GAD
   (B) panic disorder with agoraphobia
   (C) separation anxiety disorder
   (D) social phobia
   (E) specific phobia

47. Which of the following would be the most appropriate treatment to initiate?

(A) alprazolam
(B) lithium
(C) propranolol
(D) sertraline
(E) tranylcypromine (Parnate)

Questions 48 and 49

A 36-year-old woman with no former psychiatric history is referred to you by a dermatologist for evaluation of her chronically chapped hands. She says she has been seeing her dermatologist for approximately 5 years for this problem and treated with a variety of topical agents with limited success. Over the past 3 weeks, her hands have become worse, to the point where they are always cracked and bleeding. Reluctantly, she confides in you that she has had a longstanding fear of germs, but since her colleague at work has been sick, she has been washing her hands at least 40 times per day because she is afraid of contracting the disease. She also refuses to touch anything that might infect her without using a handkerchief. She admits to being very tidy at home, as well. She spends about 2½ hours in the morning getting showered. She realizes her fears of contamination are irrational, but every time she tries to stop washing her hands she becomes increasingly anxious.

48. Which of the following diagnoses would be most likely?

(A) GAD
(B) MDD
(C) OCD
(D) panic disorder
(E) somatization disorder

49. Which of the following treatments would be most appropriate for this patient?

(A) cognitive-behavioral therapy
(B) ECT
(C) lithium
(D) psychodynamic psychotherapy
(E) risperidone

50. A 47-year-old secretary comes to your office complaining, "I'm always worried." She says that she worries about her job, her kids, her housework, and her husband. She is seeking help now because she has been having an increasingly difficult time concentrating at work and has been more irritable with people around her. Her sleep has been "okay," but she does not feel rested when she gets up in the morning. She has been more aware of these feelings over the last 2 years and they occur almost every day. She denies any discrete episodes of increased anxiety. Which of the following diagnoses is the most likely in this patient?

(A) GAD
(B) OCD
(C) social phobia disorder
(D) panic disorder
(E) schizophrenia

51. A 28-year-old woman with no previous psychiatric or medical history is admitted to the neurology service for evaluation of acute onset of numbness and weakness of the right side of her face and right arm and leg. Physical examination shows symmetrical 2/4 reflexes in all distributions, downgoing plantar reflexes bilaterally, and 2/5 strength in the right upper and lower extremity in all muscle groups. No atrophy or fasciculations are noted. Her gait is ataxic and staggering with extreme exaggerated movements of her arms; however, she does not fall when ambulating without assistance. Given the severity of her deficits, she seems unconcerned by her level of disability. Which of the following diagnoses would be the most appropriate?

(A) conversion disorder
(B) factitious disorder
(C) malingering
(D) somatization disorder
(E) undiagnosed neurologic disease

52. A 54-year-old woman with a past medical history of hypothyroidism is admitted with a septic right knee. The surgery team asks you to evaluate the patient because they found that the fluid aspirate from the knee was growing a pathogen found primarily in the human mouth. They suspect the patient was injecting saliva into her knee. You evaluate the patient and find her to be pleasant and cooperative. She tells you that she has had a very tough time lately because her husband has recently been sick. Fortunately, she is a nurse and has been able to care for him at home. Lately, she admits to feeling overwhelmed and not appreciated. She has no idea what has caused the problem with her knee. You talk to the family and they tell you the patient is in no financial difficulty and continues to enjoy work as a nurse. After working closely with you for several weeks, she eventually admits to injecting her knee although cannot understand why she did it. Which of the following is the most appropriate diagnosis?

(A) conversion disorder
(B) factitious disorder
(C) hypochondriasis
(D) malingering
(E) somatization disorder

Questions 53 and 54

An 18-year-old woman in her first year of college comes to see you for evaluation of depression, after her roommates encouraged her to seek help. She reports difficulty falling asleep and early morning awakenings, poor concentration, fatigue, and anxiety over the past month since arriving for the fall semester. She tells you that her parents are very strict and she is worried that she will not "get straight As." On examination, she is a calm, thin woman dressed in a very baggy jogging suit. You comment on her thinness, and she tells you she prides herself on her appearance and tries to stay slim by exercising about 4 hours a day along with a good diet. She denies problems with eating too much or too little and claims that only diet and exercise help her to control her weight. Despite your concerns, she admits that she would like to lose a few more pounds. Upon further questioning, she informs you she has not had a regular menstrual period for over a year.

53. Which of the following would be the most likely working diagnosis?

(A) anorexia nervosa
(B) anxiety disorder
(C) body dysmorphic disorder
(D) bulimia nervosa
(E) MDD

54. Which of the following tests would be most helpful in supporting your provisional diagnosis?

(A) ECG
(B) serum amylase
(C) serum magnesium level
(D) serum potassium level
(E) weight and height

Questions 55 and 56

A 5-year-old boy is referred to you by his pediatrician for evaluation of aggressive behavior. His medical and extensive neurologic workup was negative. An interview with the patient reveals a restless boy who is able to engage in conversation. He tells you he gets angry and frustrated in school as he "thinks it's boring." His parents report that he is currently repeating kindergarten due to poor performance and difficulty socializing with other children. His aggressive outbursts at school seem to occur at times when he does not understand the schoolwork. His mother tells you that she still has to help him pick out his clothes for school and get dressed. His family history is positive for two paternal uncles with learning disabilities.

55. Which of the following tests would be most helpful in the evaluation of this patient?

(A) Goodenough-Harris Draw-A-Person Test
(B) Kohs Block Test
(C) Minnesota Multiphasic Personality Inventory-2 (MMPI-2)
(D) Peabody Vocabulary Test
(E) Wechsler Intelligence Scale for Children (WISC)

56. A score of 69 on this test would be most consistent with which of the following diagnoses?

(A) borderline intellectual functioning
(B) mild mental retardation
(C) moderate mental retardation
(D) severe mental retardation
(E) profound mental retardation

Questions 57 and 58

An 8-year-old boy is brought into your office by his mother because she is concerned that he cannot stop blinking his eyes and shrugging his shoulders. She tells you that this occurs almost everyday and has been this way for the past year and a half. She tells her son to stop doing this while he is in your office, and he does stop. You notice, however, that he starts sniffing and coughing repeatedly.

57. Which of the following medications should be used to treat the patient's condition?

(A) atomoxetine
(B) clonidine
(C) lamotrigine
(D) lorazepam
(E) valproic acid

58. You begin the appropriate medication and 2 months later the boy and his mother return for a follow-up visit. She tells you that while the eye blinking and shoulder shrugging have gotten better, he is now falling asleep in his classes at school. What is the next most appropriate step in the management?

(A) Add another medication to keep the boy awake.
(B) Educate the mother about proper sleep hygiene.
(C) Discontinue the medication.
(D) Reduce the dosage.
(E) Switch to another medication.

59. A 17-year-old boy with a history of attention-deficit hyperactivity disorder (ADHD) presents with odd behavior, confusion, a blood pressure of 128/85 mm Hg, and a heart rate of 68 beats/min. His parents report that at times they have observed him repetitively touching his stomach and rapidly blinking his eyes. On examination, he appears dazed and unable to concentrate. Which of the following is the most likely diagnosis?

(A) amphetamine toxicosis
(B) epilepsy
(C) hypoglycemia
(D) MDD
(E) somatization disorder

60. A 50-year-old man with a long history of IV drug use is brought to the hospital by police after a local homeless shelter worker noted him to be confused and "walking funny." While at the shelter, he became very suspicious of the workers and accused them of taking his belongings. On examination, you observe that he has a left pupil that accommodates but does not react, depressed deep tendon reflexes in all distributions, and loss of position sense at the great toes bilaterally. Although the patient was treated with antipsychotic medications in the past, he denies currently taking any medication. Which of the following diagnoses best accounts for this patient's symptoms?

(A) Korsakoff psychosis
(B) neuroleptic-induced dyskinesia
(C) neuroleptic malignant syndrome
(D) neurosyphilis
(E) Wernicke encephalopathy

61. A 57-year-old woman with no previous psychiatric history complains of increasing anxiety over the last 2 months. Today she reports that it became "very bad." She also notes that with these periods of anxiety she gets a pounding headache and once fainted. She continues to feel "shaky." When you check her vital signs, her heart rate is 170 beats/min and her blood pressure is 230/130 mm Hg. She is diaphoretic and tremulous. Given this patient's symptoms, which of the following conditions is most likely?

(A) acute alcohol intoxication
(B) hypercalcemia
(C) hypothyroidism
(D) pheochromocytoma
(E) posterior circulation stroke

DIRECTIONS (Questions 62 through 67): For each patient vignette, select the one lettered option that is *most* closely associated with it. Each lettered option may be used once, multiple times, or not at all.

(A) conversion disorder

(B) hepatic encephalopathy

(C) human immunodeficiency virus (HIV)

(D) hyperthyroidism

(E) hypoglycemia

(F) pheochromocytoma

(G) systemic lupus erythematosus (SLE)

(H) somatization disorder

62. A 55-year-old man is admitted to the hospital. His wife reports that he's changed over the last year, is becoming very forgetful, and has periods when he becomes very upset. On examination, he has significant memory impairment, asterixis, palmar erythema, and a large ecchymotic area on his right scapula. He was initially cooperative, but now is very agitated and demands to leave.

63. A 52-year-old man with a history of IV drug use is brought to the emergency department by his social worker from a homeless shelter. She has known the patient for 10 years but has seen a drastic change in him over the last year. While previously jovial and interactive, he is now disengaged and subdued. He has been increasingly forgetful, today having difficulty using his eating utensils. He has lost at least 40 lb in the last 6 months and complained about feeling weak and losing his balance. He scores a 20/30 on the MMSE.

64. A 33-year-old woman is brought to the emergency department by her husband, who tells you that over the last few months she has been increasingly tearful, irritable, restless, as well as having difficulty paying bills and balancing her checkbook. She has occasional "hot flashes." On examination, she continuously changes position in her seat. She has difficulty with simple arithmetic and short-term memory. Her deep tendon reflexes are brisk symmetrically throughout. She has a fine resting tremor of her hands and difficulty rising from a seated position.

65. A 33-year-old woman presents with a 1-year history of tension headaches, recently worsening with blurry vision, despite a negative neurologic evaluation. She volunteers that she has been sick most of her life, beginning at age 16 when she had surgery for presumed endometriosis, which has left her unable to have sexual relations. Since the surgery, she has intermittent abdominal cramping, bloating, and diarrhea. Three months ago, she saw a rheumatologist for knee, back, and eye pain.

66. A 30-year-old woman is brought to the hospital by her fiancé. He says that over the last 2 weeks, she has been "a totally different person." She has not been eating or sleeping, and has been irritable and angry. Earlier in the month, she complained of headaches, pain in her hands and feet, and a fever. On examination, she looks tired; she is fully oriented but has difficulty relating the events of the last month. Occasionally, she seems to become confused.

67. A 42-year-old woman in the emergency department appears confused and will not allow blood to be drawn. She is not oriented to time or place. She takes medications for "a condition," but cannot elaborate further. The only vital signs that were taken show a heart rate of 140 beats/min and a blood pressure of 172/98 mm Hg. Physical examination is remarkable for a fine tremor of her hands bilaterally and diaphoresis. Five minutes later, the patient has a seizure.

DIRECTIONS (Questions 68 through 73): For each patient vignette, select the one lettered option that is *most* closely associated with it. Each lettered option may be used once, multiple times, or not at all.

(A) Alzheimer disease

(B) Cruetzfeld-Jacob disease

(C) delirium

(D) Huntington disease

(E) Lewy body dementia

(F) MDD (pseudodementia)

(G) Pick disease

(H) vascular dementia

68. A 71-year-old female is brought in by her husband. Over the past few years, he has noticed that she has been having memory problems. She often forgets where she put her keys or purse. He no longer lets her drive because she gets lost easily. On MMSE, she has particular problems with the day of the week, date, three item recall, and naming a pencil.   A

69. A 68-year-old male with no psychiatric history is brought by his daughter because, despite multiple reassurances, he continues to insist someone else is in the house. The patient states he sees a small man every day just inside of the door. She has also noticed that he has problems with his memory. On examination, he has a shuffling gait and a blunted affect, which the daughter states began at the same time as the visual hallucinations.   E

70. A 55-year-old male is brought by his wife because she has noticed changes in his behavior. Lately, his food preferences have changed and he is now cursing loudly in public. On examination, he is easily agitated. Neurologic examination demonstrates a positive Babinski response and a snout reflex. An MRI shows atrophy in the frontal and temporal lobes.   G

71. An 86-year-old female is brought to the ED after the nursing home staff noticed a sudden change in her behavior over the last several days. On history and physical examination, it is difficult to elicit information as the patient keeps falling asleep. Her vital signs show a temperature of 101.2°F and a heart rate of 101 beats/min. Urinalysis is positive for ketones.   C

72. A 59-year-old female is brought in by her son with whom she lives. He states that over the past couple of months his mother has been isolative, no longer spends her time reading which she used to enjoy. She will remain awake late at night and early in the morning, and her appetite has decreased. He is also concerned because she will sometimes remember minor details from the day before, but other times will not recall what she had for breakfast. Mental status examination is significant for

increased speech latency, depressed mood and affect, and trouble recalling 2/3 items after several minutes.   F

73. A 39-year-old male with no previous psychiatric history presents with complaints of feeling "very depressed lately." His family notes that he has been much more irritable recently, often yelling with little provocation and seemingly talking to himself. On MSE, he is noted to have quick, sudden, but involuntary jerking movements of his arms.   D

DIRECTIONS (Questions 74 through 89): For each of the multiple choice questions in this section, select the lettered answer that is the one *best* response in each case.

74. A 56-year-old man presents to your office at the request of his wife, who says that he drinks too much. What would be the most important strategy in evaluating this patient for alcoholism?

    (A) Ascertain how often he drinks.
    (B) Ask him how frequently he gets drunk.
    (C) Ask him what his family and friends say about his drinking.
    (D) Perform a complete laboratory investigation.
    (E) Quantify the average amount he drinks.

75. A patient presents to your office stating that for the past 7 months he has been worrying about financial and work-related problems. He states that more often than not, he is worrying about these issues throughout the day. He has a difficult time staying asleep, he feels tired all day long, and he can no longer concentrate adequately at work due to the worrying. He also tells you that he feels very tense in his shoulder and back. Which of the following is the most appropriate diagnosis?

    (A) dependent personality disorder
    (B) generalized anxiety disorder (GAD)
    (C) major depressive disorder (MDD)
    (D) panic disorder
    (E) separation anxiety

Questions 76 and 77

You are interviewing a 54-year-old married woman who has been urged to "see a shrink" by her family. She describes symptoms of feeling ineffectual, believing that the world is always hostile to her, and knowing that things will never change.

76. This triad of symptoms is most associated with which of the following disorders?

    (A) depressive disorders
    (B) dissociative disorder
    (C) GAD
    (D) panic disorder
    (E) schizophrenia

77. Which of the following treatments would best target these symptoms?

    (A) behavioral therapy
    (B) cognitive therapy
    (C) couples therapy
    (D) interpersonal therapy
    (E) paradoxical therapy

Questions 78 and 79

A 55-year-old male with a history of alcohol dependence presents to your office because he would like to stop drinking alcohol. He believes he drinks because he is depressed and wishes to also get treatment for his depression. After further history is obtained, it is recommended that the first step is to stop the alcohol as alcohol can cause depression. He agrees to with this plan.

78. What is the likelihood of his remaining depressed if he is able to refrain from using alcohol for 1 month?

    (A) 5%
    (B) 15%
    (C) 25%
    (D) 33%
    (E) 50%

79. The above patient returns after 6 weeks of maintaining sobriety from alcohol. He tells you that he has continued to feel depressed. He has

problems sleeping at night, feels tired throughout the day, has poor appetite, and he no longer derives pleasure from playing with his dogs? Which of the following medications would be the most appropriate to begin at this time?

(A) amitriptyline (Elavil)
(B) buspirone (BuSpar)
(C) lithium (Eskalith)
(D) lorazepam (Ativan)
(E) sertraline (Zoloft)

Questions 80 and 81

A 52-year-old male with a longstanding history of alcoholism is brought into the ED intoxicated with alcohol. Basic labs are done and he is found to be dehydrated, so he is given IV fluids along with glucose. About an hour later, the physician reevaluates the patient and finds that his speech is more slurred, he is more confused, and he now has nystagmus.

80. Which of the following is the next most appropriate step in the management of this patient?

    (A) Administer antibiotics.
    (B) Administer benzodiazepine.
    (C) Administer heparin.
    (D) Administer thiamine.
    (E) Administer tissue plasminogen activator.

81. You chose the correct medication to administer and the patient improves significantly. His family arrives the next morning and they tell you that he has recently been starting to make up facts about his life. You order an MRI of his brain and discover lesions in his mammillary bodies. Which of the following diagnoses would best explain these symptoms?

    (A) Alzheimer disease
    (B) conversion disorder
    (C) delirium
    (D) Korsakoff syndrome
    (E) malingering

Questions 82 and 83

A 27-year-old man complains that he has felt "down in the dumps" for months and is feeling guilty because he has been having an extramarital affair. In recent weeks, he has started to believe that his wife is poisoning his food and the rest of his family is involved in an elaborate plot to drive him from the house.

82. Assuming his thinking is delusional, how would his delusions be best characterized?

    (A) bizarre
    (B) ego-syntonic
    (C) mood congruent
    (D) mood incongruent
    (E) somatic

83. Which of the following diagnoses would most likely be responsible for the above delusions?

    (A) adjustment disorder
    (B) dysthymia
    (C) MDD
    (D) mania
    (E) schizophrenia

84. A 45-year-old man is in the emergency department because of a diabetic foot ulcer. In gathering a history, the physician learns that this man lives alone and works nights as a security guard. He says he has no friends but that this does not bother him. He has never been hospitalized or received any psychiatric help. His affect is flat. Although he answers questions and seems to trust the judgment of the doctors, he has little interest in the interview. He exhibits no signs or symptoms of psychosis or depression. What is the most likely diagnosis?

    (A) MDD
    (B) paranoid personality disorder
    (C) schizoid personality disorder
    (D) schizophrenia
    (E) schizotypal personality disorder

85. The identified patient is a 30-year-old separated female brought into the emergency room by her identical twin sister. The patient's history is notable for a prior episode of depression 5 years ago successfully treated with venlafaxine. The patient has been staying with her sister since her separation 1 month ago. For the past 2 weeks, she has been pacing around the house, not sleeping more than 2 to 3 hours per night. Despite her feeling "sad" immediately after the separation, the patient now feels "wonderful, like I can accomplish anything!" In fact, she has been attempting to remodel her sister's bathroom, even though she has no training or experience. Her sister has been extremely concerned about her, but she has been unable to talk to her about it as, "I can't get a word in edgewise, and she doesn't always make sense." The patient is only taking oral contraceptives and omeprazole for acid reflux. Her sister is concerned that she, herself, may eventually develop this illness. What is her approximate risk of developing this disease?

    (A) 40% to 50%
    (B) 50% to 60%
    (C) 60% to 70%
    (D) 70% to 80%
    (E) 80% to 90%

86. A 19-year-old man is admitted to a psychiatric hospital for the first time and eventually discharged with a diagnosis of schizophrenia. When he returns to the hospital a month later for follow-up, the patient's speech is logical and he is able to sit and talk with the interviewer, becoming relatively engaged in the examination. He says that he has been hearing voices since his discharge and he believes his every word is being recorded by a tape recorder inside his mouth. What is the most likely type of schizophrenia in this patient?

    (A) catatonic
    (B) disorganized
    (C) paranoid
    (D) residual
    (E) undifferentiated

87. A 33-year-old woman with a history of paranoid schizophrenia tells you she has been hearing voices for the past 5 years. She has a baseline auditory hallucination that she cannot understand most of the time. During periods where

the voices become worse, she typically hears command auditory hallucinations. Which of the following is the most important information to obtain regarding her auditory hallucinations?

(A) whether the voices come from inside or outside her head

(B) how loud the voices are

(C) how long she has been hearing voices

(D) what the voices are saying

(E) whether she recognizes the voices

88. A 38-year-old man complains that for the past 2 years he has required several naps over the course of the day; he finds the naps quite refreshing, but sees his doctor because lately, as he is waking up, he feels momentarily "paralyzed." He is currently not on any medications. He denies the use of any illicit substances. Which of the following is the most likely diagnosis?

(A) advanced sleep phase syndrome

(B) delayed sleep phase syndrome

(C) idiopathic hypersomnolence

(D) narcolepsy

(E) parasomnia

89. A 45-year-old male with a history of heroin dependence presents to your office complaining of problems with sleep. He claims that he has been sober from heroin for the past 10 years. He asks to be started on a medication for his insomnia. Which of the following medications would be the best choice for this patient?

(A) alprazolam (Xanax)

(B) codeine (Brontex)

(C) diphenhydramine (Benadryl)

(D) quetiapine (Seroquel)

(E) zolpidem (Ambien)

DIRECTIONS (Questions 90 through 101): For each of the following patients , choose the axis used. Each lettered option may be used once, multiple times, or not at all.

(A) Axis I

(B) Axis II

(C) Axis III

(D) Axis IV

(E) Axis V

90. A 32-year-old woman has been sleeping on the street for 6 months.

91. A 57-year-old man who comes to see you for a consultation has diabetes that is difficult to control.

92. A 12-year-old boy has an intelligence quotient (IQ) of 72.

93. A 34-year-old woman has just gone through a divorce.

94. A 45-year-old woman carries a diagnosis of borderline personality disorder.

95. A 32-year-old man carries a diagnosis of schizophrenia.

96. A 46-year-old man is diagnosed with MDD.

97. A 43-year-old woman has just been diagnosed with late-stage breast cancer.

98. A 34-year-old woman carries a diagnosis of bipolar I disorder.

99. A 32-year-old man who suffers from chronic paranoia is given a diagnosis of paranoid personality disorder.

100. A 78-year-old man is being seen after the death of his wife.

101. An 18-year-old man has a history of heroin dependence.

Answers and Explanations

1. **(C)** The most likely diagnosis in this case is schizoaffective disorder. The patient has prominent psychotic symptoms, including auditory hallucinations which are a running commentary of her behaviors, but also concurrent mood symptoms, including depressed mood, decreased sleep, anhedonia, and poor appetite. Also important, the patient's hallucinations have occurred in the absence of mood symptoms, and her mood symptoms appear to have been present for a substantial portion of the total duration of her illness. The presence of prominent psychotic symptoms in the absence of mood symptoms makes major depression with psychotic features unlikely. A diagnosis of schizophrenia alone would not adequately account for this patient's mood symptoms. Bipolar II disorder is not a valid choice since there is no clear history of a hypomanic episode. Schizoid personality disorder is unlikely because that diagnosis would not account for the patient's psychotic and mood symptoms.

2. **(E)** In schizoaffective disorder, it is important to treat both the mood and psychotic symptoms. Because the patient's symptoms mainly consist of depression and psychosis, a combination of an antipsychotic and antidepressant medication would be a reasonable approach. Mirtazapine, citalopram, fluoxetine, and sertraline are antidepressant medications, while ziprasidone, haloperidol, and perphenazine are antipsychotic medications. Lorazepam and diazepam are benzodiazepines. Divalproex sodium is a mood stabilizer and is used for bipolar disorder.

3. **(C)** The patient most likely has a diagnosis of postpartum depression with psychotic features as the depression started after she gave birth to her son. Hearing a child crying is a common psychotic symptom of postpartum depression. While the patient has been having psychotic symptoms, diagnosing her with a brief psychotic disorder would not fully account for her mood symptoms. In order to meet the diagnosis of schizoaffective disorder, a patient must have psychotic symptoms during a period when there are no mood symptoms present. Adjustment disorder would not account for her psychotic symptoms. Postpartum obsessive compulsive disorder would usually present as a mother with a significant amount of anxiety due to an egodystonic thought.

4. **(A)** The patient would best be treated by initiating an antidepressant such as an SSRI and an antipsychotic to address her hallucinations. Hospitalizing this patient would be premature because the mother is still taking care of her child and is not having any thoughts of wanting to hurt the child or herself. Lithium is indicated as a mood stabilizer for someone who has a diagnosis of bipolar disorder. Haloperidol alone would help treat her psychosis, but would do nothing to address her depression. Providing supportive therapy could help the patient, however, considering the severity of her illness, medications would need to be initiated.

5. **(E)** This patient presents with the signs of Wernicke encephalopathy, which results from thiamine (vitamin B_1) deficiency. It is

characterized by bilateral abducens nerve palsy, horizontal nystagmus, ataxia, and a global confusion accompanied by apathy. Each of the other choices is possible and should be actively ruled out. Alcohol withdrawal usually presents with unstable vital signs, tremulousness, and agitation. Folic acid deficiency presents with diarrhea, cheilosis, and glossitis; neurologic abnormalities are usually not seen. NPH is associated with the classic triad of dementia, incontinence, and gait disturbance. An acute subdural hematoma would typically present after a trauma to the head. Depending on the location of the hematoma, patients can have problems with speech, altered mental status, hemiplegia, and/or a nonreactive pupil.

6. **(C)** If Wernicke is suspected, emergent administration of IV thiamine is essential, because many sequelae of thiamine deficiency are reversible with this treatment; mistaken administration of thiamine is rarely harmful. A CT scan of the head should be ordered immediately in this case; optimally, the IV thiamine would be started as the CT was being arranged. The remaining choices do not address the urgent need to replete thiamine. It should also be noted that giving this patient any glucose prior to administering thiamine can result in a worsening of the Wernicke encephalopathy.

7. **(A)** Delusional disorders typically present with a delusion that is not bizarre. These patients otherwise have an organized thought process and function well in other aspects of their life. In order to have a diagnosis of schizophrenia, the delusion would need to be bizarre, or they should have additional first rank symptoms such as auditory hallucinations, thought withdrawal, or thought broadcasting. This patient does not have any characteristics of bipolar disorder or depression and therefore should not be given a diagnosis of schizoaffective disorder. Paranoid personality disorder could be diagnosed if the paranoia were a longstanding problem that affected multiple aspects of the patient's life but never reached a psychotic (delusional) level. In this case, the only psychotic symptom described is body odor. Patients with obsessive compulsive disorder

have anxiety over particular thoughts that they know are not rational (obsessions), and they perform ritualized behaviors to relieve their anxiety (compulsions).

8. **(D)** Delusional disorders are typically treated with an antipsychotic. Of the choices listed, the only antipsychotic is olanzapine. Fluoxetine is an SSRI and is most commonly used for depression and/or anxiety. Tegretol is an antiepileptic that is also used to treat bipolar disorder. ECT can be used for the management of acute psychosis, but has not been shown to be beneficial in the treatment of delusional disorder. Lithium is a mood stabilizer and is not used as a treatment for delusional disorder.

9. **(D)** NMS is characterized by severe ("lead pipe") rigidity, change in mental status, autonomic instability, elevated CPK, and elevated white blood count; a slight elevation in cerebrospinal fluid protein count is possible. NMS may be induced by any neuroleptic including the newer atypical antipsychotics. No one symptom is necessary for the diagnosis; instead, a constellation of symptoms and their severity, in a setting of neuroleptic exposure, makes the diagnosis more or less likely. Anticholinergic syndrome, resulting from overdosing on anticholinergic medications, does not produce rigidity and an elevated CPK. Malignant hyperthermia, an acute muscular pathologic process, resembles NMS, but follows the administration of inhaled anesthetic agents, as in general surgery. A diagnosis of CNS infection would be better supported by findings on the lumbar puncture and CT or MRI scan; an elevated CPK would be possible if the CNS infection caused seizures. Prolonged immobilization could result in an elevated CPK, but would not account for the other findings.

10. **(C)** Command auditory hallucinations are a psychiatric emergency and most clinicians would agree that this patient should be restarted on a neuroleptic. Because they are long-acting (ie, with a long half-life), depot injections of a neuroleptic are not a first choice. Because the patient is not violent, physical restraints should be avoided. ECT

has some efficacy in treatment-resistant schizophrenia but is not a first-line therapy.

11. **(B)** Command auditory hallucinations to perform suicidal attempts such as overdosing on medications are a psychiatric emergency and usually require psychiatric admission. We are given no clues that there is a necessity to admit the patient to a medical unit; however, she will need a complete medical workup to rule out medical causes of depression. This can usually be accomplished on a psychiatric unit. We are given no indication, such as violent behavior, that this patient needs to be restrained.

12. **(D)** This patient requires an antidepressant and antipsychotic. In fact, either an antidepressant or an antipsychotic would not treat this condition as well as both together. A TCA would not be the first choice. First, there is a suggestion that this patient has some cardiac history and the tricyclics can have a proarrhythmia effect. Second, unlike SSRIs, tricyclics can be lethal in overdose and this patient has risk factors for a suicide attempt, such as a recent breakup with her boyfriend, command auditory hallucinations, and feelings of helplessness. Lithium does have some antidepressant effects, but in the absence of convincing evidence that this patient has a bipolar disorder lithium is not the appropriate choice. (If this patient has only a partial response to the SSRI, lithium may at some point in the future be added for augmentation.) Although a benzodiazepine may help this patient's irritability, as a sole agent it is a poor choice for treating her depression and psychosis.

13. **(A)** The patient most likely has bipolar disorder and is currently in a manic state as characterized by his poor sleep, grandiose ideas, irritable mood, pressured speech, and delusions. Initial medications in this case are aimed at the target symptoms of agitation, delusional thinking, and disruptive behavior and could reasonably include an antipsychotic and a benzodiazepine. While a mood stabilizer such as lithium or carbamazepine could work as well, these are not expected to start showing an effect for at least a week and are not the important medications to start emergently. SSRIs must be used with

extreme caution in bipolar illness because they can incite or exacerbate mania. Buspirone is an anxiolytic used mostly in generalized anxiety disorder. It is of extremely limited use in bipolar disorder and does not adequately address the target symptoms seen in this case.

14. **(A)** When the patient returns for his first follow-up visit, his lithium level is therapeutic at 0.8 mEq/L and is not in need of adjustment. However, his muscle stiffness is a parkinsonian side effect of haloperidol. This is normally treated by lowering the dose of the neuroleptic or with anticholinergic medication, not with a muscle relaxant such as baclofen. The patient would have to be followed closely for reemergence of psychotic symptoms.

15. **(A)** Acute stress disorder is a reaction that may occur in a patient who witnesses or experiences a traumatic event. The event must involve death, threatened death, or serious injury. The typical symptoms include hyperarousal states, dissociative states, and intrusive reexperiencing of the event (eg, flashbacks and avoidance behaviors). PTSD is similar in most respects to acute distress disorder, but in PTSD the symptoms persist for at least 4 weeks following the trauma; a shorter duration suggests a diagnosis of acute distress disorder. The patient does not appear to be suffering from any of the typical criteria for MDD or adjustment disorder, except for guilt. Although she is suffering from agoraphobia, a symptom consistent with an acute stress reaction, there is no evidence of panic attacks or panic disorder.

16. **(C)** While the patient initially had symptoms consistent with acute stress disorder, all of these symptoms resolved with psychotherapy. Had these symptoms persisted over 1 month, she would have met criteria for PTSD. When she presents again a year later, she displays symptoms consistent with MDD such as depressed mood, anhedonia, poor sleep and appetite, and feeling tired all day long. Adjustment disorder should not be diagnosed when a diagnosis of MDD can be made. The patient does not appear to have any panic attacks and she does not describe

fears of having another panic attack which would be consistent with a diagnosis of panic disorder.

17. **(B)** Oculogyric crisis is a specific example of an acute dystonic reaction in which there is spasm of the muscles of extraocular motion. Torticollis and retrocollis refer to muscle spasms that cause abnormal positioning of the head. Trismus is a spasm of the jaw muscles. NMS, also a reaction to neuroleptic medications, is characterized by dystonia, autonomic instability, and usually some degree of delirium.

18. **(B)** Benzodiazepines, SSRIs, and cognitive-behavioral therapy each have a place in treatment of the anxiety disorders. In this case, while the patient does have a history of GAD, she does not have a history of panic attacks. It would be uncommon for a 59-year-old woman to suddenly develop panic attacks. Therefore, a further medical workup is necessary. A short differential diagnosis list would include arrhythmia, hypoglycemia, angina, seizure, and orthostatic hypotension.

19. **(B)** Regardless of a patient's past psychiatric diagnosis, medical causes of physical signs and symptoms must always be ruled out. The anxiety disorders, although intensely distressing and uncomfortable to patients, rarely, if ever, result in unconsciousness. Many aspects of the patient's story seem to be related to anxiety and could in fact occur during a panic attack; however this patient's presentation is more consistent with ischemic heart disease which should prompt a cardiac workup.

20. **(B)** Paraphilias are defined as having intense sexual fantasies or urges toward nonhuman objects, involving humiliation or pain, or toward nonconsenting persons. Paraphilias are further differentiated based on what behavior provides the urges or fantasies. Frotteurism is the desire to rub one's genitals against a nonconsenting person. Voyeurism is the desire to watch people undress without their consent. Masochism is the desire to be humiliated by another person. Sadism is the desire to inflict pain on another person. Exhibitionism is the desire to expose one's genitals to a nonconsenting person.

21. **(E)** While any of these side effects can occur with the use of SSRIs, most of these side effects will go away with time. Sexual dysfunction, either manifesting as delayed orgasm or decreased libido, can remain a side effect in up to 35% to 45% of patients after 3 months of treatment.

22. **(A)** The most common cause of death with a tricyclic antidepressant overdose is a cardiac arrhythmia. Seizures, shock, respiratory failure, and coma can also occur, but are not the most common causes of death. Strokes are typically not caused by overdosing on tricyclic antidepressants.

23. **(E)** The key points in this case presentation are the absence of a previous psychiatric history and the duration of symptoms. Before diagnosing a mental illness, it is necessary to rule out the effects of a substance. A urine toxicology screen usually includes opiates, cocaine, and PCP. Amphetamines, cocaine, and PCP intoxication can mimic symptoms of schizophrenia. Although a CT scan is helpful to rule out a mass lesion or bleeding, these are not likely given his age group or the non-focal neurologic examination. Liver function tests, CBC, and ESR are unlikely to aid in the diagnosis.

24. **(D)** Delusions, hallucinations, and disorganized behavior are some of the hallmark symptoms of schizophrenia. Because the symptoms have been present for more than 1 month but less than 6 months (and there is no previous psychiatric history), the most appropriate diagnosis is schizophreniform disorder. There is no history suggestive of a mood disorder and thus major depression with psychotic features is not as likely. The toxicology screen is negative, so the diagnosis of substance-induced psychotic disorder is less likely. Delusional disorder usually manifests in a middle-aged individual who, while functional in society, experiences a circumscribed delusion of the jealous, erotomanic, grandiose, persecutory, or somatic type. As this patient is also suffering from auditory hallucinations, this also excludes the diagnosis of delusional disorder.

25. **(C)** The patient is most likely experiencing alcohol withdrawal as demonstrated by the fact that since being hospitalized 2 days ago (his last drink) he has had an increase in his blood pressure, heart rate, and has increased anxiety. Often times, patients can also become febrile. Benzodiazepines are the treatment of choice for alcohol withdrawal. Any benzodiazepine can be used—the choice depends on the desired route of delivery or the presence of liver dysfunction. With decreased liver function, lorazepam (Ativan) or oxazepam (Serax) are preferable because they are primarily metabolized and eliminated renally instead of through the liver as are the other benzodiazepines. Additionally, lorazepam may be chosen because it can be given IV, intramuscularly (IM), or by mouth (PO). Methadone or clonidine may be used for opiate withdrawal. Carbamazepine in conjunction with propranolol has been advocated in some settings for alcohol withdrawal, but carbamazepine is not used as single-agent therapy. Naltrexone has been used to help maintain abstinence from alcohol but has no efficacy in withdrawal.

26. **(E)** Alcohol withdrawal can be life-threatening. Tremors begin about 6 to 8 hours after cessation, followed within 8 to 12 hours by psychotic and perceptual abnormalities (hallucinosis). Seizures may follow anywhere from 12 to 72 hours after cessation. Delirium tremens (DTs) may occur any time in the first week of abstinence. Untreated DTs have a mortality rate of approximately 20%. Fatty liver and cirrhosis are long-term consequences of alcohol abuse. Abdominal pain and muscle cramps can be symptoms of opiate withdrawal.

27. **(E)** This patient is experiencing acute intoxication with PCP as illustrated by his agitation, psychosis, vital sign instability, and tics. A toxicology screen is the best way to diagnose this condition. Often, a urine toxicology screen includes opiates, cocaine, and PCP, but this varies depending on individual institutions. There is no indication for an EEG at this time because no seizure history is elicited and the patient does not appear postictal. Although

structural brain lesions can cause psychotic symptoms, substance-induced symptoms are more common in this age group. A nonfocal neurologic examination would further decrease the likelihood that imaging studies would alter the diagnosis or treatment plan in this case.

28. **(A)** Unless the patient is extremely agitated and at risk for hurting himself or others, the best choice for treatment would be to place him in a quiet, dark (low stimulation) room. If the patient is violent and/or psychotic, a combination of neuroleptics and benzodiazepines could be used to keep the patient safe. Methylphenidate is a stimulant. Benztropine, used to prevent extrapyramidal symptoms associated with neuroleptic use, might worsen the patient's delirium. Because the patient is not suffering a seizure or is not at risk for seizures, phenytoin is not indicated.

29. **(E)** The first part of the vignette illustrates some of the features of opiate intoxication, namely pupillary constriction, drowsiness, impaired attention and memory, and slurred speech. In the second interaction, the patient shows signs and symptoms of opiate withdrawal. Yawning, muscle aches, diarrhea, lacrimation or rhinorrhea, and fever are all typical of opiate withdrawal. Additionally, mildly elevated vital signs may occur; however, significant tachycardia and hypertension should always signal possible alcohol withdrawal. Pharmacologic management of withdrawal can include clonidine, a centrally acting alpha-2-agonist; and methadone, a synthetic long-acting opiate. Lorazepam can be used to treat elevated vital signs and loperamide can be used to treat diarrhea.

30. **(E)** Triazolam is a short-acting benzodiazepine. Sudden discontinuation of any sedative, hypnotic, or anxiolytic agent, such as benzodiazepines, can cause significant withdrawal symptoms, including seizures. Thioridazine and fluphenazine are neuroleptics, and nortriptyline and imipramine are TCAs. Neither TCAs nor neuroleptics cause life-threatening withdrawal symptoms.

31. **(B)** As with the sudden discontinuation of alcohol, benzodiazepine or barbiturate withdrawal can be life-threatening. Withdrawal symptoms include tremors, anxiety, auditory, visual, and tactile hallucinations, autonomic hyperactivity, and seizures. The onset of symptoms depends on the half-life of the medication, the dose, and duration of use. The most concerning discontinuation side effect is seizures.

32. **(B)** The patient is exhibiting typical signs of delirium, including an impaired level of consciousness and difficulty with cognition, manifested as drowsiness and disorientation. Classically, these symptoms may fluctuate during the day. Patients who meet criteria for delirium may appear depressed with a decreased level of arousal or may appear overly active and energetic, with the depressed type occurring more commonly. Patients also show cognitive and memory impairments, which may be manifested as disorientation or decreased capacity to register, retain, and recall information. An MMSE may also be low due to an underlying dementia or depressive illness. In this setting, it would be important to gather information from family or other individuals who know the patient in order to evaluate for a possible coexisting dementia or major depression. Risk factors for delirium are extremes of age, prior history of delirium, alcohol dependence, sensory impairment (auditory or visual), and preexisting brain damage. There is a broad etiologic differential for delirium. In this case, causative factors may be infection, hypoxia, metabolic abnormalities, and current medications.

33. **(D)** Haloperidol is the drug of choice for managing the agitated or confused patient with delirium. Thioridazine, benztropine, and diphenhydramine all have anticholinergic properties that may actually worsen the delirium. Lorazepam, especially in older patients, may have a paradoxical disinhibiting effect and exacerbate agitation and confusion. Haloperidol in low doses, such as 0.5 mg every 8 hours, helps to manage the agitated patient. It has the advantage of IM, IV, or PO administration.

34. **(B)** The cluster B categories of personality disorders are characterized as the dramatic and emotional personality group. Borderline personality disorder (PD) manifests as a longstanding pattern of instability in many aspects of their lives. They see things in either black or white, contributing to a great deal of affect dysregulation. Self-mutilation such as superficial cutting or burning is common. Histrionic PD patients typically display dramatic but superficial emotions, with oversexualized behaviors. Narcissistic PD patients display an overvalued sense of self, entitlement, and rage. Bipolar disorder and major depression are affective disorders that present as having periods of good functioning along with periods of impairment or distress during the acute episodes (eg, during manic or depressed phases).

35. **(A)** Dialectical behavioral therapy is considered the treatment of choice for patients with borderline personality disorder. Psychoanalysis can be used for different psychiatric illnesses; however, it is not considered a first-line treatment for borderline personality disorder. Medications, especially SSRIs, can be affective for borderline personality disorder, however, medications tend to be more useful in conjunction with psychotherapy and should be tailored to specific symptoms.

36. **(C)** This patient is exhibiting signs and symptoms consistent with major depressive disorder (MDD) with psychotic features. For more than 2 weeks, the patient has displayed depressed mood, loss of interest in pleasurable activities, weight loss, inability to concentrate, poor sleep, and guilt about her current depressive state. She is also suffering delusional concerns about bodily functioning and infection. If the patient were complaining of contamination fears and performing multiple compulsive tasks to rid herself of the pathogens, a diagnosis of OCD with comorbid depression could be considered. Somatization disorder is a chronic condition characterized by a myriad of somatic complaints, including four pain symptoms, and at least one neurologic and sexual symptom. Dysthymia presents with a chronic moderate

level of depressive symptoms, but this patient is describing an acute episodic decompensation over the last month.

37. **(E)** Because of the delusional quality to her presentation, the treatment of choice is both an antidepressant and an antipsychotic, or electroconvulsive therapy (ECT). Antidepressants alone with or without benzodiazepines would not help with her psychotic symptoms. Lithium and divalproex sodium are used as mood stabilizers in bipolar depression or mania but not commonly in the treatment of unipolar depression.

38. **(A)** Brief psychotic disorder is diagnosed when symptoms have been persistent for more than 1 day but less than 1 month. Delusional disorder is a condition usually beginning in middle age in which the primary symptom is a non-bizarre delusion; that is, it could possibly occur. Delusional disorder is further classified into subtypes, including grandiose, jealous, persecutory, somatic, erotomanic, and unspecified. There are no symptoms of a mood disorder such as a depressed, irritable, or elevated mood. Schizophrenia would be diagnosed if the patient's symptoms occurred for longer than 6 months, and schizophreniform disorder would be diagnosed if these symptoms persisted for greater than 1 month but fewer than 6 months.

39. **(E)** The most helpful test would be a urine toxicology screen, since intoxication with a variety of substances, including cocaine, PCP, or amphetamines may mimic the symptoms of schizophrenia. It is necessary to first rule out these intoxication syndromes prior to making a diagnosis of a primary psychotic illness, such as schizophrenia. A CT scan may help to rule out a mass lesion or a bleed, but his age and a nonfocal neurologic examination make this unlikely to be contributing to this presentation. Similarly, because the patient does not present with signs or symptoms of a seizure disorder, an EEG is unlikely to provide information that will impact the diagnosis. There is no specific diagnostic utility for a CBC or electrolytes for any of the primary psychotic disorders.

40. **(B)** The patient has a diagnosis of MDD as characterized by the depressed mood, poor concentration, poor sleep, poor appetite, and guilty feelings. The diagnosis of normal bereavement should not be made because of the thoughts of suicide. There are two choices for antidepressants in this group. Phenelzine, an MAOI, is not the first choice of antidepressant because the SSRIs have a more favorable side effect profile, are safer in overdose, and have similar efficacy in the treatment of MDD. Fluoxetine, therefore, is the best choice at this time. Triazolam is a benzodiazepine, flumazenil is a benzodiazepine antagonist used for the treatment of benzodiazepine overdose, and fluphenazine is an antipsychotic.

41. **(D)** SSRIs have a number of side effects, including diarrhea, constipation, nausea, headache, sexual dysfunction, and agitation. A frequent, initial side effect is insomnia, which is also a common symptom of depression. Most of the above side effects improve after several days. Constipation and akathisia are also common side effects of antipsychotics.

42. **(B)** Normal bereavement can appear similar to a major depressive episode (MDE), but there are ways to distinguish between the two. MDE should be considered if the depressive symptoms last for longer than 2 months after the person died, if the survivor has guilt surrounding anything other than actions they should have taken to prevent the death, if the survivor has prominent hallucinations (except for occasional experiences where they can see or hear the deceased), psychomotor retardation, or thoughts of wanting to end their life. Schizophrenia would not be an appropriate diagnosis because the patient does not have a previous psychiatric history and the hallucinations are better accounted for by bereavement. A diagnosis of dysthymic disorder should be considered for patients who have depressive symptoms more often than not for 2 years. The recent death excludes the diagnosis of adjustment disorder.

43. **(E)** At this time, the person meets criteria for normal bereavement and no further interventions at this time are necessary. Should the

symptoms continue for a longer period of time, worsen, or the patient becomes less functional, initiating an antidepressant such as fluoxetine or amitriptyline would be appropriate. Lithium is indicated for bipolar disorder. The patient's auditory hallucinations are still considered to be a normal part of bereavement at this time, so an antipsychotic should not be initiated unless the voices become more distressing and pervasive.

44. **(B)** Adjustment disorder is characterized by the onset of emotional or behavioral disturbances within 3 months of a significant life event that may manifest as marked change in an individual's ability to function in school, work, or interpersonal relationships. The disturbances are not so severe, however, as to suggest the diagnosis of another disorder such as MDD. The differential diagnosis for adjustment disorder includes mood disorders such as MDD and anxiety disorders such as PTSD, GAD, and acute stress disorder. In this case, the patient may be suffering from depressed mood but does not have other neurovegetative signs of depression. Acute stress disorder is usually diagnosed when an individual who has experienced an extreme stressor has dissociative experiences and anxiety shortly after the traumatic experience. Similarly, PTSD usually requires exposure to or witnessing of a life-threatening event, with episodes of reexperiencing the event, hyperarousal states, and efforts to avoid settings that remind the patient of the experience. In this case, the patient has experienced a significant stressor, but it is not a life-threatening event as is required for the diagnosis of acute stress disorder or PTSD. In addition, this patient is not describing these symptoms. Bereavement is the normal response to the loss or death of an individual close to the patient.

45. **(D)** The diagnosis of adjustment disorder does not usually require pharmacotherapeutic intervention, but instead may respond to supportive, individual, or group psychotherapy. Risperidone is an atypical antipsychotic. Fluoxetine is an SSRI, and nortriptyline is a TCA, both antidepressants. Alprazolam is a benzodiazepine used for the treatment of anxiety.

46. **(B)** This patient is describing symptoms associated with panic disorder. This disorder begins in late adolescence or early adulthood and is more common in women than in men. People typically describe feelings of fear, dread, or intense discomfort associated with a variety of somatic symptoms, including tachycardia, chest pain, shortness of breath, tremulousness, diaphoresis, nausea, fear of dying, paresthesias, light headedness, and hot or cold flashes. The diagnosis of agoraphobia is made when fears of having an attack or being unable to escape during an attack force patients to remain in familiar places. The medical workup for panic disorder includes CBC, electrolytes, fasting glucose, calcium, liver function tests, BUN, creatinine, urinalysis, toxicology screen, ECG, and thyroid function studies. A careful substance abuse and caffeine intake history should also be obtained. Social phobia or social anxiety disorder occurs in the context of public appearances or performances, where individuals experience anxiety and fear. These feelings cause great distress and may cause people to avoid these settings. This disorder differs from panic disorder by having an identifiable trigger. Specific phobias also have an identifiable trigger. Separation anxiety disorder is usually diagnosed in young children who display excessive anxiety when separated from their primary caregiver. GAD occurs in individuals experiencing continued anxiety and worry over several events lasting for greater than 6 months. In contrast to panic disorder, there are not discrete episodes in GAD.

47. **(D)** A variety of medications, including SSRIs (sertraline), TCAs, MAOIs (tranylcypromine), and benzodiazepines (alprazolam) have been used to treat panic disorder. Although all have shown some efficacy in the treatment of panic, SSRIs are usually the first agent of choice because they are generally well-tolerated, with fewer side effects than TCAs or MAOIs, and lack the dependency potential of benzodiazepines. Common side effects include sexual dysfunction, gastrointestinal disturbances, and insomnia. Lithium is used in the treatment of bipolar disorder, and propranolol can be used for social phobia.

48. **(C)** The patient likely has obsessive-compulsive disorder (OCD) as she suffers from recurrent, intrusive, unwanted thoughts or images (obsessions) and repetitive behaviors or mental acts (compulsions) that are performed in response to these obsessions. Patients realize that the obsessions and compulsions are unreasonable, and they cause marked impairment in their lives. Many patients with OCD hide their symptoms and may first come to the attention of other medical specialists. Somatization disorder presents with numerous somatic complaints that cannot be fully explained by the results of medical investigations. GAD is a suitable diagnosis in individuals who have worries and concerns that are not limited to any particular aspect of their lives, but with the anxiety significantly impairing their ability to function. Panic disorder manifests as recurrent, discrete episodes of extreme anxiety and fear that occur unexpectedly and remit spontaneously.

49. **(A)** A widespread and effective treatment for OCD is cognitive-behavioral therapy, during which the patient is exposed to the threat or fear (obsession) with the response (hand washing) prevented for progressively longer periods of time until the behavior is extinguished. SSRIs have also been successful in the treatment of OCD. Risperidone is an atypical neuroleptic that is used to treat psychotic disorders. Lithium is used in the treatment of bipolar disorder and has not been shown to be effective in the treatment of OCD. Psychodynamic psychotherapy is intensive, long-term therapy that may be helpful for people who wish to better understand the nature of their relationship with others, but it has not demonstrated significant efficacy in OCD.

50. **(A)** Symptoms of excessive worry and anxiety occurring for over 6 months without discrete episodes are best characterized by the diagnosis of GAD. Other symptoms of GAD include sleep difficulties, irritability, and difficulty concentrating. Patients with GAD may also suffer from muscle tension, fatigue, and restlessness. Although this patient does admit to anxiety, it does not occur in an episodic fashion or in response to public performances, as with panic disorder or social phobia, respectively. Similarly, although the symptoms of anxiety and worry are in excess of what would be expected, they do not reach the magnitude characteristic for OCD, nor are any specific obsessions or compulsions elicited. There is no evidence of psychosis in this patient.

51. **(A)** The diagnosis of conversion disorder is most likely given that the primary symptoms are neurologic and the workup is negative for evidence of pathology that would account for the deficits. Neurologic deficits in conversion disorder involve either motor or sensory modalities and are believed to be a result of underlying, unconscious psychological conflicts or stressors. Had the symptoms been intentionally produced, the diagnosis of factitious disorder or malingering would be appropriate. If the primary incentive for the behavior was to assume the sick role, the diagnosis would be factitious disorder. If the symptoms are feigned or exaggerated in order to gain monetary reimbursement, the diagnosis would be malingering. Somatization disorder is not appropriate in this case because the number and types of complaints do not extend past the neurologic complaints. An undiagnosed neurologic condition is a possibility, but given the presentation and physical examination, it is less likely. It is important to note that as many as 25% to 50% of those diagnosed with conversion disorder are eventually diagnosed with a neurologic condition that could have produced the initial symptoms.

52. **(B)** Factitious disorder is an appropriate diagnosis when physical or psychological symptoms are intentionally produced in order to assume the sick role. It must be clear that these symptoms are not intentionally produced for other reasons, such as avoiding work, gaining monetary compensation, or avoiding legal issues. If any of these reasons are present, the diagnosis is malingering. Somatization disorder presents with multiple complaints of pain, gastrointestinal symptoms, sexual dysfunction, and pseudoneurological symptoms. The diagnosis of hypochondriasis is not appropriate as this patient is not preoccupied with the idea of

having a severe disease that is unrecognized despite repeated reassurances by medical personnel. Classically, people with factitious disorder are more likely to be female and to have experience in health care. Often, these patients will have numerous admissions to many different hospitals with a variety of symptoms. The psychological factors underlying this disorder are not well understood. No effective form of psychotherapy or pharmacotherapy has been identified for the treatment of factitious disorder.

53. **(A)** The most likely diagnosis in this patient is anorexia nervosa and is supported by the fact that she appears very underweight and continues to feel that she needs to lose more weight, her excessive exercising, and her lack of a menstrual period. Bulimia nervosa can be excluded because she does not have a regular menstrual period and she appears underweight. While the patient does have symptoms suggestive of MDD such as problems with sleep, poor concentration, and fatigue, it does not mention any problem with her mood or with anhedonia, which are required for a diagnosis of MDD. Patients with body dysmorphic disorder generally focus on one specific defect rather than something as general as weight. While the patient does have some anxiety, it is not clear if her anxiety has reached to a level that it is causing any type of dysfunction in her daily activities.

54. **(E)** Obtaining height and weight is crucial for establishing the diagnosis of anorexia nervosa as patients with anorexia nervosa are unable to achieve or maintain greater than 85% of expected body weight for height and frame structure. Additionally, they have continued concerns about thinness and body image despite being underweight. In contrast, most patients with bulimia nervosa are of normal height and weight or are slightly overweight.

55. **(E)** Given the patient's history of anger and aggressive outbursts when not understanding schoolwork, difficulties with socialization and caring for himself, as well as a family history of learning disabilities, you suspect the diagnosis

of mental retardation. A diagnosis of mental retardation includes subnormal functioning with an IQ of less than 70. Either the WISC or the Stanford-Binet Intelligence Scale is an adequate instrument for estimating IQ. The MMPI-2 is frequently used to assess personality structure. The Goodenough-Harris Draw-A-Person Test and Kohs Block Test assess visual-motor coordination. The Peabody-Vocabulary Test is used when patients suffer from a language barrier.

56. **(B)** Mental retardation is classified according to severity based on IQ scores: mild mental retardation is 50 to 70; moderate is 35 to 49; severe is 20 to 34; and profound is less than 20. Borderline intellectual functioning refers to an IQ score in the 71 to 84 range.

57. **(B)** This patient suffers from Tourette disorder, a syndrome of multiple motor and vocal tics that occur daily for at least 1 year, with the onset before age 18. Tourette disorder occurs more commonly in boys than girls. First-line treatment for mild to moderate Tourette disorder is clonidine. An antipsychotic can be used to treat the disorder, but is usually reserved for patients with more severe cases. Lorazepam is a benzodiazepine and is typically used for anxiety disorders and sleep. Valproic acid and lamotrigine are mood stabilizer used for the treatment of bipolar disorder. Atomoxetine is a selective norepinephrine reuptake inhibitor that has been used for the treatment of ADHD. It can be effective for children who develop tics after using stimulants, but is not a first-line agent.

58. **(D)** Given the significant improvement due to the medication, it would not be appropriate at this time to discontinue or switch medications. Sedation is the most common side effect of clonidine and will often go away after a few weeks. However, if it continues or interferes in functioning, a dosage reduction should be attempted before making any other changes.

59. **(B)** Epilepsy is a complex set of disorders that may initially come to the attention of a psychiatrist because of unusual behaviors. Complex partial seizures, in particular, may be associated

with a wide range of symptoms, including sensory auras and automatic behaviors. Prior to the seizure, the patient may notice a bad smell, an unusual taste, or gastrointestinal symptoms. During the event, the patient may look dazed or frightened and may exhibit a number of automatisms such as lip smacking, eye blinking, and fumbling with his or her clothes. Additionally, there is impairment of consciousness. Complex partial seizures are usually associated with temporal lobe epilepsy but can also result from lesions elsewhere in the brain. In this particular case, another diagnosis to rule out is amphetamine intoxication. Amphetamines are commonly used to treat ADHD and may be drugs of abuse in this age group. Intoxication with amphetamines may present as seizures and can be easily ruled out by a urine toxicology screen.

60. **(D)** Although syphilitic infections have been on the decline since World War I, they must still be considered in the differential for a wide variety of psychiatric disorders, especially when combined with neurologic abnormalities. In this case, two forms of neurosyphilis (tabes dorsalis and general paresis) are combined in one patient. Patients demonstrate sensory ataxia with a wide-based gait, a positive Romberg sign, and a loss of vibratory and proprioceptive senses initially in the lower extremities. Deep tendon reflexes are decreased and pupil abnormalities are common, although the full Argyll-Robertson pupil (a pupil that accommodates but does not react to light) is infrequent. General paresis is usually associated with a dementing process along with neurologic symptoms such as pupil abnormalities, tremors, dyscoordination, and spasticity in the lower extremities. Testing for neurosyphilis should include a blood test for VDRL and fluorescent treponemal antibody absorption test (FTA-ABS). Consideration should also be given to performing a lumbar puncture to test cerebrospinal fluid for evidence of treponemal infection. Although this patient has some symptoms of Wernicke encephalopathy and Korsakoff psychosis, neither diagnosis alone would account for this patient's constellation of neuropsychiatric symptoms. A diagnosis of NMS should not be entertained because he is currently not taking an antipsychotic medication.

61. **(D)** Pheochromocytoma is a tumor of the chromaffin cells, usually occurring in the adrenal medulla. Symptoms may differ according to the predominant catecholamine released. As norepinephrine-secreting tumors are the most common, baseline hypertension with paroxysmal exacerbations are frequent. Anxiety, fear, and palpitations may accompany exacerbations of hypertension. Because this may mimic symptoms of a panic attack or GAD, it is essential to consider this in the differential diagnosis when patients present with anxiety coupled with physiologic changes.

62. **(B)** Hepatic encephalopathy can present in many ways and may have a fluctuating course making it difficult to diagnose without peripheral stigmata. Neurologically, the patient may exhibit asterixis, which, although characteristic for hepatic encephalopathy, is not specific for the disorder. Patients may display 6- to 9-Hz tremors, mildly increased deep tendon reflexes, and an altered sensorium. Typical psychiatric symptoms may include changes in personality, abrupt mood swings, and changes in cognitive ability. In an acute decompensation, depression, catatonia, psychosis, and delirium may develop. Physical stigmata reflecting changes in liver function can include ecchymosis, peripheral edema, ascites formation, palmar erythema, and spider angiomas.

63. **(C)** HIV can produce a spectrum of neuropsychiatric manifestations as a result of opportunistic infections, neoplasms, or direct invasion of the CNS by the virus. HIV-associated dementia is one of the most common manifestations of primary CNS invasion. Criteria for dementia include memory impairment plus the presence of at least one cognitive disturbance, such as aphasia, apraxia, agnosia, or disturbance in executive function. It may present in a variety of ways, including motor abnormalities, cognitive decline, or behavioral changes. This case describes typical behavioral changes, for example, lethargy and social withdrawal. HIV dementia may also include neurologic abnormalities such as weakness, imbalance, or ataxia, as well as with irritability and apathy. The results of the MMSE support the diagnosis of dementia.

64. (D) This case illustrates a presentation of hyperthyroidism with depression, irritability, and cognitive difficulty. Hyperthyroidism may present with symptoms consistent with a variety of psychiatric disorders, including depression, anxiety, psychosis, mania, and, at an extreme, delirium. Patients may report hot flashes and/or increased sensitivity to heat. Hyperthyroidism may also cause mild cognitive deficits in calculation and recent memory. Neurologically, patients may demonstrate a fine 8- to 12-Hz tremor, lid lag, brisk deep tendon reflexes, proximal myopathy with muscle wasting, and myalgias.

65. (H) Somatization disorder is characterized by a variety of somatic complaints that cannot be verified by laboratory and physical findings. The disorder has its onset before age 30 and is more common in women than in men. Diagnosis is based on the occurrence of four pain symptoms, two gastrointestinal symptoms, one sexual symptom, and one pseudoneurologic symptom. It is important to determine that these symptoms are not intentionally produced or feigned for other purposes. Similarly, it is important to ensure that the patient has received the appropriate medical workup because a number of disease processes may present with a constellation of symptoms. Basic tests that could be ordered include blood tests, ECG, colonoscopy, and gynecological examinations.

66. (G) Depression is a common symptom of SLE. Although neuropsychiatric conditions may arise at any time during the course of the disease, they are most frequent during acute exacerbations or late in the disease process. Other symptoms include delirium, personality changes, anxiety, and psychosis. Patients may also exhibit cognitive impairment on neuropsychological testing. Neurologically, patients can present with seizures, stroke, cranial nerve abnormalities, and headache.

67. (E) This patient is exhibiting signs and symptoms consistent with delirium secondary to hypoglycemia. Signs of hypoglycemia manifested by this patient include tachycardia, tremor, hypertension, and seizure. Delirious

states should receive immediate workup for an etiology as they carry a significant rate of morbidity and mortality. A standard workup consists of a CBC with differential, electrolytes, BUN, creatinine, VDRL, vitamin B_{12}, folate, urinalysis, thyroid-stimulating hormone (TSH), calcium, magnesium, phosphorus, glucose, urine toxicology screen, liver function tests, peripheral oxygen saturation, chest x-ray, ECG, as well as mental status and physical examination.

68. (A) Patients with Alzheimer disease typically present with memory problems which gradually worsen, as well as either an aphasia, apraxia, agnosia, or disturbances in executive functioning. In this case, she demonstrates memory problems and an agnosia (unable to name a pencil).

69. (E) Lewy body dementia typically presents as well-formed visual hallucinations (peduncular hallucinosis or Lilliputionism) late in life without previous psychiatric disturbances. Motor disturbances are similar to that of Parkinson disease but tend to occur at the same time as the cognitive deficits. Motor problems include cogwheel rigidity, shuffling gait, and reduced arm swing. The typical pill-rolling tremor of Parkinson disease is less common.

70. (G) Pick disease is characterized by changes in personality early in the illness. Primitive reflexes are seen, such as the suck, Babinski, and snout. Other features of dementia such as aphasia, apraxia, and agnosia typically occur late in the disease. Imaging is usually characterized by preferential atrophy of the frontal and temporal lobes. Confirmation of the diagnosis is made via biopsy or autopsy and reveals Pick inclusion bodies.

71. (C) Delirium is a syndrome consisting of a fluctuation in the level of attention and consciousness, symptoms of which can wax and wane. It is essential to look for one or more underlying causes, such as electrolyte abnormalities, infections, and side effects of medications. In contrast to dementia, delirium has an acute onset of symptoms and is typically reversible once the underlying etiology is corrected.

72. **(F)** Pseudodementia is a term referring to the cognitive disturbances ("dementia") caused by a depressive illness, such as major depression. Patients typically present with depressed affect, neurovegetative symptoms, and memory problems. During examination, patients demonstrate poor concentration and motivation such that they have difficulty completing questioning. Pseudodementia is reversible once the depression is treated.

73. **(D)** Huntington disease is an autosomal dominant disease caused by a CAG repeat on the short arm of chromosome number 4. The disease typically causes psychiatric disturbances such as depression or anxiety, hallucinations, memory problems, and choreiform movements. On imaging, patients may have boxcar ventricles that appear as having corners rather than rounded edges.

74. **(C)** Because the defense mechanism of denial is primary in alcoholism, the best approach in evaluating a patient is to explore how alcohol affects his life, rather than direct questions about drinking behavior. Hearing about his drinking from his friends and family may provide a more accurate description of a patient's alcoholism than the alcoholic would provide of himself. Although laboratory work might provide clues to the presence of alcoholism, it cannot be relied on to make the diagnosis.

75. **(B)** GAD is defined by excessive anxiety or worry occurring for at least 6 months. Associated symptoms include feeling restless, fatigued, or irritable; muscle tension; difficulty with concentration; and sleep disturbance. Patients with panic disorder are usually more disabled by their symptoms and seek help much earlier than patients with GAD. The onset of anxiety with panic disorder is more sudden and intense, with the fear of choking or dying more common, and the panic attacks are recurrent and unexpected. Although depression and dysthymia share some symptoms with GAD, the depressive symptoms are more severe in the mood disorders than with the anxiety disorders. Separation anxiety

requires the onset of symptoms before the age of 18, and dependent personality disorder represents a pattern of the pervasive need to be taken care of, leading to submissive, clinging behavior that begins in early childhood.

76. **(A)** Negative thoughts regarding the self, the world, and the future are known as the Beck cognitive triad. Beck, who developed the Beck Depression Inventory, pioneered the use of cognitive therapy for depressive disorders. This triad of symptoms is helpful in understanding and treating depression with cognitive therapy and is not characteristically seen in other disorders.

77. **(B)** Cognitive therapy can help to target these negative ways of perceiving the self and the environment. In paradoxical therapy, developed by Bateson, the therapist suggests that the patient engage in the behavior with negative connotations (eg, a phobia or compulsion). Behavioral therapy is focused on behaviors, not on underlying factors (such as cognitive errors) that cause behaviors. Couples therapy would be less efficacious than cognitive therapy given this patient's symptoms. The major focus of interpersonal psychotherapy is communication analysis and one's role in relationships.

78. **(A)** About 40% of alcoholics will become severely depressed within the first week of abstaining from alcohol. However, if they are able to abstain from alcohol for a total of 4 weeks, only 5% of people will continue to have symptoms of depression.

79. **(E)** This patient continues to experience a depressed mood and neurovegetative symptoms (insomnia, anergia, poor concentration) 6 weeks after the cessation of alcohol. Depressive symptoms during the first 4 weeks of stopping the use of alcohol are more likely to be substance-induced. However, the fact that the depressive episode has lasted longer than 4 weeks after the cessation of alcohol points to an underlying (comorbid) mood disorder such as a major depressive disorder (MDD) rather than a substance-induced mood disorder.

Sertraline is an SSRI and is a first-line agent for the treatment for MDD. While amitriptyline (a tricyclic antidepressant) is an option, because of its side effect profile and lethality in overdose, it is typically not used as a first-line agent for depression. Buspirone is an anxiolytic used for the treatment of generalized anxiety disorder. Lithium is a mood stabilizer typically used for bipolar disorder (mania) and not commonly for unipolar depression. Lorazepam (a benzodiazepine) is also an anxiolytic, but it would not address the patient's depressive symptoms and can cause dependence, especially in this patient with a history of alcohol addiction.

80. **(D)** This patient is experiencing an acute Wernicke encephalopathy caused by administration of glucose without thiamine. In alcoholics who are likely to have low levels of thiamine, giving glucose prior to giving thiamine can often precipitate this condition because glucose oxidation requires a lot of thiamine, depleting the remaining stores of thiamine in the body. This depletion can cause a rapid drop in the thiamine levels which causes the encephalopathy.

81. **(D)** Korsakoff syndrome is an anterograde amnestic disorder caused by chronic thiamine deficiency, which classically presents with confabulation where the patients make up aspects of their life that they cannot remember. It is caused by damage to the mammillary bodies. Conversion disorder should only be made when there is no other reasonable explanation for neurologic symptoms. In this case, the patient is not faking his symptoms for a secondary gain making the diagnosis of malingering incorrect. Delirium is a problem of attention, not memory. Alzheimer disease, which does present with memory disturbances, does not present so acutely.

82. **(C)** Mood-congruent delusions are compatible and consistent with the state of mind of the patient. In this case, the patient feels guilty and presumably believes he deserves punishment. His delusions express these thoughts.

If he described delusions of grandiosity, that would be an example of a mood-incongruent delusion. Bizarre delusions describe circumstances that are impossible to be true, for example, a schizophrenic patient believing a computer chip is implanted in his brain. The delusions in this question, however unlikely, are in some sense conceivable. Somatic delusions focus on bodily functions and integrity. Ego-syntonic delusions are experienced by the sufferer as acceptable; for example, the manic patient believing he is the greatest actor in the world. This patient's delusions are ego-dystonic, experienced as unacceptable and unpleasant.

83. **(C)** Often, the nature of the delusion and its relation to mood state can provide clues to a diagnosis. Delusions arising out of a severe depression, as in this case, are frequently mood congruent. The delusions of schizophrenic patients can be bizarre and are often unrelated to mood state. Mania produces delusions that are grandiose, usually related to a sense of inflated self-esteem. The presence of delusions rules out dysthymia and adjustment disorder as these affective illnesses do not reach a severity that includes delusional thinking.

84. **(C)** Patients with schizoid personality disorder are typically socially isolated and distinctly inept at forming and carrying on interpersonal relationships. They often come to the attention of physicians as a result of some other issue, as seen in this case. Their apparent apathy and indifference may resemble the negative symptoms of schizophrenia, and indeed, that is in the differential here; but it would be difficult to make a diagnosis of schizophrenia without evidence of psychosis. This patient lacks the actively odd and peculiar mannerisms or eccentric way of thinking seen in schizotypal personality disorder. He exhibits none of the mistrust and suspiciousness seen in paranoid personality disorder. Although he may be depressed, we are given no direct evidence of this.

85. **(E)** Bipolar disorder has one of the largest genetic components of all the mental illnesses. Having a monozygotic twin with bipolar disorder increases the risk of developing bipolar disorder to 80% to 90%.

86. **(C)** Schizophrenia is commonly classified according to types, which try to descriptively capture the symptoms that dominate the clinical picture. In the paranoid type, the patient is preoccupied with delusions, typically persecutory in nature, and often has auditory hallucinations. Speech and behavior appear relatively organized. The disorganized type is characterized by disorganized speech and behavior as well as a flat or inappropriate affect. In catatonic type, motor activity is retarded to the point of immobility, or else excessive, purposeless, and unrelated to external events. A diagnosis of undifferentiated type indicates that the patient meets criteria for schizophrenia, but does not meet criteria for paranoid, disorganized, or catatonic types. The residual type describes an absence of positive symptoms and a preponderance of negative symptoms.

87. **(D)** From a safety standpoint, the most important feature of voices heard by a patient with schizophrenia is the nature of what the voices are saying. Command auditory hallucinations telling a patient to harm or kill him or herself or someone else are almost always a psychiatric emergency, often requiring hospitalization. A possible exception may be where an experienced clinician knows the patient well and believes the situation to be safe. All of the other choices in this question speak to important characteristics of auditory hallucinations that should be evaluated, but the presence of command auditory hallucinations requires immediate attention.

88. **(D)** Narcolepsy is characterized by persistent daytime hypersomnolence that is temporarily relieved by brief naps. Narcolepsy is often accompanied by phenomena commonly associated with inappropriate REM sleep, including hypnagogic or hypnopompic hallucinations (vivid hallucinations upon falling asleep or waking up), cataplexy (a sudden dramatic loss of muscle tone, usually following an intense emotional reaction), and sleep paralysis (a loss of voluntary muscle tone at the beginning or end of sleep, as seen in this case). Idiopathic hypersomnolence is also characterized by persistent sleepiness but can be distinguished from narcolepsy by the fact that the naps accompanying it are often long and unrefreshing. Advanced sleep-phase syndrome refers to people whose social/occupational functioning is disturbed by their drowsiness during the evening. Delayed sleep-phase syndrome refers to those whose social/occupational functioning is disturbed by drowsiness in the morning and alertness in the evening. Parasomnias are behaviors that are worsened or only occur during sleep.

89. **(C)** The patient in this question has a previous substance abuse history. Because of this, choosing nonaddictive medications would be preferred over addictive medications. Diphenhydramine is a histamine blocker and is not addictive. It can be helpful for patients with insomnia. Alprazolam and zolpidem, while they can be beneficial, do have an addictive potential. Codeine is an opiate, and, while one side effect is sedation, it should be used for the relief of pain. Quetiapine is an antipsychotic which causes sedation. However, due to its side effect profile such as movement disorders, weight gain, increased cholesterol, and increased fasting sugars, it should not be used as a first-line agent for insomnia.

90–101. **[90 (D), 91 (C), 92 (B), 93 (D), 94 (B), 95 (A), 96 (A), 97 (C), 98 (A), 99 (B), 100 (D), 101 (A)]** It is useful to distinguish the various axes of the *Diagnostic and Statistical Manual of Mental Disorders* (DSM's) multiaxial classification system from one another, particularly on the wards when it is necessary to write notes. The system is used to categorize and organize the diagnoses utilizing a biopsychosocial formulation. Axis I includes all mental illnesses, including substance abuse and developmental disorders, *except* personality disorders and mental retardation, which are coded on Axis II. Axis III includes general medical conditions, and Axis IV includes psychosocial and environmental factors that may be contributing to the mental illness. The Global Assessment of Functioning, a scale from 0 to 100, is used to rate the level of psychological, social, and occupational functioning, and it is coded on Axis V.

CHAPTER 7

Practice Test 1
Questions

DIRECTIONS (Questions 1 through 107): For each of the multiple choice questions in this section, select the lettered answer that is the one *best* response in each case.

Questions 1 and 2

A 29-year-old man with a history of bipolar disorder presents to the psychiatric emergency department saying that he is the king of "Pumbar" and needs everyone's allegiance for the upcoming war with the Martians. In the past few days, he has slept a total of 3 hours but says that he is not tired. He has spent all of his money soliciting phone sex. Now, he is agitated, demanding, and threatening.

1. Which of the following is the best treatment for this patient in the acute setting?

    (A) carbamazepine (Tegretol)
    (B) divalproex sodium (Depakote)
    (C) haloperidol (Haldol)
    (D) hydroxyzine (Atarax)
    (E) lithium

2. After treating the patient acutely, a medication is required for ongoing treatment of his bipolar disorder. You find that he has a history of agranulocytosis. Which of the following is the best choice for his treatment ?

    (A) antipsychotic medication
    (B) carbamazepine
    (C) divalproex sodium
    (D) lithium
    (E) lorazepam (Ativan)

Questions 3 and 4

A 44-year-old woman presents to her primary care doctor with multiple complaints, including weakness in her lower extremities, bloating, headaches, intermittent loss of appetite, and back pain. A careful review of symptoms reveals many other vague symptoms. Her complaints date back to adolescence and she has seen many doctors. Thorough workups, including an exploratory laparotomy, have failed to uncover any clear, anatomic or physiologic cause.

3. Which of the following is the best approach to this patient?

    (A) Tell her any physical workup is unnecessary.
    (B) Tell her to come back in 1 month and, if the symptoms are still present, you will initiate a physical workup.
    (C) Tactfully ask her why she is inventing symptoms.
    (D) Assess her for other psychiatric illnesses.
    (E) Initiate a physical workup and arrange for follow-up in a year's time.

4. Which of the following personality disorders would most likely be comorbid in the above patient?

    (A) avoidant
    (B) histrionic
    (C) obsessive-compulsive
    (D) paranoid
    (E) schizotypal

Questions 5 and 6

A 50-year-old man is a concern to his neighbors. He works at a comic-book store, dresses in odd, outdated clothes, and displays poor eye contact. Although he tends to keep to himself, he has told neighborhood children that there are witches who live down the street.

5. Which of the following is the most likely diagnosis?

   (A) bipolar disorder
   (B) borderline personality disorder
   (C) schizoid personality disorder
   (D) schizophrenia
   (E) schizotypal personality disorder

6. The patient's brother brings him to a doctor after the death of their mother. Since then, the patient's paranoia has caused him to question his neighbors' activities. He has since moved into a hotel that he could not afford in order to get away from the "spies" living next to him. Which of the following is the most appropriate intervention?

   (A) antipsychotic
   (B) benzodiazepine
   (C) no treatment
   (D) psychodynamic psychotherapy
   (E) selective serotonin reuptake inhibitor (SSRI)

Questions 7 and 8

A 25-year-old female college graduate is brought to her doctor by her mother. Described as "odd" since she lost her job a year ago, the patient has complained of hearing voices and believes that her body is a receiving antenna for a foreign spy operation. Her mother notes she has been isolating herself in her room. She is alert and oriented but suspicious and guarded on examination. Her affect is flat and her speech reveals loose associations. A complete medical workup is negative.

7. Which of the following symptoms is considered a "negative symptom" in this patient's presentation?

   (A) auditory hallucinations
   (B) delusions
   (C) flat affect
   (D) loose associations
   (E) paranoia

8. The patient is started on medication and many of her symptoms improve. She begins a new job and does well. One year later, she is brought to her doctor floridly psychotic, actively hearing voices, and extremely paranoid. She thinks her boss is trying to kill her. She has an upper respiratory viral illness that she believes to be the work of a foreign government. She discontinued her medication 4 weeks ago because she felt too sedated. In the past year, her cigarette smoking habit has decreased to one pack per day. What is the most likely cause of her exacerbation?

   (A) stress from work
   (B) a reaction to the viral illness
   (C) medication noncompliance
   (D) medication side effects
   (E) decreased cigarette smoking

Questions 9 and 10

A 44-year-old man complains to his doctor that he is always tired and is having difficulty getting out of bed in the morning. Upon questioning, he reveals he has three or four drinks each night and perhaps more on the weekends, but denies he has any problem with alcohol. A diagnosis of alcohol dependence is made and the patient comes to your office in acute alcohol withdrawal. He subsequently has a withdrawal seizure and is admitted to the intensive care unit.

9. Which of the following laboratory findings would be most likely found in this patient?

   (A) decreased prothrombin time
   (B) elevated or depressed liver enzymes
   (C) high blood-alcohol level
   (D) hypermagnesemia
   (E) thrombocytosis

10. Which of the following medications would be most important to administer?

(A) diazepam

(B) haloperidol

(C) lorazepam

(D) phenytoin

(E) valproic acid

11. A 28-year-old woman is brought to the emergency department for active suicidal ideation with a plan to overdose on acetaminophen. She has no history of a psychiatric illness but endorses many criteria for major depressive disorder (MDD), including poor sleep for the past 2 weeks. She recently lost her job and fears that she may not be able to pay her rent. Attempts to obtain collateral information have been unsuccessful. You believe the patient requires inpatient evaluation but her health maintenance organization (HMO) denies authorization for inpatient care, alternatively authorizing eight outpatient visits with a psychiatrist. You speak to the weekend on-call physician-reviewer and report that the patient remains unsafe and wishes to be discharged. Upon learning that the patient does not have a history of psychiatric illness, the reviewer fails to authorize inpatient care, despite your assessment. Which of the following is the most appropriate intervention?

(A) Begin antidepressant therapy and arrange for outpatient follow-up the next day.

(B) Admit the patient on an emergency certificate to an inpatient facility.

(C) Administer an antipsychotic medication and reevaluate the patient in 1 hour.

(D) Explain to the patient that her HMO did not authorize hospitalization and discharge her with follow-up care.

(E) Prescribe a medication to help her sleep, discharge her, and arrange for follow-up care.

Questions 12 and 13

A 34-year-old woman suffering from severe major depressive disorder is admitted to the hospital due to worsening depressive symptoms and acute suicidality.

She has had multiple trials of medications without significant improvement. It is decided to perform a course of electroconvulsive therapy (ECT).

12. While undergoing the ECT, the treatment team wishes to monitor improvement in her depression. Which of the following tests has the greatest reliability and validity for this purpose?

(A) Beck Depression Inventory

(B) Draw-A-Person Test

(C) Halstead-Reitan Neuropsychological Battery

(D) Rorschach Test

(E) Thematic Apperception Test (TAT)

13. After one of her treatments, the patient complaints of memory impairment. Which of the following tests would be the most appropriate to assess her complaint?

(A) Beck Depression Inventory

(B) Brown-Peterson Task

(C) Bulimia Test—Revised

(D) Eating Disorder Inventory 2 (EDI-2)

(E) State-Trait Anxiety Inventory

14. A 67-year-old woman with a history of depression presents to your office for evaluation. Her symptoms of poor appetite, insomnia, low energy, and feelings of hopelessness have worsened recently. She has been on several different serotonin-specific reuptake inhibitors (SSRIs), which you learn have not resulted in complete remission of her symptoms. Which of the following medications would be most appropriate to prescribe?

(A) citalopram

(B) fluvoxamine

(C) paroxetine

(D) sertraline

(E) venlafaxine

Questions 15 and 16

A 29-year-old woman presents to the emergency department with her 3-year-old child reporting that the child suffered a seizure while at home. Hospital records verify that this is the third emergency department visit in as many weeks for the same presentation. Neurologic workup for seizure disorder was negative. Initiation of an anticonvulsant has been ineffective. The mother becomes very frustrated, demanding that her son be admitted to the hospital for further testing.

15. Based on the above presentation, which of the following diagnoses is most likely in the child?

    (A) conversion disorder
    (B) factitious disorder
    (C) no diagnosis
    (D) seizure disorder
    (E) separation anxiety disorder

16. The mother is additionally most likely to suffer from which of the following?

    (A) bipolar disorder
    (B) depression
    (C) epilepsy
    (D) posttraumatic stress disorder (PTSD)
    (E) schizophrenia

Questions 17 and 18

A 26-year-old man is being evaluated in the emergency department for sudden onset of chest pressure and dyspnea. This is his third emergency department visit for similar symptoms for which he reports "I feel like I'm going to die." An electrocardiogram (ECG) and stress test were normal. The patient denies risk factors for heart disease and does not have a family history of heart disease. Urine toxicology was negative.

17. Which of the following is the most likely diagnosis?

    (A) acute myocardial infarction
    (B) acute stress disorder
    (C) delirium
    (D) hypochondriasis
    (E) panic disorder

18. Which of the following medications is the most efficacious in the treatment of this disorder?

    (A) clonidine (Catapres)
    (B) haloperidol
    (C) lithium
    (D) propranolol
    (E) sertraline (Zoloft)

19. A woman being treated for major depression is brought to the emergency department after being found unconscious by a neighbor. The neighbor states that over the past few days the woman had been complaining of severe headaches. She also mentions that the woman often enjoys red wine. The woman's blood pressure is recorded as 220/110 mm Hg. Which of the following should be administered intravenously?

    (A) alpha-blocker
    (B) beta-blocker
    (C) bromocriptine (Parlodel)
    (D) calcium channel blocker
    (E) dantrolene sodium (Dantrium)

Questions 20 and 21

A 28-year-old man recently began taking clozapine (Clozaril) to treat symptoms of schizophrenia. He does not suffer from any medical illness.

20. Which of the following adverse effects is associated with this medication?

    (A) bradycardia
    (B) galactorrhea
    (C) hypertension
    (D) seizures
    (E) weight loss

21. Which of the following blood tests will require frequent, regular monitoring for this patient?

    (A) calcium level
    (B) complete blood count with differential
    (C) electrolytes
    (D) thyroid function tests
    (E) urinalysis

Questions 22 and 23

You admit an 83-year-old widowed female for further evaluation as she is no longer able to care for herself at home. She has lost 30 lb in the past year, has poor hygiene, and admits to increasing forgetfulness.

22. Which of the following tests would best help to make the correct diagnosis?

    (A) Blessed Rating Scale
    (B) Folstein Mini-Mental State Examination (MMSE)
    (C) Geriatric Rating Scale
    (D) Glasgow Coma Scale
    (E) Mental Status Examination (MSE)

23. Which of the following disorders would be most important to rule out as a cause of her clinical presentation?

    (A) generalized anxiety disorder
    (B) major depressive disorder
    (C) obsessive-compulsive disorder
    (D) panic disorder
    (E) post-traumatic stress disorder

24. A 35-year-old patient is encouraged to seek "professional help" by his coworkers. He denies pervasive depression or anxiety, but upon interview he is oddly dressed, expresses unusual beliefs and thinking, some paranoia regarding his coworkers motivations, and has few close friends. He denies delusions or hallucinations, and there is no suicidal or homicidal ideation. Which of the following diagnoses is the most appropriate to consider?

    (A) avoidant personality disorder
    (B) narcissistic personality disorder
    (C) paranoid personality disorder
    (D) schizoid personality disorder
    (E) schizotypal personality disorder

25. A 28-year-old separated woman is referred from her primary care doctor for depression. While she admits to occasional periods of dysphoria, she claims to "always feel empty inside." Upon further questioning she demonstrates a pervasive pattern of unstable relationships, poor self-image, impulsiveness, and irritability. Which of the following diagnoses is the most appropriate to consider?

    (A) antisocial personality disorder
    (B) borderline personality disorder
    (C) dependent personality disorder
    (D) histrionic personality disorder
    (E) schizoid personality disorder

Questions 26 and 27

A 28-year-old single man with a long history of schizophrenia has been taking his medications regularly. He now presents with worsening hallucinations and prominent thought disorganization.

26. Which of the following neuropsychological tests would best determine his ability to organize and correctly process information?

    (A) Bender Gestalt Test
    (B) Draw-A-Person Test
    (C) Luria-Nebraska Neuropsychological Battery
    (D) Mini-Mental State Examination
    (E) Wisconsin Card Sorting Test (WCST)

27. The above test measures functioning at which of the following lobes of the brain?

    (A) cerebellar
    (B) frontal
    (C) occipital
    (D) parietal
    (E) temporal

Questions 28 and 29

A 30-year-old woman without prior psychiatric history is brought to the emergency department by the police after being arrested for breach of the peace. The woman was observed acting irrationally at a local business where she demanded to speak with the president of the company claiming that she had new ideas for product development. The patient reports that she has not slept for days and that her mood is "fabulous." Urine human chorionic gonadotropin is positive. Illicit substances were not detected.

28. Which of the following additional findings would most likely be present in her history or mental status examination (MSE)?

    (A) visual hallucinations
    (B) daytime sleepiness
    (C) depressed affect
    (D) racing thoughts
    (E) weight loss

29. Which of the following medical disorders can present with similar symptoms?

    (A) cirrhosis
    (B) diabetes mellitus
    (C) hyperglycemia
    (D) rheumatoid arthritis
    (E) thyroid disorder

Questions 30 and 31

A 24-year-old man with a history of seizure disorder and polysubstance abuse has been incarcerated for assaultive behavior. The patient is evaluated by a neurologist, who prescribes phenytoin (Dilantin).

30. Which of the following side effects is most likely associated with this medication?

    (A) Ebstein anomaly
    (B) gingival hyperplasia
    (C) hepatic failure
    (D) hypertension
    (E) leukocytosis

31. The patient returns 1 month later for a follow-up examination and reports that he experienced a generalized seizure. Laboratory investigation reveals that the phenytoin level is 6.5 mg/dL (normal, 10-20 mg/dL). Which of the following is the most appropriate intervention at this time?

    (A) Increase the phenytoin dose.
    (B) Discontinue phenytoin and begin divalproex sodium.
    (C) Add a benzodiazepine.
    (D) Assess compliance.
    (E) Add phenobarbital.

32. A 24-year-old woman with a history of schizophrenia tells you that she would like to become pregnant. Her husband has no history of mental illness. What do you tell her is the chance of her offspring developing schizophrenia?

    (A) 1%
    (B) 2%
    (C) 5%
    (D) 8%
    (E) 12%

33. A 28-year-old married female patient is admitted to the hospital with bizarre behavior and disorganized thinking. Consideration is given to a diagnosis of schizophreniform disorder. To help with the diagnosis, the patient is administered a test that consists of viewing a set of 10 inkblots sequentially. The examiner scores the patient's responses to the blots by noting the content of the perception, the area of the blot that forms the basis of the response, and the aspects of the area that are used to form the response.

    In which of the following classes does this projective test belong?

    (A) associations
    (B) choice of ordering
    (C) completions
    (D) constructions
    (E) self-expression

34. A mother and her 17-year-old son present to your psychiatric clinic seeking family therapy. The mother reports that she and her son have a tumultuous relationship and are constantly arguing with each other. The son admits that about a year ago he disclosed to his mother that he is gay. He feels that because of his mother's strong religious beliefs, she has not accepted his sexuality and this has been the source of tension in their relationship. The mother firmly believes that her son is "just confused" and needs counseling. She has heard of a particular therapy that can change the sexual orientation of an individual and asks that you conduct this on her son. Which of the following is the appropriate next step?

(A) Ask the son if he is willing to pursue this treatment.

(B) Engage the son in this therapy based off on what you know.

(C) Inform the mother that such therapy is unethical.

(D) Learn more about the treatment first and ask the family to return when you are knowledge able enough to conduct this.

(E) Refer the family to a therapist who specializes in such treatments.

35. An 18-year-old man is referred to his college counseling center due to failing grades. It is determined that he has stopped attending classes, preferring to remain in his dorm room. His roommates claim that he stays up "all night," with little apparent sleep. The patient claims that he has discovered something that will make him a millionaire. On mental status examination he appears diaphoretic with psychomotor agitation. His speech is rapid, and his affect is euphoric. He denies suicidal or homicidal ideation but displays significant grandiosity. His insight is poor. Which of the is the most likely diagnosis?

(A) cannabis dependence

(B) cocaine dependence

(C) MDD with psychotic features

(D) schizoaffective disorder

(E) schizophrenia, paranoid type

36. An 89-year-old married woman with no prior psychiatric history but a history of multiple medical problems is admitted for failure to thrive. Upon history, the patient does not seem acclimated to her surroundings. Which of the following tests would best help to determine her level of confusion?

(A) Fargo Map Test

(B) Spatial Orientation Memory Test

(C) Stroop Test

(D) Temporal Orientation Test

(E) Wisconsin Card Sorting Test

37. A Malaysian man is brought into custody by the police after murdering his friend. While he does not remember committing the act, he does recall being insulted by him at an earlier time. Which of the following conditions is most associated with this presentation?

(A) amok

(B) dhat

(C) Ganser syndrome

(D) koro

(E) latah

Questions 38 and 39

A 26-year-old woman is diagnosed with schizophrenia. The psychiatrist decides to treat her symptoms with a high-potency antipsychotic medication. While her symptoms appear to improve on the medication, she develops acute, painful muscle spasms of her jaw.

38. Which of the following medications should be added?

(A) benztropine (Cogentin)

(B) cholinergic agonist

(C) clozapine

(D) methylphenidate (Ritalin)

(E) risperidone (Risperdal)

39. Despite compliance with the above regimen, the patient continues to suffer with extrapyramidal symptoms. As a result of this, she abruptly stops taking her antipsychotic medication. It is decided to switch to another medication. Which of the following is the most appropriate choice?

(A) haloperidol

(B) loxapine (Loxitane)

(C) perphenazine (Trilafon)

(D) pimozide (Orap)

(E) quetiapine

Questions 40 and 41

A 30-year-old woman presents with a history of chronic feelings of depression, low-self esteem, chronic suicidal ideation, as well as frequent but brief sexual relationships, anger outbursts, and self-mutilation.

40. Which of the following disorders is this patient most likely to be suffering from?

    (A) avoidant personality disorder
    (B) bipolar disorder
    (C) borderline personality disorder
    (D) dependent personality disorder
    (E) narcissistic personality disorder

41. The above patient is referred for dialectical behavioral therapy (DBT). Which of the following techniques is the most important in her therapy?

    (A) aversion
    (B) eye-movement desensitization and reprocessing (EMDR).
    (C) flooding
    (D) homework
    (E) systematic desensitization

42. A 21-year-old man presents with a 4-week history of bizarre behavior, paranoid delusions, and auditory hallucinations that comment on his appearance. After a thorough evaluation, you diagnose him with schizophrenia, paranoid type, and prescribe haloperidol 5 mg bid. One week later, the patient returns for a follow-up examination and reports that, although his symptoms have improved, he now experiences muscle stiffness in his arms and neck. You prescribe benztropine 1 mg bid and schedule a follow-up appointment in 2 weeks. One week later, the patient's mother calls you and reports that her son is more agitated and confused. Physical examination reveals tachycardia, dilated pupils, and flushed skin. Which of the following would be the most appropriate next step?

    (A) Discontinue benztropine and prescribe amantadine (Symmetrel).
    (B) Increase haloperidol to 5 mg tid.

    (C) Increase benztropine to 2 mg bid.
    (D) Discontinue haloperidol and prescribe risperidone.
    (E) Prescribe lorazepam 1 mg bid.

Questions 43 and 44

A 25-year-old single woman who carries the provisional diagnosis of dependent personality disorder is referred for psychological testing. You decide to administer the Rorschach.

43. Which of the following aspects of this type of psychological testing would be the most important in this case?

    (A) Ask specific questions with itemized responses.
    (B) Determine how a patient feels about you.
    (C) Lack of structure allows for a variety of responses.
    (D) Provide numerical scores.
    (E) Results allow for easy statistical analysis.

44. You additionally decide to administer the Minnesota Multiphasic Personality Inventory 2 (MMPI-2). Which of the following aspects of this type of psychological testing would be the most important in this case?

    (A) Assesses test-taking attitudes.
    (B) Instructions are unambiguous in nature.
    (C) Items designed to separate normal subjects from those with psychiatric illness.
    (D) More sensitive in picking up gender-specific issues.
    (E) Most researched and with normative data.

45. A 28-year-old male medical student is found to have an enlarged testicle during a routine physical examination. The student reports that it has been gradually enlarging for several months. The physician asks why he did not report these findings earlier. "I'm sure it's nothing," the student replies. Which of the following types of responses does this most represent?

    (A) confidence
    (B) immature defense

(C) mature defense

(D) narcissistic defense

(E) neurotic defense

46. A 45-year-old Asian-American woman is brought to the emergency department by her husband, who reports that for the past 3 days his wife has not been sleeping well, has been experiencing bad dreams, and appears "in a daze" with a sense of feeling "numb." The patient endorses feeling anxious but does not know why. She has been unable to perform her usual activities of daily living. One week ago, the patient was discharged from the hospital after experiencing an anaphylactic reaction to IV contrast dye while undergoing an imaging procedure for sinusitis. Although she cannot recall specifics, her husband verifies the history, adding that the doctors "thought she was going to die." Upon returning to the hospital, she experiences intense fear about revisiting the same hospital from which she was recently discharged. Which of the following is the most appropriate diagnosis?

(A) acute stress disorder

(B) adjustment disorder

(C) generalized anxiety disorder (GAD)

(D) major depressive disorder (MDD)

(E) posttraumatic stress disorder (PTSD)

47. A 40-year-old woman without past psychiatric history is admitted to the hospital for treatment of depression. During morning rounds, the patient appears unresponsive and does not respond to verbal stimuli. There are no signs of trauma or overdose. A review of her chart reveals that the patient was well the night before and went to sleep without incident. You determine that the patient's unresponsiveness is psychogenic. Which of the following findings is most likely to be apparent on her examination?

(A) abnormal electroencephalogram (EEG)

(B) cold-caloric-induced nystagmus

(C) decreased respirations

(D) elevated temperature

(E) nonsaccadic eye movements

48. A 24-year-old woman is referred by her family practice doctor after the Christmas holiday. She gives a significant history of fatigue, weight gain, and hyperphagia during the winter months. She describes a "sad mood" and "can't wait" until her vacation to Florida. Which of the following is the most likely diagnosis?

(A) acute stress disorder

(B) dysthymic disorder

(C) generalized anxiety disorder

(D) seasonal affective disorder

(E) sundowning syndrome

49. A 27-year-old woman is brought to the emergency department by her parents, who report that their daughter is unable to recall her name. The emergency department physician reports that a complete neurologic workup is within normal limits. Collateral information reveals that the patient had episodes in which she would take unplanned trips, sometimes for days or weeks, without notice, and would return unable to recall the episode. A review of her medical chart notes a past history of possible sexual abuse as a child. Urine toxicology is negative and she does not take any medications. Which of the following is the most likely diagnosis?

(A) delirium

(B) dissociative fugue

(C) major depressive disorder

(D) partial complex seizures

(E) posttraumatic stress disorder

Questions 50 and 51

A 20-year-old college student is referred for testing to evaluate poor academic performance. He reports that he has always "struggled" to pass his classes despite studying for many hours. He attends all of his lectures and is able to pay attention, yet he does not seem to be able to adequately learn the material. You suspect he has a learning disability.

50. Which of the following tests would be the most appropriate to help determine this patient's problem?

   (A) Draw-A-Person Test
   (B) Minnesota Multiphasic Personality Inventory 2 (MMPI-2)
   (C) Wechsler Adult Intelligence Scale—Revised (WAIS-R)
   (D) Wechsler Intelligence Scale for Children (WISC)
   (E) Wechsler Memory Test (WMT)

51 Which of the following formulas is used to calculate the intelligence quotient (IQ)?

   (A) actual IQ/theoretical IQ × 100
   (B) chronological age/performance IQ × 100
   (C) mental age/chronological age × 100
   (D) mental age/full-scale IQ × 100
   (E) performance IQ/verbal IQ × 100

52. A 26-year-old female graduate student reports to you a 4-week history of a depressed mood that has caused her significant difficulty in attending her classes. The patient reports difficulty falling asleep at night, reduced appetite and weight loss, poor energy, and passive suicidal ideation. A careful review of her history reveals that for the past 2 years she also experienced brief and distinct periods of an elevated and expansive mood, a decreased need for sleep, and an increase in activities, although she was still able to function adequately. Which of the following is the most likely diagnosis?

   (A) bipolar I disorder
   (B) bipolar II disorder
   (C) cyclothymic disorder
   (D) dysthymic disorder
   (E) major depressive disorder

53. You are asked to evaluate a 30-year-old male prisoner who reports a depressed mood and suicidal ideation. During your interview and mental status examination, you note that the prisoner doesn't give correct or specific answers, responding instead to your questions with approximate answers. Which of the following is the most appropriate diagnosis?

   (A) Capgras syndrome
   (B) dementia
   (C) fugue state
   (D) Ganser syndrome
   (E) Munchausen syndrome

54. A 75-year-old man is admitted to the hospital following a serious suicide attempt. The patient exhibits clinical features of depression with severe neurovegetative symptoms and has a past history of suicide attempts. The medical chart reveals that he is prescribed levodopa/carbidopa, digoxin, aspirin, and a medication for cardiac arrhythmia. He remains extremely helpless and hopeless, with little appetite, and ongoing suicidal ideation with several lethal plans. Which of the following treatments would be the most appropriate?

   (A) diazepam (Valium)
   (B) electroconvulsive therapy (ECT)
   (C) nortriptyline (Pamelor)
   (D) risperidone
   (E) supportive psychotherapy

55. A 38-year-old woman presents to your office with an 8-week history of symptoms of depressed mood with an increased appetite and 10 lb weight gain, hypersomnia, a "heavy feeling" in her body, and rejection sensitivity. Upon further questioning she admits to being able to brighten when spending time in activities she usually enjoys. She reports to you that she recently enrolled in graduate school and is having trouble with many of her classes. Which of the following diagnoses is the most appropriate?

   (A) adjustment disorder
   (B) dysthymic disorder
   (C) major depression with atypical features
   (D) major depression with melancholic features
   (E) sleep disorder

56. A 33-year-old man changes his first name to honor a musician whom he idolizes. He recently bought the same guitar as the musician and formed a rock band to play his music.

During practice, the man dresses like his idol. Which of the following defense mechanisms does this behavior best represent?

(A) fixation
(B) idealization
(C) identification
(D) projection
(E) regression

57. A 60-year-old man with schizophrenia sits motionless in his chair. The patient is mute and reacts very little to his environment. His eyes appear fixated on a distant object. At times, he assumes bizarre postures and imitates the movements of others. Which of the following is the best description of his behavior?

(A) absence seizure
(B) catalepsy
(C) cataplexy
(D) catatonia
(E) partial complex seizure

58. During an examination to evaluate muscle rigidity, a male bipolar patient is seen in a bizarre posture. He is somewhat resistant to movement of his arms but maintains the arm in the position in which you place it. This is an example of which of the following?

(A) catalepsy
(B) cataplexy
(C) dystonia
(D) malingering
(E) rigidity

Questions 59 and 60

A 42-year-old healthy man is undergoing a lot of stress at his work. As a result, he is having a difficult time falling and staying asleep. His primary care doctor has since prescribed him a medication to help with his insomnia. While he is sleeping better, he calls one morning several weeks later with complaints of a very painful, persistent penile erection which has lasted throughout the evening.

59. Which of the following medications has most likely been prescribed?

(A) fluoxetine (Prozac)
(B) nortriptyline (Pamelor)
(C) paroxetine (Paxil)
(D) sertraline (Zoloft)
(E) trazodone (Desyrel)

60. Which of the following is the most appropriate next step?

(A) Tell him to decrease the dose.
(B) Tell him to stop the medication and restart in 3 days.
(C) Tell him to stop the medication and monitor his condition.
(D) Tell him to stop the medication and go immediately to the emergency room.
(E) Tell him to stop the medication and have sexual intercourse or masturbate.

Questions 61 and 62

A 66-year-old man reports a history of excessive worry about his daughter since she moved away from the area 1 year ago. His wife of 43 years verifies his complaint, adding "he worries about everything." Recently, his wife made plans to travel abroad to visit friends. The patient is unable to accompany his wife because of chronic obstructive pulmonary disease caused by years of heavy smoking and is very anxious about her leaving. He reports subsequent difficulty falling asleep, excessive daytime fatigue, and trouble concentrating at work.

61. Which of the following medications would be the most appropriate to treat his symptoms?

(A) alprazolam (Xanax)
(B) buspirone (BuSpar)
(C) diazepam (Valium)
(D) lorazepam (Ativan)
(E) propranolol (Inderal)

62. Several weeks later, the patient reports that the medication you prescribed has helped everything but his difficulty falling asleep. He reports that during the past week he has slept only 4 hours per night. After careful consideration, you decide to begin a trial of a 1-week supply of medication to help his insomnia. Which of the following medications would be most appropriate to prescribe?

    (A) clorazepate (Tranxene)
    (B) diphenhydramine (Benadryl)
    (C) oxazepam (Serax)
    (D) temazepam (Restoril)
    (E) zolpidem (Ambien)

Questions 63 and 64

A 25-year-old woman with a history of major depressive disorder, single episode, in remission is admitted to the hospital for removal of a fibroid. Her procedure is completed without difficulty, but upon discharge, she is still experiencing significant pain. She has no other medical problems or allergies. She is currently taking oral contraceptives and a monoamine oxidase inhibitor (MAOI) for her depression.

63. Which of the following analgesics should be most avoided in this patient?

    (A) acetaminophen
    (B) codeine
    (C) ibuprofen
    (D) meperidine (Demerol)
    (E) oxycodone

64. Two months later the patient returns for a follow-up visit and reports that she is pregnant. Which of the following interventions is most appropriate?

    (A) Continue the MAOI.
    (B) Discontinue the MAOI.
    (C) Discontinue the MAOI and initiate treatment with fluoxetine after 2 weeks.
    (D) Discontinue the MAOI during the first trimester only.
    (E) Discontinue the MAOI and begin maintenance ECT.

65. A 62-year-old homeless man presents to the emergency department with confusion, agitation, impaired gait, and nystagmus. His vital signs are stable and an ophthalmologic examination is within normal limits. The patient is unable to recall the date and has difficulty sustaining attention. Which of the following is the most appropriate initial intervention?

    (A) Administer IV dextrose.
    (B) Administer parenteral thiamine.
    (C) Obtain a computed tomographic scan of the brain.
    (D) Perform a breathalyzer.
    (E) Perform a lumbar puncture.

66. You are a community psychiatrist who is seeing a patient for the first time. The patient informs that he has just moved into the area and needs to establish himself with a psychiatrist to continue his treatment for depression and anxiety. On further evaluation, you learn that he was previously arrested for child pornography and served several years in prison. He is currently in therapy to address this issue. You are surprised to find that after the disclosure, you feel angry toward the patient as you have two young daughters of your own. You are concerned about whether it may be difficult for you to treat the patient in an unbiased, nonjudgmental manner because of his criminal history. Which of the following is the next most appropriate step?

    (A) Continue to see the patient but limit the time spent with him.
    (B) Immediately refer the patient to another physician in your clinic.
    (C) Inform the patient that you are unable to see him and refer him back to the community.
    (D) Obtain the patient's therapy records so that you are aware of his progress.
    (E) Seek a consultation with an experienced colleague regarding your feelings toward the patient.

67. A 39-year-old executive without psychiatric history but a history of hypertension reports drinking up to six cups of caffeinated coffee per day. He boards a plane scheduled for an 18-hour flight on which only decaffeinated beverages are served. Which of the following symptoms is he most likely to experience?

   (A) depressed mood
   (B) headache
   (C) irritability
   (D) muscle cramping
   (E) nausea

Questions 68 and 69

A 25-year-old man with a history of schizophrenia presents to the emergency department with severe muscle stiffness and an elevated temperature. His caseworker claims that he is compliant with his medications and denies that he uses alcohol or drugs. His vital signs demonstrate elevated temperature, blood pressure, and pulse. The patient appears confused and is diaphoretic. A urine toxicology screen is negative.

68. Which of the following is the most essential intervention?

   (A) Administer bromocriptine.
   (B) Administer IV dantrolene sodium.
   (C) Administer naloxone (Narcan).
   (D) Apply cooling blankets.
   (E) Discontinue medications.

69. Which of the following laboratory abnormalities is most likely to be present in this patient?

   (A) anemia
   (B) elevated blood urea nitrogen (BUN)
   (C) elevated creatine phosphokinase (CPK)
   (D) decreased transaminases
   (E) leukopenia

70. An 18-year-old man is brought to the emergency department by the paramedics after being involved in a motor vehicle accident.

His medical chart reports a history of substance use. Which of the following tests can most likely confirm the diagnosis of substance dependence?

   (A) breath analysis
   (B) elevated heart rate
   (C) naloxone injection
   (D) serum liver function studies
   (E) urine toxicology screen

71. A 72-year-old man without prior psychiatric history presents to the outpatient clinic with a recent history of memory difficulty. The patient has had a stable level of consciousness and denies any current or past substance abuse. He has not been prescribed any new medications. The medical chart reveals a history of megaloblastic anemia and a subtotal gastrectomy for severe peptic ulcer disease. Which of the following initial interventions is most appropriate?

   (A) Discuss long-term extended-care facility admission.
   (B) Obtain a forensic examination to evaluate competency.
   (C) Obtain a neurologic consult.
   (D) Order a magnetic resonance imaging scan of the brain to confirm dementia, Alzheimer type.
   (E) Order a reversible workup for dementia.

72. A 37-year-old woman presents to the emergency department complaining of severe diarrhea, nausea, and a coarse tremor. The medical chart notes a history of bipolar I disorder. Which of the following would be the most appropriate initial intervention?

   (A) Obtain renal function studies.
   (B) Obtain a serum medication level.
   (C) Obtain a urine pregnancy test.
   (D) Obtain a urine toxicology screen.
   (E) Prescribe antidiarrheal medication.

Questions 73 and 74

A 72-year-old man is brought into the emergency room via ambulance after suffering what is suspected to be a stroke in his right parietal region.

73. Which of the following areas would be most likely to have deficits due to the stroke?

   (A) long-term implicit memory
   (B) long-term procedural memory
   (C) tactile memory
   (D) verbal memory
   (E) visual nonverbal memory

74. Which of the following tests would best identify the abnormality in that region?

   (A) Minnesota Multiphasic Personality Inventory 2
   (B) Rey-Osterrieth Test
   (C) Rorschach Test
   (D) Wechsler Intelligence Scales
   (E) Wisconsin Card Sorting Test

75. A 32-year-old married man is diagnosed with bipolar I disorder. Various treatment options are discussed, and he agrees to begin lithium carbonate to treat his symptoms of mania. Which of the following tests should be obtained before initiating treatment with lithium?

   (A) creatinine clearance
   (B) EEG
   (C) liver function studies
   (D) thyroid-stimulating hormone
   (E) 24-hour urine volume

76. A 27-year-old woman has been prescribed fluoxetine for depression for the past year. She comes to you complaining of medication side effects and wishes to discontinue her antidepressant. As her physician, you discuss with her the appropriate risks and benefits, and you discontinue her treatment. Two weeks later, she returns complaining of depressive symptoms characterized by sleep and appetite changes, poor concentration, and a depressed mood for most of the day. You determine that she is experiencing a recurrent major depressive episode

and decide to prescribe her a different class of medication to treat her symptoms. After discussing the appropriate precautions with her, you prescribe an MAOI. Within 1 week, she begins experiencing irritability, abdominal pain and diarrhea, and autonomic instability characterized by hypertension and tachycardia. Her temperature is 103.5°F. The patient also reports experiencing jerking of her muscles and vivid visual hallucinations of colorful flowers spinning toward the sky. She states that she has followed your directions carefully while taking this medication. Which of the following conditions most likely account for this presentation?

   (A) hallucinogen abuse
   (B) malignant hyperthermia
   (C) neuroleptic malignant syndrome (NMS)
   (D) serotonin syndrome
   (E) tyramine-induced hypertensive crisis

Questions 77 and 78

A 17-year-old girl is referred to the school nurse for frequent episodes of vomiting in the bathroom during lunch breaks. Her friends report that, despite always talking about wanting to loose weight, she eats "twice as much as anybody else." The parents are called to the school and recall that a recent bill from their charge account at the local pharmacy indicated a large number of laxative purchases. The girl reports that her mood is fine, and her records at school indicate that she is an above-average student.

77. Which of the following medical complications would be most likely in this patient?

   (A) acidosis
   (B) dental carries
   (C) diarrhea
   (D) hyperkalemia
   (E) hyperchloremia

78. Which of the following medications is the most appropriate initial treatment for her symptoms?

   (A) antianxiety agents
   (B) antidepressants
   (C) antiemetics

(D) appetite stimulants

(E) sedative-hypnotic medications

79. A 70-year-old man with multiple medical problems is suspected to have had a stroke, affecting his ability to speak. Which of the following tests would best assess the nature of his speech difficulty?

(A) Bender Gestalt Test

(B) Boston Diagnostic Aphasia Examination

(C) Folstein MMSE

(D) Sentence Completion Test

(E) Stroop Test

Questions 80 and 81

A 16-year-old female high school student is referred by her parents for an evaluation. One year prior to the evaluation, the girl began restricting her food intake and started a rigorous exercise program to improve her appearance. Aspiring to be a model, the girl lost 25 lb but remained preoccupied with her appearance despite weighing only 85 lb. Her friends reported that she constantly referred to herself as being "fat" and did not seem interested in dating. The girl continued to lose weight and was reluctant to discuss her condition.

80. Which of the following complications would be most likely in this patient?

(A) diarrhea

(B) heat intolerance

(C) leukocytosis

(D) menorrhagia

(E) osteoporosis

81. Which of the following is the most accurate upper end of the mortality rate associated with this disorder?

(A) 5%

(B) 10%

(C) 20%

(D) 25%

(E) 30%

Questions 82 and 83

A 50-year-old woman reports a depressed mood, poor appetite, and weight loss 1 month following the death of her husband. After his death, she began to feel that she would be "better off dead." At times, she believes that she can hear his voice calling to her. She denies any feelings of worthlessness but feels guilty about not being able to do the right things for him before he died. When talking with others, she believes that her feelings are normal.

82. Which of the following is the most likely diagnosis?

(A) adjustment disorder with depressed mood

(B) complicated bereavement

(C) dysthymic disorder

(D) major depressive episode

(E) uncomplicated bereavement

83. Which of the following is the most appropriate course of action?

(A) Admission to a hospital.

(B) Evaluate for a sleep disorder.

(C) No treatment.

(D) Prescribe antidepressant medication.

(E) Prescribe sedative-hypnotic medication.

84. A 25-year-old man reports a 5-year history of excessive hand washing and a preoccupation with feeling clean. The thought of contracting an infectious disease persists throughout the day even though he makes attempts to ignore it. His condition has progressively worsened and has caused significant impairment while at work and at home. Which of the following medications is the best initial choice to treat his symptoms?

(A) antidepressant

(B) antiepileptic

(C) antipsychotic

(D) benzodiazepine

(E) lithium

85. A 28-year-old woman with no psychiatric history is arrested for shoplifting. She claims she does not remember details of the crime, and that for "a while" she has had trouble recalling details from things she's recently read. You are called to assess her, but want to ensure she'll give good effort on testing. Which of the following tests would be the most appropriate to administer?

(A) Benton Visual Retention Test
(B) Clock Drawing
(C) Test of Memory Malingering
(D) Wechsler Intelligence Scale
(E) Wisconsin Card Sorting Test

Questions 86 and 87

A 52-year-old obese man experiences excessive daytime sleepiness and a depressed mood. His wife reports that he snores loudly and is restless while sleeping. There is no evidence of substance abuse, and the patient does not have a prior psychiatric history.

86. Which of the following is the most likely cause of his symptoms?

(A) abnormal circadian rhythm
(B) airway obstruction
(C) depressive disorder
(D) nocturnal myoclonus
(E) periodic limb movements of sleep

87. Which of the following is the treatment of choice for his symptoms?

(A) antidepressant medication
(B) benzodiazepine medication
(C) breathing air under positive pressure
(D) nasal surgery
(E) uvulopalatoplasty

Questions 88 and 89

A patient with chronic paranoid schizophrenia who has been stable for years on a low-potency antipsychotic agent begins experiencing parkinsonian-like side effects. His physician prescribes a drug to alleviate some of these side effects. One week later, the patient is seen in the emergency department with dilated pupils, dry mouth, warm skin, and tachycardia.

He is also experiencing the new onset of visual hallucinations.

88. Which of the following would be the most appropriate medication to administer?

(A) anticholinesterase
(B) atropine
(C) benzodiazepine
(D) dantrolene sodium
(E) haloperidol

89. After the appropriate intervention, the patient experiences nausea and vomiting and subsequently has a seizure. Which of the following medications should be administered next?

(A) atropine
(B) epinephrine
(C) lorazepam
(D) physostigmine
(E) prochlorperazine (Compazine)

90. A 40-year-old woman complains of 3 to 4 months of feeling sad, with trouble falling asleep, decreased appetite and some weight loss, difficulty concentrating at work, and fatigue. She admits to suicidal ideation without specific plan or intent. There is no history of mania. She also mentions long-standing and repetitive thoughts were she worries about "germs." As a result, she washes her hands very frequently, sometimes ending up with cracked and chapped skin. She realizes that her worries are unrealistic, but she cannot keep from doing it. Which of the following medications would be the most appropriate to prescribe?

(A) buspirone
(B) clomipramine (Anafranil)
(C) doxepin (Sinequan)
(D) fluvoxamine (Luvox)
(E) phenelzine (Nardil)

Questions 91 and 92

A 56-year-old man with a long history of alcohol dependence and liver disease is ordered by the court to enroll in an inpatient detoxification program for alcohol dependence. After 2 days in treatment, he begins to experience tremors, sweating, flushing, and anxiety.

91. Which of the following medications would be the most appropriate to prescribe?

(A) alprazolam
(B) chlordiazepoxide (Librium)
(C) disulfiram (Antabuse)
(D) lorazepam
(E) phenobarbital

92. Shortly after this time, the man begins to report visual hallucinations and becomes agitated. Which of the following medications should be prescribed to treat these symptoms?

(A) fluoxetine
(B) haloperidol
(C) lithium
(D) lorazepam
(E) sertraline

93. A 48-year-old woman successfully completes an inpatient program for alcohol detoxification for which she was prescribed chlordiazepoxide. Upon discharge, the patient is prescribed disulfiram. Soon after discharge, the patient attends an office party where she admits to having a few drinks. She has been compliant with her prescribed medication and does not have any active medical problems. Which of the following symptoms is she most likely to experience?

(A) blurred vision
(B) euphoria
(C) high blood pressure
(D) urinary retention
(E) vomiting

94. A 22-year-old man with a history of bipolar disorder is prescribed lithium carbonate to treat his symptoms. During a weekend rugby tournament, he hurts his knee and an orthopedic physician prescribes a medication to reduce his

symptoms of pain and swelling. Although the patient reports relief from this medication, he begins to experience abdominal pain, diarrhea, and drowsiness. Which of the following medications would most likely contribute to the production of these symptoms?

(A) acetaminophen
(B) aspirin
(C) codeine
(D) ibuprofen
(E) meperidine

95. A 32-year-old, newly married man with a past history of major depressive disorder presents with a 4-week history of depression, insomnia, anergia, poor concentration, and anhedonia. He has had passive suicidal ideation without a plan, as well. He has not taken citalopram for several years, and, despite remission of his symptoms, he had significant sexual dysfunction when taking it. He wishes to restart a medication but is greatly concerned about the impact on his marriage. Which of the following medications would be the most appropriate?

(A) citalopram
(B) fluvoxamine
(C) paroxetine
(D) mirtazapine
(E) venlafaxine

96. A patient who is human immunodeficiency virus (HIV)-positive reports 4 weeks of a depressed mood, low energy, poor sleep, and hopelessness. His appetite is negligible, and he has been refusing to eat or drink anything for 2 days. Which of the following medications would be the most appropriate to prescribe?

(A) bupropion
(B) buspirone
(C) fluoxetine
(D) methylphenidate
(E) nefazodone (Serzone)

97. A 43-year-old woman presents with a new history of depressive symptoms, including insomnia, poor appetite and weight loss, low energy, and distractibility. On mental status examination she is asked to count backward by 7s, beginning at 100. Which of the following aspects is being assessed by this test?

    (A) attention
    (B) fund of knowledge
    (C) mathematics skills
    (D) remote memory
    (E) verbal memory

Questions 98 and 99

A college-aged man reports that he and his friends have been experimenting with the new drug craze on campus called "huffing." His roommate reports that he has been accumulating typewriter correction fluid, nail polish remover, and model airplane glue.

98. Which of the following would he most likely experience during intoxication?

    (A) conjunctival injection
    (B) depressed reflexes
    (C) diminished response to pain
    (D) increased appetite
    (E) staring into space

99. Which of the following is the most effective treatment for this type of drug abuse?

    (A) abstinence
    (B) antidepressant agents
    (C) antipsychotic agents
    (D) dialectic behavioral therapy
    (E) exposure and response prevention

100. A 30-year-old man with chronic schizophrenia continues to exhibit pervasive symptoms and poor functioning despite continued compliance with antipsychotic medication. Which of the following symptoms would be most consistent with the diagnosis of the paranoid subtype?

    (A) disorganized speech
    (B) immobility

    (C) inappropriate affect
    (D) posturing
    (E) prominent hallucinations

101. You are treating a 32-year-old woman for bipolar I disorder with a combination of medications. She develops hair loss which eventually resolves on its own. Which of the following medications is most likely responsible for this side effect?

    (A) carbamazepine
    (B) clozapine
    (C) divalproex sodium
    (D) olanzapine (Zyprexa)
    (E) ziprasidone (Geodon)

102. A 34-year-old man is referred by his internist for depression. For the past 2 months he has been suffering from anhedonia, crying spells, frequent awakenings, poor appetite, and low energy. He is subsequently diagnosed with a major depressive episode and recommended to begin citalopram 20 mg daily. After discussion of the risks and benefits of the medication, he expresses concern about possible sexual dysfunction as he is currently in a new relationship with a coworker. Which of the following symptoms are most likely with this medication?

    (A) decreased libido
    (B) premature ejaculation
    (C) priapism
    (D) retrograde ejaculation
    (E) vaginismus

Questions 103 and 104

A 21-year-old male college student without prior medical or psychiatric history is evaluated for poor work performance. The student reports to the dean that he finds it hard to follow through with assignments and is easily distracted by environmental stimuli. The dean comments to the student about how frequently he interrupts others during conversations and observes that it seems that the student is not paying attention to what he is saying. Overall, his grades are poor except in the class he considers "the most interesting class I have ever had." He often forgets required materials for classes and his assignments are frequently late. The student's parents report that he was evaluated for similar difficulties while in public school, but he seemed to improve when the family moved out of the area and he attended private school.

103. Which of the following is the most likely diagnosis?

(A) attention-deficit hyperactivity disorder (ADHD)
(B) bipolar I disorder
(C) bipolar II disorder
(D) conduct disorder
(E) learning disability

104. The patient is prescribed methylphenidate for the above symptoms. After an adequate trial and dose, he continues to display some symptoms which interfere with his school functioning. Which of the following actions would be the most appropriate next step?

(A) Add a low-dose amphetamine.
(B) Add an antidepressant.
(C) Add an anxiolytic medication.
(D) Discontinue methylphenidate and prescribe a mixed amphetamine compound.
(E) Discontinue methylphenidate and prescribe an antidepressant.

105. A 35-year-old woman presents with episodic anxiety and complains of the occasional feeling when hearing something that she has heard before. She expresses her concern that she is "going crazy." Which of the following terms best describes this phenomenon?

(A) déjà entendu
(B) déjà vu
(C) folie à deux
(D) jamais vu
(E) la belle indifférence

106. A 19-year-old man is brought to the emergency department by the police for an evaluation. The written police report states that the patient has been calling 911 for the past 5 weeks reporting that he is being spied on by aliens from a distant planet. The patient reports that he is receiving messages from the aliens through his radio and that he hears voices in his head commenting on his appearance. He has not been sleeping well at night because he has been "guarding his bedroom." You note that his affect is flat, and he appears tired during your examination. A urine toxicology screen is negative. Which of the following is the most likely diagnosis?

(A) bipolar I disorder with psychotic features
(B) brief psychotic disorder
(C) major depressive disorder (MDD) with psychotic features
(D) schizoaffective disorder
(E) schizophreniform disorder

107. An 18-year-old woman with recently diagnosed schizophrenia is acutely psychotic and in labor with her first child. The obstetrics service requests a psychiatric consultation for an appropriate and safe medication to use in order to control the patient's psychotic symptoms. Which of the following would be the best choice?

(A) chlorpromazine (Thorazine)
(B) droperidol (Inapsine)
(C) haloperidol
(D) perphenazine (Trilafon)
(E) thioridazine (Mellaril)

DIRECTIONS (Questions 108 through 116): The following group of questions are preceded by a list of lettered options. For each questions, select the one lettered option that is *most* closely associated with it. Each lettered option may be used once, multiple times, or not at all.

Questions 108 through 111

Match the clinical presentation with the appropriate neuropsychological test.

- (A) Beck Depression Inventory
- (B) Bender Gestalt Test
- (C) Blessed Rating Scale
- (D) Boston Diagnostic Aphasia Examination
- (E) Mini-Mental state Examination (MMSE)
- (F) Minnesota Multiphasic Personality Inventory 2 (MMPI-2)
- (G) Rey-Osterrieth Test
- (H) Rorschach Test
- (I) Wada Test
- (J) Wechsler Adult Intelligence Scale—Revised (WAIS-R)
- (K) Wechsler Intelligence Scale for Children (WISC)

108. A 65-year-old female physician who is now concerned about memory difficulties.

109. A 35-year-old woman with a protein S deficiency shows evidence of left side hemineglect.

110. A 7-year-old boy with difficulty in school needs further evaluation of academic potential.

111. You would like to address the deficits of a 69-year-old man with nonfluent speech and formulate a specific treatment plan.

Questions 112 through 116

Select the drug most likely to cause the associated symptoms.

- (A) cocaine
- (B) lysergic acid diethylamine (LSD)
- (C) marijuana
- (D) nicotine
- (E) opiates
- (F) phencyclidine (PCP)

112. An 18-year-old high school student with conjunctival redness, increased appetite, dry mouth, tachycardia, and a sensation of slowed time.

113. A 31-year-old man with miosis, bradycardia, hypotension, hypothermia, and constipation.

114. An assaultive 26-year-old man with vertical nystagmus, echolalia, paranoid ideation, and hallucinations.

115. A 16-year-old girl with abdominal cramps, confusion, palpitations, and muscle twitching.

116. A 21-year-old man with tachycardia, dilated pupils, hallucinations, and complaints of chest pain.

Answers and Explanations

1. **(C)** Antipsychotics are indicated for acute treatment of agitation and violence sometimes seen in manic patients. Haloperidol works relatively quickly (20-30 minutes). Doses of 2 to 5 mg by mouth (PO) or intramuscularly (IM) are usual, although it may be given IV as well, especially in the intensive care unit (ICU). Hydroxyzine is an antihistamine; it is not effective in mania. Lithium, divalproex sodium, and carbamazepine have all been shown to control mood fluctuations in manic patients. However, these agents take days to work and are not effective in the immediate management of this patient.

2. **(D)** Lithium is not associated with significant blood dyscrasias, although it can cause a modest benign increase in the white blood cell (WBC) count. Carbamazepine is commonly associated with a benign reduction in WBC count, but severe blood dyscrasias only occur in approximately 1 in 125,000 patients. Agranulocytosis is also a rare complication with divalproex sodium, although a benign thrombocytopenia is more common. Agranulocytosis can also occur in the setting of antipsychotic medication use in rare cases (clozapine has a higher incidence). Lorazepam is not associated with WBC abnormalities but is not a mood stabilizer.

3. **(D)** This patient is most likely suffering from somatization disorder, which often coexists with other psychiatric illnesses such as anxiety, depressive, and personality disorders. The suspected presence of a somatization disorder should prompt a search for other treatable illnesses. In managing patients with somatization disorder, it is important to accept that symptoms are not consciously produced and to let patients know that you realize their symptoms are a source of great consternation. Regardless of history, any patient presenting to a physician with physical complaints deserves a reasonable physical investigation; patients with somatization disorder are as likely, if not more likely, to develop identifiable medical conditions. However, rather than repeat tests, it may be necessary to contact previous treaters. Sending this patient away for a year would not be helpful; rather regular, frequent checkups and fostering a therapeutic alliance and support are in order.

4. **(B)** Individuals with somatization disorder frequently (up to 50%) have additional psychiatric illnesses; personality traits or a disorder are not uncommon. Histrionic personality disorder is the most likely in female patients while antisocial is more common in male patients.

5. **(E)** This patient is most likely suffering from schizotypal personal disorder, which as with all personality disorders, represents a lifelong maladaptive approach to life and do not suddenly develop in adulthood. Schizotypal personality disorder with its attendant social isolation and subtle distortions of reality may indeed resemble schizophrenia; the diagnosis can be sorted out by a thorough history. Frank hallucinations of any type are uncommon; only subtle distortion of environmental cues is seen. There is no evidence of mania to justify a diagnosis of bipolar disorder. While under stress, patients with borderline personality disorder can have so-called "micropsychotic episodes," they display chronic feelings of emptiness, mood/affect lability, self-mutilation, and intense anger and

impulsivity. Schizoid personality disorder may appear similar to schizotypal personality disorder, although it is characterized more by feelings of detachment, lack of friends, choosing solitary activities, and anhedonia.

6. **(A)** In schizotypal personality disorder, the subtle disconnection from reality, which may be exacerbated in times of stress as in this case, can be treated with low doses of antipsychotic medication. These patients lack the capability, stable sense of self, and trust to be able to engage in, or benefit from, psychodynamic psychotherapy. Antidepressant medication of any type, including tricyclics and SSRIs, are helpful in the schizotypal patient who displays significant affective (mood) symptoms, which is not seen in this case. Benzodiazepines are not indicated in this case as there is no evidence of anxiety.

7. **(C)** This patient is most likely suffering from schizophrenia. Symptoms of schizophrenia are commonly divided into positive and negative symptoms. Flat affect, a negative symptom, represents an absence of a normally reactive and variable affect. Auditory hallucinations, delusions (including paranoid delusions), and loose associations are all positive symptoms.

8. **(C)** The exacerbation seen is most likely precipitated by medication noncompliance. Stress from work or a viral illness may indeed contribute to a relapse, but they are less strongly predictive of a reemergence of psychotic symptoms than medication noncompliance. Nicotine has been shown to lower neuroleptic levels, which has been offered as a reason cigarette smoking is rampant among patients with schizophrenia. However, this patient's smoking decreased, which if anything would be expected to increase antipsychotic levels.

9. **(B)** Classically, patients with hepatitis secondary to alcohol abuse or dependence have elevated liver enzymes (such as gamma-glutamyl transpeptidase, aspartate transaminase, or alanine transaminase). However, in advanced alcoholism, the liver may be "burnt out" and

liver function tests may reveal low or normal levels of these enzymes. As a result of liver damage, prothrombin time is typically increased. Hypomagnesemia, not hypermagnesemia, is more likely to be found in alcoholism, usually as a result of dietary deficiency. In the patient having a withdrawal seizure, the problem is absence, not presence, of alcohol. His blood alcohol is expected to be zero. The alcoholic is more likely to have thrombocytopenia rather than thrombocytosis.

10. **(C)** The patient has alcohol dependence and has suffered a withdrawal seizure. The mainstay of alcohol detoxification remains benzodiazepines, which may be administered parenterally. Lorazepam is commonly used, since it can be given PO, IM, or IV, and it is not dependent on adequate liver functioning (which may be compromised in alcoholics) for its metabolism. While diazepam (Valium) can be used, it has erratic absorption when given IM, and, in a patient with liver damage, its prolonged half-life can create a large buildup and subsequent oversedation and potential respiratory depression. Haloperidol is an antipsychotic medication which may help with agitation seen in alcohol withdrawal, but doesn't actually treat the underlying problem and may further lower the seizure threshold. While carbamazepine has been shown to be as effective as benzodiazepines in the management of alcohol withdrawal, the other anti-seizure medications are not appropriate treatment.

11. **(B)** While the patient does not have a history of mental illness, which provides information about past behaviors, she is actively suicidal with a plan, and attempts to contact collaterals have been unsuccessful. Collateral information would be helpful to validate the present history as well as to provide data about baseline mental status. Given the absence of collateral input and the fact that she remains suicidal, the patient should not be discharged from the emergency department and should be involuntarily admitted under certificate and petition. The patient does not exhibit psychotic behavior and is not a management problem; the administration of an antipsychotic medication can

cause side effects and may affect future compliance with psychotropic medications. The other choices do not adequately address her safety.

12. **(A)** The Beck Depression Inventory is a widely used test that allows clinicians to follow the severity of previously diagnosed depression. The Draw-A-Person Test, Rorschach Test, and TAT are all types of projective testing. Projective tests, although useful clinical tools, often suffer low reliability and validity. Projective tests require a person skilled at this type of evaluation and do not always have rigorous empirical data and group comparison. The evaluation of depression using the Halstead-Reitan Test is limited by the fact that many depressed patients fail to show deficits on such classic neuropsychological batteries. In addition, these tests, even when demonstrating deficits in cognitive domains such as attention and learning, still have very limited usefulness in evaluating the severity of the depression.

13. **(B)** The Brown-Peterson Task is a test specifically designed to evaluate short-term memory, a capacity that can be affected during ECT. The Bulimia Test—Revised and the EDI-2 are both useful for the evaluation of bulimia and eating disorders, respectively. The Beck Depression Inventory and State-Trait Anxiety Inventory are used to evaluate depression and anxiety disorders, respectively.

14. **(E)** The patient has multiple episodes of depression, unfortunately without remission despite several medication trials with SSRIs. Utilizing an antidepressant with a different mechanism of action (affecting different neurotransmitters) may be beneficial. Venlafaxine is a serotonin and norepinephrine reuptake inhibitor, which, in higher doses, will increase the intrasynaptic levels of both neurotransmitters. All the other choices are SSRIs.

15. **(C)** This scenario represents a case of factitious disorder by proxy, in which one person feigns illness in another to vicariously gain medical attention. Commonly, the victim is a child and the perpetrator is the child's mother. Apparent bleeding, seizures, and central nervous system

(CNS) depression are typical presentations. The disorder is underdiagnosed due both to the elusive and crafty planning of the perpetrator and the unwillingness of health care providers to accuse the ostensibly caring parent. Given the age of the child, it is extremely unlikely that the child, himself, is intentionally producing the symptoms, and there is no evidence that he is experiencing physiologic seizures. Conversion disorder is characterized by the presence of one or more neurologic symptoms that are left unexplained by a known medical or neurologic disorder. Paralysis, blindness, and mutism are the most common conversion disorder symptoms. The diagnosis requires the association of psychological factors to the initiation and exacerbation of conversion symptoms. Separation anxiety disorder is characterized by excessive and inappropriate anxiety concerning separation from home or to whom individuals are attached.

16. **(B)** Mothers with factitious disorder by proxy have been variously described as depressed, anxious, and suicidal; therefore, of the choices listed, depression is the most likely. Borderline and histrionic personality disorders are the most common Axis II diagnoses associated with factitious disorder by proxy. Bipolar disorder and PTSD have not been clearly described in the literature. Epilepsy is not associated with the disorder to any significant extent, and schizophrenia has been reported in only a few cases.

17. **(E)** Panic disorder is characterized by the sudden unexpected occurrence of panic attacks (periods of intense anxiety or fear accompanied by somatic symptoms), commonly causing the misdiagnosis of a medical illness such as myocardial infarction. The frequency of panic attacks varies widely from many per day to a few per year. Panic disorder is often associated with agoraphobia, the fear of being in places where escape is difficult. The lifetime prevalence is up to 3%. Concerns of death from cardiac or respiratory disorders occur frequently. Acute stress disorder is diagnosed in individuals who have experienced a traumatic event and subsequently develop symptoms within 4 weeks of the event that remit after 1 month. The traumatic event must be reexperienced by

the patient, and this causes the patient to avoid stimuli that arouse recollections of the trauma. Other criteria necessary for the diagnosis are the presence of dissociative symptoms and marked anxiety or increased arousal not better accounted for by other medical or psychiatric illnesses. Delirium is characterized by the sudden onset of a disturbance of consciousness with cognitive changes caused by a general medical condition.

18. **(E)** Of the choices listed, sertraline, an SSRI, is the most efficacious. In addition, tricyclic antidepressants, MAOIs, and the benzodiazepines are also effective in the treatment of panic disorder. Beta-adrenergic drugs like propranolol are not effective for the treatment of panic disorder. Haloperidol, an antipsychotic agent; lithium, a mood stabilizer; and clonidine, an alpha-2-adrenergic agonist, are ineffective.

19. **(A)** Hypertensive crisis is a potentially life-threatening complication that occurs when patients taking an MAOI eat tyramine-containing foods such as wine, beer, pickled foods, and aged cheese. Clinical features include hypertension, severe occipital headache, stiff neck, nausea, vomiting, and sweating. IV phentolamine, an alpha-adrenergic receptor blocker, is given to control the hypertension. It has been shown to be more effective than beta-blockers or calcium channel blockers. Admission to an ICU and supportive measures are indicated. Although muscle rigidity can occur, the use of dantrolene, a muscle relaxant, is not indicated.

20. **(D)** Clozapine is an effective antipsychotic medication that has been associated with fewer extrapyramidal side effects than the conventional antipsychotics (which primarily act by blocking dopamine type 2 receptors). About 5% of patients taking more than 600 mg/d of clozapine experience clozapine-associated seizures. Tachycardia, hypotension, sedation, fatigue, and weight gain have all been associated with clozapine treatment. Clozapine, unlike the conventional antipsychotic agents, does not affect prolactin secretion and thus does not cause galactorrhea.

21. **(B)** Agranulocytosis is a potentially life-threatening side effect of clozapine treatment. It is defined as a decrease in the number of WBCs, with a specific decrease in the number of neutrophil granulocytes. It occurs in 1% to 2% of all patients treated with clozapine. Therefore, a complete blood count with differential is required weekly in the beginning of treatment and frequently thereafter. Routine monitoring with the other tests are not required or necessary with clozapine treatment.

22. **(B)** The Folstein MMSE is a frequently used screening assessment for dementia (although more in depth and formal neuropsychological testing should be performed at some point). It is a 30-point scale with deductions for incorrect answers. Scores less than 25 are suggestive of cognitive impairment. Scores less than 20 indicate definitive impairment. The Blessed Rating Scale is a tool that typically asks a patient's friends or relatives to assess the ability of the patient to function in his or her current environment. The Geriatric Rating Scale is a rating scale for nonprofessional staff to evaluate patients' abilities to perform their activities of daily living and interact with others. It may be most helpful in evaluation of the moderately to severely demented individual. The Glasgow Coma Scale is an easy-to-perform instrument that evaluates level of consciousness. There are three general categories that the examiner tests: eye opening, verbal response, and best motor response. Each category receives a number for patient response. Overall scores range from 3 to 15, with lower scores reflecting more severely impaired consciousness. A mental status examination is the formal psychiatric examination that includes many items such as appearance, behavior, speech, assessment of mood and affect, presence of psychosis, and evaluation of insight and judgment. It is not a substitute for the Folstein MMSE.

23. **(B)** When evaluating the MMSE score in elderly patients, it is critical to consider that depression (also known as "pseudodementia") may produce similar impairments in cognition. The other diagnoses listed would not commonly reduce the Folstein MMSE score.

24. **(E)** Schizotypal personality disorder is characterized by a pervasive pattern of social and interpersonal deficits. Individuals demonstrate a reduced capacity to establish any close relationships, and eccentric behavior is present. The presence of odd beliefs or magical thinking separates schizotypal personality disorder from schizoid personality disorder. Paranoid ideation is common in both schizotypal and paranoid personality disorders but not in the others. Avoidant personality disorder represents a pervasive pattern of behavior characterized by social inhibition, feelings of inadequacy, and hypersensitivity to negative evaluation. Narcissistic personality disorder represents a pervasive pattern of grandiosity, lack of empathy, and a need for admiration. Schizoid personality disorder represents a pervasive pattern of detachment from social relationships and a restricted range of expressed emotions.

25. **(B)** Borderline personality disorder is a pervasive pattern of instability of interpersonal relationships, self-image, affect, and marked impulsivity. Antisocial personality disorder describes individuals with long histories of disregard for the rights of others and often dishonesty used in attempts to gain something for themselves. Patients with dependent personality disorder require an excessive amount of advice, reassurance, and approval from others. Individuals with histrionic personality disorder, like those with borderline personality disorder, may display excessive emotionality and attention-seeking behavior, but their core symptoms center around superficial seductiveness and theatricality. Schizoid personality disorder represents a pervasive pattern of detachment from social relationships and a restricted range of expressed emotions.

26. **(E)** In the WCST, examinees are asked to sort cards depicting various pictures and symbols according to a variety of different criteria that change over time without the subject's knowing. The WCST assesses a person's ability to switch sets, reason abstractly, and solve problems. These capacities are also known as executive functions and are localized in the frontal lobes. Current research regarding the psychopathology of schizophrenia suggests that there are abnormalities in the frontal lobes, specifically in the dorsolateral prefrontal cortex, that are reflected in poor performance on the WCST. People with schizophrenia perform more poorly on the WCST than people without schizophrenia; however, individuals with damage to their frontal lobes from a variety of causes also show executive function deficits. The Bender Gestalt Test involves copying figures, which helps determine if organic brain disease is present. The Draw-A-Person Test requires the examinee to draw a person. It was initially devised to test intelligence in children, but is now used primarily as a screening test for brain damage. The Luria-Nebraska Neuropsychological Battery is a comprehensive set of neuropsychological tests used to assess specific cortical areas and aids in assessment of hemispheric dominance. The Mini-Mental State Examination is a commonly used scale to assess the possibility of dementia.

27. **(B)** The WCST assesses a person's ability to switch sets, reason abstractly, and solve problems. These capacities are also known as executive functions and are localized in the frontal lobes. The cerebellum is responsible for coordination. The occipital lobe is dedicated to the sense of sight. The parietal lobe handles sensory input, motor output, and visuospatial processing. The temporal lobe is responsible for the sense of sound, taste, and memory storage.

28. **(D)** This patient is most likely suffering from bipolar I disorder. Racing thoughts, pressured speech, expansive mood, a decreased need for sleep, and an increase in goal-directed activity are all common manifestations of mania. The patient is usually energized during the day even after only a few hours of sleep. Visual hallucinations could be present in severe cases of mania but are more commonly a symptom of a primary psychotic disorder such as schizophrenia. Weight loss and depressed mood are more characteristic of a depressive disorder.

29. **(E)** Many disorders can mimic symptoms of mania. A complete history, physical examination, and routine laboratory tests can sufficiently

rule out most medical causes of mania. They include endocrine disorders such as thyrotox-icosis and Cushing syndrome, hypoglycemia, electrolyte disorders, substance abuse and withdrawal, medications such as steroids and anticholinergic agents, nutritional deficiencies, and CNS insults.

30. **(B)** Gingival hyperplasia is associated with administration of phenytoin. Other, dose-related symptoms include nystagmus, dizzi-ness, slurred speech, ataxia, mental confusion, and decreased coordination. Ebstein anomaly is associated with lithium therapy, and hepatic failure is associated with divalproex sodium.

31. **(D)** Before any pharmacologic changes are considered, the physician must assess compli-ance with medications. The subtherapeutic phenytoin level may be due to patient non-compliance, especially if side effects are being experienced.

32. **(E)** The risk of schizophrenia among first-degree relatives where one parent has schizo-phrenia may be as high as 12%, compared with a 1% risk in the general population.

33. **(A)** The patient is being evaluated with the Rorschach Test, which was developed in 1921 by Hermann Rorschach. It consists of showing a subject a set of 10 inkblot stimuli in a sequen-tial manner while noting (1) the responses in relationship to the content of the perception; (2) the area of the blot that forms the basis of the response; and (3) the aspects of the area that are used to form the response. In 1961, Lindzey proposed a method of classifying pro-jective tests based on the type of activity. The Rorschach is classified in the category of asso-ciations. Another test in this category is the Word Association Test. In the choice of ordering category, patients place objects in a rank order with respect to preference. Tests such as the Sentence Completion Test fall into the category of completions, in which a person completes an uncompleted stimulus. The construction cate-gory requires the subject to construct con-tent based on a stimulus, such as a story in the Thematic Apperception Test. The self-expression category consists of tests such as the Draw-A-Person Test, in which the subject produces a response without a stimulus.

34. **(C)** It is not ethical to engage in therapy (ie, conversion therapy) to the change the sexual orientation of a patient. According to the APA's ethics committee "any treatment that is based on an assumption that homosexuality per se is a mental disorder, or is based on an assumption that the patient should change his or her sexual orientation, is by its nature unethical, as it vio-lates numerous ethics principles. Such so-called treatment ignores established scientific evi-dence, demeans the dignity of the patient, suc-cumbs to individual and social prejudice and stigma, and has often been significantly harm-ful to patients, families, others, and their rela-tionships." Ultimately, per APA's principles of medical ethics "a psychiatrist should not be a party to any type of policy that excludes, seg-regates, or demeans the dignity of any patient because of ethnic origin, race, sex, creed, age, socioeconomic status, or sexual orientation." All the other choices would be considered unethical.

35. **(B)** Cocaine intoxication can appear similar to a manic episode associated with bipolar I disor-der with an increase in energy, euphoria, grandiosity, pressured speech, and impaired judgment. While cannabis intoxication can pres-ent with euphoria, paranoia, and impaired judgment (in association with physical symp-toms of conjunctival injection, increased appetite, dry mouth, and tachycardia), a decreased need for sleep, diaphoresis, and rapid speech do not suggest cannabis intoxication. The acute onset of symptoms makes the diagno-sis of major depression unlikely. A diagnosis of schizoaffective disorder requires that during the period of illness there are symptoms that suggest a both schizophrenia and a mood disorder (major depressive episode, manic episode, or a mixed episode). Schizophrenia requires the presence of significant psychotic symptoms during a 1-month period, which is not evident in this case; the patient experienced euphoria which is not characteristic of schizo-phrenia. Negative symptoms (eg, flattened

affect, avolition, alogia) are also more common in schizophrenia.

36. **(D)** The Temporal Orientation Test asks the patient to identify the appropriate day, month, day of the week, and current time. Deviation from the correct response is differentially scored in each category. Total score and the data incorrectly identified separate the patients into two groups: patients with brain damage and patients without brain damage. The Temporal Orientation Test is also sensitive to cognitive abnormalities in dementing illnesses. The Fargo Map Test assesses recent and remote spatial memory and visuospatial orientation by using maps of the United States and different regions within it. Patients are asked to identify certain areas. Education level and age influence the score on this test. The Spatial Orientation Memory Test evaluates the ability to immediately recall the orientation of figures and is used to evaluate immediate memory. The Stroop Test has a number of different formats, but the general concept is that it takes longer to correctly identify a color than to read words and longer yet to correctly identify a word (eg, name of a color) when that word is in a color different from that word. This test seems to be primarily an assessment of ability to concentrate. The WCST is used to evaluate executive functioning of the brain.

37. **(A)** Culture-bound syndromes denote recurrent, locality-specific patterns of behavior. The syndrome of amok is a culture-bound syndrome of Malaysian origin that refers to a violent or furious outburst with homicidal intent. Four defining characteristics are prodromal brooding, a homicidal outburst, persistence in reckless killing without an apparent motive, and a claim of amnesia. The attack typically results in multiple casualties and is most common in young men whose self-esteem has been injured. Dhat is an Indian term referring to anxiety regarding the discharge of semen. Ganser syndrome is characterized by a patient who responds to questions by giving approximate or outright ridiculous answers. Additional features may also include altered consciousness, hallucinations, conversion phenomenon,

and amnesia for the episode. Koro is another Malaysian term that refers to sudden anxiety that the penis (or vulva in females) will recede into the body and cause death. Latah is also of Malaysian or Indonesian origin, more frequent in middle-aged women, and is characterized by sudden fear, often with dissociation and catatonic-like features (eg, echolalia, echopraxia).

38. **(A)** Neuroleptic-induced extrapyramidal side effects due to the blockade of dopamine are common in the treatment of psychosis. The higher-potency neuroleptic drugs are more likely to cause extrapyramidal side effects than the lower-potency neuroleptics. Extrapyramidal side effects include acute dystonic reactions (as in this case), akathisia (restlessness), pseudoparkinsonism, and tardive dyskinesia. Acute dystonia is treated with anticholinergic agents such as benztropine and antihistamines. Other options include reducing the dose or switching to a lower-potency agent or atypical antipsychotic (such as risperidone). Neither of these are preferable at this point as the patient's symptoms have improved.

39. **(E)** Because of this patient's continued extrapyramidal symptoms despite treatment with an anticholinergic, the most appropriate choice would be to switch to an atypical antipsychotic medication. Atypical, or second-generation antipsychotics, such as quetiapine, are believed to act on various subpopulations of dopamine receptor subtypes as well as on other neurotransmitter systems, including the serotonergic. They are considered "atypical" agents because they are associated with a lower risk of extrapyramidal symptoms. Clozapine, introduced to the United States in 1989, is the first antipsychotic to be labeled atypical. Other atypical or second-generation medications include risperidone, olanzapine, ziprasidone, and aripiprazole. The other choices are all considered to be typical antipsychotics.

40. **(C)** Borderline personality disorder is a pattern of instability in interpersonal relationships, self-image, affect, and marked impulsivity, including inappropriate anger and self-mutilation.

Avoidant personality disorder represents a pervasive pattern of behavior characterized by social inhibition, feelings of inadequacy, and hypersensitivity to negative evaluation. Bipolar disorder is an affective illness characterized by alternating periods of mania and major depression. Features of dependent personality disorder are an excessive need to be taken care of, clinging behavior, and fears of separation. Narcissistic patients demonstrate a pattern of grandiosity, need for admiration, and lack of empathy.

41. **(D)** DBT is a manualized treatment for chronically parasuicidal patients such as borderline personality disorder. It incorporates elements of cognitive, behavioral, and supportive therapies, and it includes techniques of advice, confrontation, and use of homework. Aversion therapy is a controversial technique where an aversive stimuli is paired with an undesired behavior, hopefully suppressing the unwanted behavior. EMDR is a cognitive-behavioral technique whereby a patient with posttraumatic stress disorder is told to think about a stressful event while tracking an object back and forth across their vision. Flooding is a behavioral intervention where a patient is exposed to a feared object directly. This is in contrast with systematic desensitization, where a phobic patient is gradually exposed to increasingly feared situations using a hierarchy of anxiety-provoking triggers.

42. **(A)** The patient is experiencing anticholinergic toxicity as evidenced by dilated pupils, dry or flushed skin, agitation, confusion, and tachycardia. Additional manifestations include disorientation and urinary retention. More severe toxicity may result in hyperthermia or coma. In this case, the patient reported benefit from haloperidol but experienced extrapyramidal side effects, common to the high-potency antipsychotic medications. Benztropine, an anticholinergic medication, is prescribed to alleviate extrapyramidal side effects, but in this patient it caused anticholinergic side effects. Amantadine is an antiviral medication that is also used to help alleviate extrapyramidal side effects and should be instituted to replace benztropine.

43. **(C)** Objective tests usually involve questions with lists of possible responses. These tests provide numerical scores on which statistical analyses are easily performed. Examples include the United States Medical Licensing Examinations. The main advantage to projective tests (such as the Rorschach) is that there are a variety of responses without a single correct answer. The idea behind projective tests is that when presented with an ambiguous stimulus, patients cannot help but reveal something about themselves both in how they address the stimulus as well as the content of their answers. Many of these tests, including the Rorschach Test, the Thematic Apperception Test (TAT), the Sentence Completion Test, and the Draw-A-Person Test, require specific training in giving the test and interpreting the results. Projective tests do not necessarily tell the interviewer how the patient feels about him or her.

44. **(C)** The MMPI and MMPI-2 are objective tests that have been used for over 50 years in the assessment of personality structure. They consist of more than 500 statements, which are condensed into clinical subscales. Items on the subscales were derived empirically and were chosen because data showed they could separate psychiatric patients from normal control subjects. Additionally, questions are asked at the time of examination to evaluate attitudes when taking the test. These questions help to provide information about the validity of the examination. Interpretation of the results requires an experienced evaluator. Together with the clinical history, this test provides valuable information about personality structure. Its accuracy does not depend on the patient's gender, and the results do not reflect how the examinee feels about test taking.

45. **(D)** Denial, a narcissistic defense, is an (unconscious) emotional defense mechanism used to avoid becoming aware of a painful aspect of reality. Denial can be used in both normal and pathologic states. As a defense mechanism it serves to keep internal or external reality out of the conscious to avert stress and anxiety. Regression, an immature defense, is an emotional and physical retreat from adult standards

of behavior toward an infantile level of passivity and dependence. Rationalization is a neurotic defense mechanism in which unacceptable behavior, feelings, or thoughts are logically justified by elaborate and reassuring answers. Suppression, a mature defense, is a conscious act of controlling and inhibiting unacceptable impulses, emotions, or ideas.

46. **(A)** The essential feature of acute stress disorder is the development of anxiety and dissociative symptoms within 1 month of exposure to an extremely traumatic stressor. Diagnosis should be considered if the symptoms persist at least 2 days and cause significant distress or impairment. While experiencing the stressor, the individual must experience three of these five symptoms: a subjective sense of numbing, detachment, or absence of emotional responsiveness; a reduction in awareness of surroundings; derealization; depersonalization; or dissociative amnesia. In addition, the person must reexperience the event in some way (eg, nightmares), must experience anxiety or increased arousal, and must experience a marked avoidance of the stimuli that arouse recollections of the traumatic event. The diagnosis of PTSD requires more than 1 month of the above symptoms. Adjustment disorder can be considered for those individuals who do not meet criteria for acute stress disorder but develop similar symptoms in excess of what is to be expected given the nature of the stressor. GAD is characterized by excessive anxiety and worry that occur for at least 6 months. MDD can exist in the context of an acute stress reaction. However, the symptoms are not suggestive of a depressive illness as there is no clear depressed mood, change in appetite, energy, or concentration.

47. **(B)** Psychogenic unresponsiveness can be delineated from coma by obtaining an EEG, which is normal in a psychogenic state. On the physical examination of a comatose patient, deep tendon reflexes may be suppressed. In patients who are awake, cold water introduced into the ear produces nystagmus with the fast component away from the ear. In coma, the eyes either do not react or they may slowly and smoothly deviate toward the ear in which the cold water was introduced. Voluntary eye movements called saccades are rapid and smooth. Saccadic eye movements are elicited in patients by asking them to stare at an object at one side of the visual field and then ask them to shift their gaze to the opposite visual field. Typically, eye movements in coma or persistent vegetative states are spontaneous and random. Abnormal vital signs such as temperature and respiration would not likely be affected.

48. **(D)** Seasonal affective disorder describes a seasonal pattern of symptoms associated with major depressive episodes in MDD, bipolar I disorder, and bipolar II disorder. The essential feature is the onset of depressive symptoms at characteristic times of the year. It occurs more commonly in women, and most episodes begin in the fall or winter and remit in the spring. Major depressive episodes that occur in a seasonal pattern are typically characterized by anergy, hypersomnia, overeating, weight gain, and carbohydrate craving. Age is a strong predictor, with young persons at higher risk. Acute stress disorder is characterized by the development of anxiety, dissociative, and other symptoms within 1 month of exposure to a traumatic event. Dysthymic disorder is mood disorder where the depressed mood occurs most of the time for at least 2 years. Generalized anxiety disorder patients describe chronic anxiety over a number of events lasting over 6 months. Sundowning refers to drowsiness, confusion, and falling, typically seen in demented patients when lights or other orienting cues are removed.

49. **(B)** The essential features of dissociative fugue are sudden and unexpected travel away from home or one's usual place of daily activities with a subsequent inability to recall the episode accompanied by confusion about personal identity or the assumption of a new identity. The disorder is more common in women and is often associated with a history of sexual abuse in childhood. Delirium is characterized by a disturbance of consciousness and a change in cognition that develop over a short period of time. Major depression is diagnosed

in individuals with 2 weeks of depression and neurovegetative symptoms (changes in sleep, appetite, energy). Partial complex seizures tend to be brief and do not last as long as the clinical picture presents. For the diagnosis of posttraumatic stress disorder, an individual must be exposed to a traumatic stressor, along with symptoms of reexperiencing, hyperarousal, and avoidance of reminders.

50. **(C)** The *DSM-IV-TR* recognizes four categories of learning disorders: reading disorder, mathematics disorder, disorder of written expression, and not otherwise specified. Learning disorders are identified when a patient's achievement IQ in that area is significantly lower than the overall IQ. The Wechsler Adult Intelligence Scale was initially published in 1955 and has undergone a series of revisions to reach the current scale, the WAIS-R. The test is composed of 11 different subtests—6 verbal and 5 performance—that allow for the calculation of the full-scale IQ, performance IQ, and verbal IQ. The WAIS-R has high reliability, which means that in normal subjects retesting does not lead to significantly different evaluations; therefore it can be used to follow people over time. The Draw-A-Person Test is used to evaluate for organic brain disease, and the MMPI-2 is a test used for the assessment of personality structure. The WISC is used to determine IQ in children from ages 6 to 16. The WMT was designed to evaluate a variety of aspects of memory function in adults.

51. **(C)** The IQ is calculated by dividing the mental age by the chronological age and multiplying this by 100.

52. **(B)** While this patient meets criteria for a major depressive episode, she has a history of symptoms consistent with a hypomanic episode (a distinct period of a persistently elevated, expansive, or irritable mood that lasts at least 4 days). Bipolar II disorder differs from bipolar I disorder in that, although the manic and hypomanic episodes of these two disorders have identical criteria, bipolar II disorder is not severe enough to cause marked impairment in social or occupational functioning or to cause

hospitalization and does not have psychotic symptoms. Cyclothymic disorder consists of chronic, fluctuating mood episodes of hypomania alternating with periods of depression which do not meet criteria for major depressive episodes. Dysthymic disorder is characterized by chronically depressed mood most of the time for 2 years without hypomanic or manic episodes.

53. **(D)** The hallmark of Ganser syndrome is that the patient responds to questions by giving approximate or ridiculous answers. It involves the production of answers to questions that are relative but not quite correct (eg, $4 \times 5 = 19$). Ganser syndrome is primarily described in males in the prison population. Although it may be related to malingering or factitious disorder with psychological symptoms, it is classified in the *DSM-IV-TR* as a dissociative disorder not otherwise specified. Capgras syndrome describes a content-specific delusion in which the patient believes that a significant other, usually a family member, has been replaced by an identical imposter. Dementias are cognitive disorders associated with memory deficits and problems with executive functioning. Although patients with dementia may confabulate, this patient's age is too young, and he has obvious secondary gain. Munchausen syndrome is a factitious disorder with physical symptoms, where the individual feigns an illness in order to assume the sick role.

54. **(B)** ECT provides a safe and effective treatment of MDD in the elderly, especially in a patient with a high risk of suicide or medical contraindications (eg, heart disease) to the use of certain psychotropic medications. It is also indicated when a more rapid onset of action (several days) is important (compared with several weeks for antidepressant medications). Diazepam is a benzodiazepine which is useful in the treatment of symptomatic anxiety but not for depression. Nortriptyline, a tricyclic antidepressant (TCA), is lethal in overdose and should not be prescribed in an acutely suicidal patient. Certain cardiac arrhythmias are also contraindications to TCA use. Risperidone is an antipsychotic medication used primarily for

psychotic disorders such as schizophrenia and schizoaffective disorder, as well as for bipolar disorder or major depression with psychotic features. Supportive psychotherapy may be helpful in conjunction with medications or ECT, but it is not indicated as monotherapy for severe depression with suicidality.

55. **(C)** This patient is suffering from a major depressive episode with atypical features. The specifiers of melancholic features and atypical features can be applied to a current or recent major depressive episode that occurs in the course of MDD and to a major depressive episode in bipolar I or bipolar II disorder. The atypical features specifier can also be applied to dysthymic disorder. The essential features of the atypical specifier are mood reactivity and two of the following four features: increased appetite or weight gain, hypersomnia, leaden paralysis, and rejection sensitivity. The essential feature of a major depressive episode with melancholic features is a loss of interest or pleasure in all or almost all activities or a lack of reactivity to usually pleasurable stimuli. The patient's depressive symptoms are too acute and severe for adjustment disorder, and don't last 2 years which would be necessary for dysthymic disorder. Although hypersomnia (and insomnia) may be due to a sleep disorder, the patient's symptoms are better accounted for by a major depressive disorder.

56. **(C)** Identification is an unconscious defense mechanism in which the person incorporates the characteristics and qualities of another person or object into his or her own ego system. The defense serves to strengthen the ego. Fixation refers to an overactive attachment to a person or object; idealization is the attribution of near-perfect, unrealistic attributes to that person or object. Projection is the false attribution of one's own unacceptable feelings to another. Regression, an immature defense, is an emotional and physical retreat from adult standards of behavior toward an infantile level of passivity and dependence.

57. **(D)** The essential feature of the catatonia observed in patients with schizophrenia (as well as mood disorders with psychotic features) is a marked psychomotor disturbance involving motor immobility, excessive motor activity, mutism, negativism, peculiar voluntary movements, echolalia (parrot-like senseless repetition of words or phrases), or echopraxia (imitation of movements of another person). Catalepsy, a term for an immobile position that is maintained, is one potential symptom of catatonia, and is not a complete answer. Cataplexy is a sudden and brief loss of muscle tone involving either a few muscle groups or most of the antigravity muscles of the body. His diagnosis of schizophrenia, and the fact that the patient occasionally mimics the movements of others, makes seizure activity from a seizure disorder unlikely.

58. **(A)** Catalepsy is a general term for the assumption of an immobile position that is constantly maintained, especially after an examination. It is a symptom of catatonia. Cataplexy is a sudden and brief loss of muscle tone involving either a few muscle groups or most of the muscles of the body. Dystonia is a painful stiffening of muscle groups sometimes seen after administration of typical antipsychotic medications. The patient does not seem to have a secondary gain for his symptoms making malingering unlikely. Rigidity (or catatonic rigidity) may also be seen in catatonic patients, but unlike catalepsy, it is held against all efforts to be moved.

59. **(E)** Priapism can occur with a number of antidepressant or antipsychotic agents but occurs more frequently with the use of trazodone (1 in 1000 to 1 in 10,000 incidence). The three serotonin-specific reuptake inhibitors (fluoxetine, paroxetine, and sertraline) listed can cause decreased sex drive and impotence, but are unlikely to cause priapism. Nortriptyline is a tricyclic antidepressant and not associated with priapism.

60. **(D)** While priapism usually occurs within the first 4 weeks of treatment, it can occur at any time. It is also independent of dose. Priapism, especially lasting over several hours, is a medical

emergency and may require surgery to prevent possible necrosis, scarring, and impotence. Ejaculation does not always reduce the erection. Priapism may require draining blood from the corpus cavernosum or intracavernosal injection of an alpha-adrenergic agonist to promote detumescence and constriction of veins. The offending medication should be immediately stopped and not restarted, as prior priapism predisposes to future episodes.

61. **(B)** The patient is most likely suffering from generalized anxiety disorder (GAD). Treatment of GAD includes antidepressants such as serotonin-specific reuptake inhibitors, benzodiazepines, buspirone, and cognitive-behavioral therapies. However, benzodiazepines (such as alprazolam, diazepam, and lorazepam) should be avoided in patients with respiratory compromise, because these medications can exacerbate breathing-related disorders, and they carry the risk of addiction. Buspirone, a nonbenzodiazepine anxiolytic, is a logical alternative and has been demonstrated to be effective in the treatment of GAD. Beta-blocking agents such as propranolol are effective in certain anxiety disorders, such as social phobia (social anxiety disorder), but should not be first-line therapy in patients with chronic obstructive pulmonary disease or other respiratory disorders.

62. **(E)** The long-term use of benzodiazepines (clorazepate, oxazepam, and temazepam) for sleep is controversial, especially in patients with substance abuse or breathing-related disorders. Zolpidem is not a member of the benzodiazepine class but does produce its effects at the gamma-aminobutyric acid (GABA)-benzodiazepine receptor and has a much lower risk of dependence. A nonbenzodiazepine medication is a logical alternative in cases in which respiratory function is compromised. Diphenhydramine should be avoided in the older population due to its anticholinergic effects and possible delirium.

63. **(D)** Hypertensive crisis is a life-threatening emergency that may result from the combination of meperidine and an MAOI. The combined use of these medications is absolutely contraindicated. The treatment of hypertensive crisis is with IV alpha-adrenergic blocking agents and ICU admission and support. All of the other medications are safe in combination with MAOIs.

64. **(C)** The use of any medications in pregnancy requires examining the risks and benefits of treatment. The use of MAOIs is contraindicated in pregnancy partly because they can exacerbate pregnancy-induced hypertension. Although ECT is safe in pregnancy, maintenance ECT is indicated after an initial course of ECT is completed. The safety of newer antidepressants such as paroxetine in pregnancy has not yet been completely established, but studies of fluoxetine suggest that it is relatively safe. In this case, after discontinuing the MAOI, there would have to be a 14-day washout before initiating fluoxetine. Specific recommendations regarding the course of treatment for a single episode of MDD do not exist. Many physicians find that the treatment of a single episode requires 9 to 12 months of pharmacotherapy. The return of symptoms suggests a recurrent MDD that requires longer-term pharmacotherapy. Of course, ongoing discussion with and education of the patient are essential.

65. **(B)** The patient presents with clinical symptoms of Wernicke encephalopathy, a medical emergency, characterized by ophthalmoplegia, ataxia, and delirium caused by acute thiamine deficiency. If the thiamine deficiency is not corrected, Korsakoff syndrome can emerge characterized by chronic persisting amnesia. Korsakoff syndrome results from chronic thiamine deficiency with resultant pathology in the mammillary bodies and the thalamus. A history of alcohol abuse is common but other causes of thiamine deficiency such as starvation, prolonged vomiting, and gastric carcinoma can cause this syndrome. The use of IV dextrose prior to the administration of thiamine may aggravate Wernicke encephalopathy. The other interventions may be appropriate if thiamine does not resolve the symptoms.

66. **(E)** According to the AMA's code of ethics "A physician shall be dedicated to providing competent medical service with compassion and respect for human dignity." In the event a

physician is concerned about whether he or she is able to remain impartial and provide adequate psychiatric treatment, the physician should seek a consultation with an unbiased colleague or supervisor to discuss the issues and ultimately determine what would be in the best interest of the patient. It may be that another physician in the clinic or community would better serve the patient's needs, but this would best be determined after a consultation. To limit the time spent with the patient is not appropriate and can constitute discrimination. While it is important to be aware of the patient's progress in therapy, the physician must first process his or her own partiality to determine whether a therapeutic alliance can be established and maintained.

67. **(B)** Caffeine withdrawal occurs after the abrupt cessation or a marked reduction in the use of caffeinated products. Studies estimate that up to 75% of caffeine users will experience symptoms of withdrawal at some point. Caffeine withdrawal symptoms have their onset 12 to 24 hours after the last dose, and symptoms peak in 24 to 48 hours. Symptoms typically remit in 1 week. Although all the possible choices are associated with caffeine withdrawal, up to 50% of sufferers experience headache, the most common symptom.

68. **(E)** This patient is most likely suffering from neuroleptic malignant syndrome (NMS). NMS is characterized by muscular rigidity, confusion, mutism, agitation, and elevated autonomic signs. Death is reported in up to 20% of cases, usually from a failure to recognize the syndrome or from delayed treatment. Discontinuation of the offending agent and supportive treatment in an ICU setting is imperative. IV dantrolene sodium and oral bromocriptine have been used but their benefits are unclear. Cooling measures may reduce hyperthermia. The exact frequency of NMS remains unknown, with some studies suggesting up to 2.4% of all patients treated with antipsychotics experiencing this syndrome. NMS may be more frequent in men and younger patients. Naloxone does not have a place in the treatment of NMS.

69. **(C)** An elevated serum CPK demonstrates muscle injury. Since liver transaminases (AST, ALT) are also found in muscle, these also may be elevated. Leukocytosis is also seen in NMS. Anemia is not found in NMS. Elevated BUN may occur due to dehydration resulting from NMS but is not as common as creatinine or CPK elevation.

70. **(C)** Physical dependence emphasizes the presence of tolerance or withdrawal. Naloxone injection can precipitate opiate withdrawal in dependent persons. Positive urine toxicology or breath analysis can identify only substance use, not necessarily dependence. Elevated heart rate can be present in many withdrawal syndromes or medical disorders and is not specific for any substance. Elevated liver function studies can be present in individuals who abuse alcohol but can also be present in other non-substance-related disorders.

71. **(E)** Dementia is characterized by memory deficits and cognitive disturbances without impaired consciousness. (This differentiates it from delirium characterized by a waxing and waning consciousness.) The most common type of dementia (50%-60%) is the Alzheimer type. Vascular dementia is the second most common type of dementia, occurring in 10% to 20% of cases. Other degenerative processes that cause dementia are Parkinson disease, Huntington disease, and Pick disease. Infectious, metabolic, endocrine, neoplastic, and toxic processes can also cause dementia. In this case, the history of cognitive decline without impaired consciousness suggests a diagnosis of dementia. His history reveals a megaloblastic anemia, the cause of which may be a vitamin B_{12} deficiency, likely secondary to a gastrectomy. Folate deficiency can also cause megaloblastic anemia. Vitamin deficiencies such as B_{12} and folate can cause clinical signs of dementia, but represent one of a few possible reversible causes of this process. A complete reversible workup for dementia should also include thyroid function studies and a rapid plasma reagin to test for syphilis. Alzheimer disease can only be definitively diagnosed on autopsy.

72. **(B)** Lithium, commonly used to treat bipolar disorder, can be dangerous in intoxication and can lead to death or permanent damage to the nervous system, particularly the cerebellum. Cardiovascular and renal manifestations may also be present. Lithium has a narrow therapeutic window with a therapeutic range of 0.6 to 1.2 mEq/L. Plasma concentrations above the therapeutic range, especially greater than 2.0 mEq/L, precipitate severe CNS and renal impairment. Early clinical signs of intoxication include dysarthria, coarse tremor, and ataxia. Impaired consciousness, fasciculations or myoclonus, seizures, and coma are ominous manifestations. The goal of treatment is removal of lithium from the body. Gastric lavage, rehydration, and hemodialysis are possible interventions. Given the danger of lithium intoxication, a serum drug level should be obtained before any of the other interventions.

73. **(E)** A right parietal stroke would most likely demonstrate abnormalities in visual, nonverbal memory.

74. **(B)** The Rey-Osterrieth Test is a complex figure that the patient is asked to copy while looking at the figure. The figure is then taken away and the patient is asked to draw the picture from immediate memory. The patient is again asked to draw the figure 5 minutes and 30 minutes after the figure has been removed. The tasks assess visual nonverbal memory. People with right parietal lesions usually show abnormalities in copying the figure correctly by neglecting the items in the left visual field. Conversely, a patient with a right temporal lobectomy may have no difficulty in copying the figure, but show marked abnormalities in drawing the item from memory. The Minnesota Multiphasic Personality Inventory, Rorschach Test, Wechsler Intelligence Scales, and Wisconsin Card Sorting Test would not be as useful in assessing a right parietal lesion.

75. **(D)** Baseline medical tests should be obtained and documented before starting many psychotropic medications including the mood stabilizers lithium, carbamazepine, and divalproex sodium. Assessment of thyroid function, complete blood count, electrolytes, ECG, and renal function studies (BUN, creatinine, urinalysis) are important before the initiation of lithium. Older patients may require additional tests, including EEG, thyrotropin-releasing hormone test, 24-hour urine volume determination, and creatinine clearance. Lithium-induced polyuria results from the inhibition of the effect of antidiuretic hormone. Reversible T-wave changes on the ECG are also common.

76. **(D)** The serotonin syndrome occurs when an SSRI is combined with another drug that can potentiate serotonin, such as the monoamine oxidase-inhibiting drugs, pentazocine, L-tryptophan, lithium, and carbamazepine. Symptoms of the syndrome include abdominal pain, diarrhea, diaphoresis, hyperpyrexia, tachycardia, hypertension, myoclonus, irritability, agitation, seizures, and delirium. Coma, cardiovascular collapse, and death have been reported. In this case, the serotonergic effects of fluoxetine are potentiated by the MAOI. Fluoxetine has a prolonged half-life with active metabolites that require up to 6 weeks clearance time. Treatment with the MAOI was initiated before adequate washout of the fluoxetine and resulted in the serotonin syndrome. Management involves discontinuation of the offending agent and supportive care. There is no evidence that the patient was not compliant with a tyramine-free diet, was abusing hallucinogens, or that she was taking antipsychotics that would be consistent with the remaining choices.

77. **(B)** Bulimia nervosa, more common than anorexia nervosa, consists of repeated episodes of binge eating of large amounts of food associated with the feeling of being out of control. The patient usually purges by self-induced vomiting, repeated laxative or diuretic use, or excessive amounts of exercise to prevent weight gain. Unlike individuals with anorexia nervosa, individuals with bulimia nervosa usually maintain a normal or above-normal body weight. Medical complications of bulimia nervosa are usually secondary to either chronic vomiting or laxative

abuse. They include fluid and electrolyte imbalances (such as alkalosis, hypokalemia, hypochloremia, dehydration); dental caries and enamel loss; gastrointestinal disturbances such as esophagitis, Mallory-Weiss tears, and constipation; and sore throat.

78. **(B)** Antidepressant medications reduce binge eating and purging independent of the presence of a mood disorder. Imipramine, desipramine, MAOIs, and fluoxetine have been effective in controlled studies. The other choices treat symptoms of the illness without treating the underlying disorder.

79. **(B)** The Boston Diagnostic Aphasia Examination is a comprehensive set of tests given by a skilled interviewer to evaluate aphasic disorders and to help define further interventions to improve speech. The Bender Gestalt Test is a constructional test for evaluation of brain damage and has some ability to differentiate the location of the lesion. The Folstein MMSE is used for rapid assessment of dementia and delirium. The Sentence Completion Test is a projective test used to describe personality structure. The Stroop Test aids in the evaluation of concentration.

80. **(E)** Anorexia nervosa is characterized by a deliberate self-imposed starvation in the pursuit of being thin, driven by a fear of being fat. The patient refuses to maintain accepted normal body weight appropriate for age and height. Failure to achieve 85% of expected body weight, the intense fear of being fat, a disturbed perception of the body weight or shape (or denial of the seriousness of the current low body weight), and amenorrhea in postmenarchal females are diagnostic criteria. Underdeveloped breasts, abnormal insulin secretion, endocrine disorders, and poor sexual development with a marked decreased interest in sexual activity are also associated with this disorder. For anorexia nervosa to be diagnosed, a postmenarchal female must have missed at least three consecutive periods. Complications include osteoporosis, constipation, cold intolerance, leukopenia, thyroid dysfunction, and cardiac arrhythmias.

81. **(C)** The mortality rate for anorexia nervosa ranges from 5% to 20%.

82. **(E)** Bereavement refers to the reaction to the death of a loved one. Some individuals go on to develop symptoms of a major depressive episode. For example, 50% of all widows and widowers meet criteria for major depression within the first year. The bereaved usually refers to feeling depressed as being normal. If the symptoms of a major depressive episode begin within 2 months of the loss and do not persist beyond the 2-month period, they are considered the result of bereavement unless associated with marked impairment of any of the following: thoughts of death other than feelings that they would be better off dead or should have died with the deceased person, expressing guilt other than about the actions taken or not taken by the survivor at the time of the death, a morbid preoccupation with worthlessness, marked psychomotor retardation, or hallucinations other than that he or she hears the voice of (or sees the image of) the deceased individual. Complicated bereavement is chronic and unremitting distress. Chronic grief may occur if the relationship between the bereaved and the deceased was close or ambivalent, if they were dependent on one another, or if few other support systems are available. Bereavement reactions are very intense after sudden or unexpected deaths. Prolonged denial, anger, or guilt complicates the course of bereavement. Adjustment disorder requires the development of symptoms within 3 months of an identifiable stressor, with marked distress in excess of what would be expected from experiencing the stressor: In this case, the symptoms are considered acceptable reactions to the death of a spouse. Dysthymic disorder requires 2 years of symptoms marked by a depressed mood.

83. **(C)** Most bereaved do fine without treatment. Support and reassurance usually come from family, friends, or clergy. When the bereaved feel unable to move beyond the grief, psychotherapeutic measures are appropriate. The treatment of anxiety or insomnia with medications remains controversial and no controlled

studies have established clear efficacy. However, medications may be warranted if cognitive or other higher functions of daily living are substantially affected.

84. **(A)** The treatment of patients with obsessive-compulsive disorder (OCD) requires integrating multiple treatment modalities including medications, psychotherapy, and collateral support systems. The best-studied medication to treat OCD is clomipramine, a TCA. SSRIs are also very effective in treating symptoms of OCD, but usually at doses higher than those used to treat depression. Antipsychotic agents are used in conjunction with antidepressants in very severe, intractable cases, but are not usually indicated as individual agents. Antiepileptics and lithium are not indicated for the treatment of OCD. Anxiolytic agents such as benzodiazepines are of little use in treating the obsessions or compulsions of OCD.

85. **(C)** The concern in this case is that the patient is lying about her memory problem, therefore malingering. When given tests of memory, malingerers tend to not put forth genuine effort. The Test of Memory Malingering can help assess this effort. It consists of a subject being presented 50 pictures; they are then presented cards and asked if they had seen a given card before. Performance below the odds of chance indicates high likelihood of intentionally changing a correct answer to an incorrect one in order to falsify results.

86. **(B)** Sleep apnea is defined as the cessation of respirations lasting at least 10 seconds. The presence of more than five episodes of apnea per hour of sleep is diagnostic. Sleep apnea is classified as obstructive, central, or a mixed picture of both types. Classified as a breathing-related sleep disorder, sleep apnea leads to excessive sleepiness or insomnia. Characterized by upper airway obstruction, obstructive sleep apnea is associated with snoring, morning headache, excessive movements at night, and mental dullness. The typical patient is a middle-aged obese man.

87. **(C)** Nasal continuous positive airway pressure (CPAP) is the treatment of choice for obstructive

sleep apnea. No medications are consistently effective in normalizing sleep in these patients. The use of nasal CPAP appears to prevent long-term morbidity and mortality and provides restorative sleep. Surgical procedures are reserved for CPAP treatment failures.

88. **(A)** Anticholinergic toxicity can be caused by many psychotropic medications. The low-potency agents chlorpromazine and thioridazine and the TCAs amitriptyline and imipramine are particularly anticholinergic. The syndrome often results when an anticholinergic medication, such as benztropine, is coadministered with an antipsychotic medication in order to prevent or treat extrapyramidal side effects such as parkinsonism and dystonia. Clinical features of anticholinergic toxicity include decreased secretions, agitation, dry skin, flushing of the skin, hyperthermia, tachycardia, dilated pupils, urinary retention, constipation, and hypotension. Seizures, hallucinations, and coma may result from severe intoxication. Drugs that inhibit the enzyme that breaks down acetylcholine (anticholinesterase medications such as physostigmine) reverse the syndrome and are usually administered IV with appropriate monitoring. Atropine would further increase the heart rate; benzodiazepines are reserved for use in agitation and anxiety, and haloperidol might likely worsen anticholinergic symptoms.

89. **(A)** Anticholinesterase toxicity, manifesting as nausea, vomiting, bradycardia, and seizures, results from excessive action of acetylcholine at specific receptors. Atropine, an antimuscarinic agent, can reverse the symptoms. Epinephrine would treat the bradycardia without treating the underlying condition. Physostigmine would worsen the toxicity. Although prochlorperazine would combat vomiting, it would not treat the underlying condition and also might worsen the anticholinergic toxicity.

90. **(D)** This woman appears to suffer from both a major depressive disorder (MDD), single episode, as well as obsessive-compulsive disorder (OCD). Serotonin-specific reuptake

inhibitors (SSRI) are used to treat a variety of psychiatric disorders, including both MDD and OCD. Fluvoxamine is an SSRI particularly indicated for both depression and OCD. Buspirone is a nonbenzodiazepine medication used to treat generalized anxiety disorder. Clomipramine is a tricyclic antidepressant (TCA) with significant serotonergic effects and is particularly useful in OCD; doxepin is also a TCA, but given the tolerability and side effect profile and safety in overdose, SSRIs are preferred as first-line therapy for MDD and OCD. Phenelzine is a monoamine oxidase inhibitor (MAOI) which can be used for depression. However, the drug–drug interactions and dietary restrictions make MAOIs a second- or third-line therapy.

91. **(D)** The patient is beginning to have symptoms of alcohol withdrawal. Because they act at the same GABA receptors as alcohol, the benzodiazepines are the preferred medications used in detoxification from alcohol. For uncomplicated detoxification, the long-acting benzodiazepines such as chlordiazepoxide and diazepam are appropriate because they are essentially self-tapering. The shorter-acting benzodiazepines such as lorazepam or oxazepam are used in patients with impaired liver function, such as in this case, because they are not dependent on liver function for their metabolism and do not accumulate. Patients with unstable medical problems, cognitive impairment, or old age are also candidates for the shorter-acting medications. Disulfiram, which interferes with the metabolism of alcohol, is reserved for long-term behavioral therapy of alcohol dependence. Phenobarbital was formerly used for detoxification and has been replaced by benzodiazepines due to safety concerns and the risk of respiratory depression.

92. **(D)** The patient is experiencing hallucinations likely due to alcohol withdrawal. Benzodiazepines will treat the underlying withdrawal as well as the hallucinations. The patient shows no evidence of either a depressive disorder that should be treated with sertraline or fluoxetine (SSRIs), or a bipolar disorder that would benefit from lithium, a mood stabilizer.

An antipsychotic, such as haloperidol, is unnecessary and may also reduce the seizure threshold.

93. **(E)** Ethanol is metabolized in the liver via alcohol dehydrogenase to acetaldehyde, which is then enzymatically converted to acetate by the enzyme acetaldehyde dehydrogenase. Disulfiram is a medication that irreversibly inhibits the action of aldehyde dehydrogenase. Acetaldehyde accumulates and accounts for the aversive effects associated with the disulfiram reaction. Flushing, sweating, dyspnea, hyperventilation, tachycardia, hypotension, nausea, and vomiting are common symptoms. Extreme but rare reactions can result in respiratory depression, cardiovascular collapse, myocardial infarction, seizures, and death. Blurred vision and urinary retention are anticholinergic effects associated with antipsychotic, antidepressant, and antiparkinsonian medications. Euphoria would not be experienced when alcohol is combined with disulfiram. Hypertension may be associated with but is not characteristic of the disulfiram-ethanol reaction. Disulfiram is not recommended for patients with moderate to severe liver disease, renal failure, severe cardiac disease, pregnancy, or peripheral neuropathy.

94. **(D)** Many nonsteroidal anti-inflammatory drugs can decrease the clearance of lithium and produce significant increases in serum levels. Ibuprofen, indomethacin, ketoprofen, diclofenac, phenylbutazone, naproxen, and piroxicam have all been reported to produce such potential dangerous interactions. The symptoms of abdominal pain, diarrhea, and drowsiness indicate mild to moderate (1.5-2.0 mEq/L) lithium toxicity. Acetaminophen, aspirin, and the opiates do not interfere with lithium clearance. Meperidine, however, can cause dangerous interactions with MAOIs.

95. **(D)** Given the patient's prior major depressive episode and current symptoms, treatment with antidepressants is warranted. However, the patient is concerned about sexual dysfunction, a very common side effect (up to 80% in some studies) of serotonin-specific reuptake

inhibitors such as citalopram. Mirtazapine is an antidepressant which has the effect of increasing both adrenergic and serotonergic neurotransmission, thus improving depression, but without causing appreciable sexual dysfunction. All the other medication choices equally cause problems with sexual functioning.

96. **(D)** Medically ill patients with depressive disorders may respond to psychostimulants, an excellent choice if the patient is unable to tolerate TCAs. The rapid onset of action and rapid clearance are beneficial, especially in a medically-compromised patient who is at risk of dehydration and starvation. Bupropion, fluoxetine, and nefazodone are all effective antidepressants but may take up to 4 to 6 weeks for full benefit. Buspirone is a nonbenzodiazepine anxiolytic medication not indicated in the treatment of depression as monotherapy.

97. **(A)** Attention refers to the ability to give focus to a cognitive task. Performing "serial sevens" (as in this case) and spelling world backward are tests of attention. Although a certain facility with the remaining choices is necessary to perform each task (no cognitive function is tested in absolute isolation), the serial sevens test provides a window on a patient's concentration. Fund of knowledge includes information the patient readily has available to him or her; knowledge of current events is often used to assess this. The mental status examination may contain tests of mathematics skills, but testing mathematics skills is not the purpose of the serial sevens test. Recent memory is recall of events occurring in the last several minutes. Remote memory involves the recall of events long past, for example, information from a patient's childhood. Any test of cognitive function must take into account the patient's cultural, educational, and social background.

98. **(B)** Inhalant abuse is commonly a social activity undertaken in groups. Volatile or toxic solvents such as toluene (found in glues and adhesives), trichloroethane (found in correction fluid), or hydrocarbons (gasoline) are placed in a bag and the fumes are inhaled.

The practice is known as huffing, sniffing, or bagging. Effects are almost immediate because the substances are rapidly absorbed. Signs and symptoms of intoxication include visual disturbances, dyscoordination (a drunken appearance), depressed reflexes, euphoria, and nystagmus. Conjunctival injection and increased appetite are consistent with marijuana use. A diminished response to pain, euphoria, and staring into space are characteristic of PCP abuse.

99. **(A)** Abstinence is the only treatment for inhalant abuse. Antidepressants have not shown utility in inhalant abuse or dependence. Antipsychotic agents are also not effective and may aggravate the presentations of inhalant abuse. Agitation can be managed by benzodiazepine medications such as lorazepam. Dialectical-behavioral therapy is a form of cognitive-behavioral therapy used in Borderline personality disorder. Exposure and response prevention is a behavioral therapy used in the treatment of anxiety disorders such as obsessive-compulsive disorder.

100. **(E)** The five subtypes of schizophrenia (paranoid, catatonic, residual, disorganized, and undifferentiated) are based on the presence or absence of predominant symptoms. The paranoid type is marked by prominent hallucinations or delusions; the disorganized type is marked by disorganized speech and behavior and inappropriate affect; and the catatonic type is marked by waxy flexibility or motoric immobility, excess motor activity, negativism, bizarre posturing, and echolalia or echopraxia. The residual type is marked by the absence of predominant hallucinations or delusions, disorganized speech, or catatonic behavior. The undifferentiated type is reserved for patients who meet criteria for schizophrenia but do not meet criteria for the other four types.

101. **(C)** Divalproex sodium, indicated for the treatment of seizures as well as bipolar disorder, can occasionally cause significant hair loss that is usually reversible. Other common side effects associated with divalproex sodium are nausea,

vomiting, and indigestion. Sedation and mildly elevated serum transaminase levels may also be seen. Rare occurrences of hepatic failure resulting in fatalities have happened, usually during the first 6 months of treatment. Hair loss is not associated with carbamazepine, clozapine, olanzapine, or ziprasidone, although these medications have their own side effects.

102. **(A)** Sexual dysfunction is a very common side effect associated with the serotonin-specific reuptake inhibitors, such as citalopram, with an incidence of approximately 50% to 80%. Decreased libido and delayed orgasm are the most common. Erectile dysfunction is also not uncommon. All SSRIs appear to be equally as likely to cause sexual dysfunction. Priapism is a rare but serious side effect of trazodone. Retrograde ejaculation is a known side effect of certain antipsychotic medications. Vaginismus is not a common side effect of psychotropic medications. Various pharmacologic strategies aimed at treating these side effects include the alpha-2-antagonist yohimbine; the dopamine agonists methylphenidate and amantadine; bupropion; cyproheptadine (an antihistamine with serotonin antagonist properties); and bethanechol, a cholinergic agonist.

103. **(A)** ADHD is a disorder of unclear etiology. As many as 9% of children suffer from this disorder, and up to 60% of those diagnosed carry the diagnosis into adulthood. The disorder is characterized by symptoms of inattention, hyperactivity, and impulsivity that are inappropriate for age. Although the *DSM-IV-TR* criteria suggest that symptoms must have been present before the age of 7 years, many cases are not diagnosed until adolescence or adulthood. In these cases, a retrospective history from both the patient and the family often support the presence of early life symptoms. Although some symptoms are reminiscent of the manic component of bipolar disorder, these disorders represent two separate entities. A careful history by astute physicians will secure the proper diagnosis. Depressive, anxiety, and substance-abuse disorders are common comorbid conditions that often make the diagnosis of ADHD

more difficult. The absence of prominent mood symptoms and the relative degree of impairment help distinguish ADHD from other disorders.

104. **(D)** The approach to the treatment of the core symptoms of ADHD has been the initiation of a trial of a psychostimulant medication, such as methylphenidate. Often, if one stimulant fails to treat symptoms, another stimulant is prescribed. Many patients benefit from one stimulant and not another. The appropriate choice in this case would be to try a second type of stimulant before alternative strategies are implemented.

105. **(A)** Déjà entendu is the feeling that one is hearing something one has heard before. It is usually associated with anxiety states or fatigue. Déjà vu is a similar experience, but refers to the sensation that something has been seen before. Jamais vu is the opposite of déjà vu in that it refers to something that should be familiar but seems quite unfamiliar. Folie à deux is a shared delusion aroused in one person by the influence of another. La belle indifférence is the indifference shown toward a deficit or loss of function, classically seen in a conversion disorder.

106. **(E)** The epidemiology and prognosis of schizophreniform disorder are poorly understood, although the lifetime prevalence rate is approximately 0.2% and most eventually go on to develop schizophrenia. The diagnostic criteria are similar to those of schizophrenia, but the episode lasts between 1 and 6 months. Distinguishing schizophrenia from mood disorders with psychotic symptoms (eg, bipolar I disorder with psychotic features, MDD with psychotic features) and schizoaffective disorder can often be difficult in that a mood disturbance is not uncommon during episodes of schizophrenia and schizophreniform disorders. If psychotic symptoms occur without the presence of mood symptoms, then schizophreniform disorder is more likely. Brief psychotic disorder is defined by the presence of delusions, hallucinations, disorganized speech or behavior,

or catatonic behavior lasting for at least 1 day but less than 1 month. Schizoaffective disorder describes the presence of a major depressive episode, a manic episode, or a mixed episode concurrent with symptoms that are characteristic of schizophrenia: delusions, hallucinations, disorganized speech or behavior, or negative symptoms.

107.   **(C)** In the context of pregnancy and labor, high-potency typical antipsychotics such as haloperidol are considered relatively safe to use to control psychosis. For a mother suffering from psychosis during delivery, the benefit of using high-potency antipsychotics outweighs the risk. All of the other antipsychotics are short- or medium-potency and may lower blood pressure significantly due to their alpha-blocking properties.

108–111. **[108 (E), 109 (G), 110 (D).** The MMSE is a quick, easily administered test that allows for immediate screening for dementia. Scores of less than 24 are suggestive of a dementing process. The Rey-Osterrieth figure is sensitive to deficits in copying and lack of attention to detail in people with right-sided parietal lobe lesions. It appears that this young woman may have had a stroke in this area resulting from her protein S deficiency, a hypercoagulable state. The appropriate test to evaluate the intelligent quotient (IQ) for children ages 5 to 15 is the WISC. The Boston Diagnostic Aphasia Examination is a series of tests given by an experienced clinician to evaluate and make treatment recommendations for individuals with aphasia. The Beck Depression Inventory **(A)** is a 21-item test, with three responses per item, that is an easily used screening tool to evaluate for depression. The Bender Gestalt Test **(B)** involves copying figures, which helps to determine if organic brain disease is present. The Blessed Rating Scale **(C)** is a tool that asks friends or families of the patient to assess the ability of the patient to function in his usual environment. MMPI-2 **(F)** is an objective test interpreted by skilled evaluators used in personality assessment. It is the most widely used and highly standardized test of personality structure.

The Rorschach Test **(H)** is a projective test used to assess personality structure. The Wada Test **(I)** is used to evaluate hemispheric language dominance prior to surgical amelioration of seizure focus. Whereas most right-handed individuals show left hemispheric dominance for language, left-handed individuals may either be right or left dominant. The test consists of injecting sodium amytal into the carotid artery and observing the transient effects on speech. Injection into the left carotid artery will anesthetize the left side of the brain; those with left hemispheric language dominance will show interrupted speech. The WAIS-R **(J)** is used to determine the IQ for individuals age 15 and older.

112.   **(C)** Cannabis (marijuana) is the most commonly abused illicit drug in the United States. The onset of action after smoking is immediate, and symptoms include conjunctival injection, mild sedation, dose-dependent hypothermia, dry mouth, increased appetite, tachycardia, and euphoria. A sensation of slowed time and paranoid ideation can also occur.

113.   **(E)** The onset of action for opiates can be almost immediate when smoked, about 5 minutes when injected and longer if taken orally. Symptoms include miosis, bradycardia, hypotension, hypothermia, constipation, and euphoria. Intoxication can lead to fatal respiratory depression.

114.   **(F)** PCP is a hallucinogen that produces a dissociative anesthesia. It can cause unpredictable behavior, assaultiveness, and belligerence. Agitation, nystagmus (vertical or horizontal), tachycardia, a numbed response to pain, muscle rigidity, hyperacusis, hypertension, echolalia, and anticholinergic effects are associated symptoms.

115.   **(D)** Nicotine found in tobacco smoke produces symptoms of excitement. Intoxication may produce symptoms of confusion, muscle twitching, weakness, abdominal cramps, depression, palpitations, coma, and respiratory failure.

116. (A) As a sympathomimetic agent, cocaine increases the heart rate and dilates the pupils. It can also cause constriction of the coronary arteries. The hallmark of cocaine intoxication is euphoria. Use of LSD **(B)** or other hallucinogens (eg, MDMA [3,4-methylenedioxy-*N*-methylamphetamine], or "Ecstasy") causes symptoms that usually begin 1 hour after ingestion and generally last 8 to 12 hours. Most hallucinogenic drugs have stimulant-type effects and produce elevated vital signs and increased activity. Hallucinations and a heightened sense of perception of objects and colors are typical.

CHAPTER 8

Practice Test 2
Questions

DIRECTIONS (Questions 1 through 4): For each of the following vignettes, select the one lettered option that is *most* closely associated with it. Each lettered option may be used once, multiple times, or not at all.

    (A) citalopram
    (B) fluoxetine
    (C) mirtazapine
    (D) nefazodone
    (E) paroxetine
    (F) sertraline
    (G) venlafaxine

1. A 29-year-old newly married male was recently switched to another antidepressant given prior sexual dysfunction and now develops jaundice, abdominal pain, and fatigue.

2. A 45-year-old man with severe major depression on a high-dose of an antidepressant develops increased blood pressure.

3. A 50-year-old divorced female being treated for major depression doesn't refill her prescription and 2 days later has headache, muscle aches, and nausea.

4. A 33-year-old woman with dysthymic disorder has a history of poor compliance with medications, occasionally missing doses.

DIRECTIONS (Questions 5 through 41): For each of the multiple choice questions in this section select the lettered answer that is the one *best* response in each case

5. An 18-year-old woman recently diagnosed with a first episode of schizophrenia agrees to take an antipsychotic medication to help decrease her hallucinations, but she is adamantly opposed to taking any medication that may cause her to gain excessive weight. Which of the following medications would be the most appropriate to prescribe?

    (A) clozapine (Clozaril)
    (B) olanzapine (Zyprexa)
    (C) quetiapine (Seroquel)
    (D) risperidone (Risperdal)
    (E) ziprasidone (Geodon)

6. A 40-year-old married female without past psychiatric history is referred by her internist. She has been feeling "down" for several weeks, with little ability to enjoy herself. Since that time, her sleep has been disrupted, her appetite reduced, and she's felt "tired." She has also been making mistakes at work and is worried about being fired. She admits to having thoughts of killing herself, but she denies any plan or intent to do so. She denies hallucinations or delusions. Which of the following medications would be the most appropriate for this patient?

    (A) aripiprazole
    (B) citalopram
    (C) methylphenidate
    (D) nortriptyline
    (E) tranylcypromine

7. A 25-year-old patient presents to her primary care doctor complaining of a sudden onset of intense fear and a feeling that she was going to die while stopped in traffic earlier in the week. At that time she became short of breath, diaphoretic, and tremulous, and she could feel her heart pounding. Her initial impulse was to drive to an emergency department, but her distress subsided on its own in about 20 minutes. Which of the following should be the next course of action?

(A) Conduct a thorough medical screening for heart and lung disease.

(B) Prescribe a selective-serotonin reuptake inhibitor (SSRI) and ask to see the patient back in 1 week.

(C) Prescribe a short-acting benzodiazepine as needed in case of another episode.

(D) Reassure the patient that her symptoms are most likely benign and not a cause for concern.

(E) Refer the patient to a psychiatrist.

8. You are seeing a 45-year-old man with a history of schizophrenia. He is currently taking antipsychotic medications but remains symptomatic, with auditory hallucinations and paranoia. On mental status examination (MSE), he speaks coherently and articulately, but makes no sense because many of the words he uses are of his own invention. Which of the following terms best describes this MSE sign?

(A) clang associations
(B) echolalia
(C) flight of ideas
(D) neologisms
(E) word salad

9. A 34-year-old woman presents to a psychiatrist with a 6-year-history of emptiness and depression for "most of the time," with low self-esteem, chronic insomnia, and difficulty making decisions. She denies any problems with her appetite or energy, and, while she does not feel like her condition will improve, she denies any suicidal ideation. She drinks 1 to 2 drinks once or twice per month, but no illicit drugs. She is subsequently begun on fluoxetine, which is gradually increased to 60 mg. She denies side effects, although she has not experienced a significant lessening of her depressive symptoms. How long should her current dosage be continued before switching to another medication?

(A) 3 days
(B) 1 week
(C) 2 weeks
(D) 4 weeks
(E) 8 weeks

10. A 56-year-old woman with chronic undifferentiated schizophrenia has been stable on haloperidol for years. She denies any current psychiatric complaints and has been compliant with her medications. She presents for a routine follow-up appointment. Which of the following tests should be administered?

(A) Abnormal Involuntary Movement Scale (AIMS)
(B) Beck Depression Inventory (BDI)
(C) Brief Psychiatric Rating Scale (BPRS)
(D) Patient Health Questionnaire (PHQ)
(E) Positive and Negative Symptom Scale (PANSS)

11. A man brings his schizophrenic wife to the doctor because she has become more symptomatic over the past several weeks since stopping her medications. She has made threats toward her husband because she believes that he is really an impostor who looks exactly like her husband. Which of the following terms best describes this symptom?

(A) amok
(B) Capgras syndrome
(C) Cotard syndrome
(D) Couvade syndrome
(E) koro

12. A 69-year-old woman without prior psychiatric history is seen by her primary care physician due to "crying spells." She states that she has felt sad since the sudden death of her husband 5 weeks ago. Since that time, she has had difficulty sleeping and fatigue. She has also lost

several pounds due to not enjoying her food. She is able to cheer up when spending time with her children, but feels especially lonely at night. She is somewhat anxious because she occasionally hears her deceased husband's voice, especially early in the morning or late in the evening. While she feels her future is "bleak," she denies any suicidal ideation or plan. Which of the following diagnoses is most likely?

(A) bereavement
(B) bipolar disorder
(C) dysthymic disorder
(D) major depressive disorder (MDD)
(E) schizoaffective disorder

Questions 13 and 14

You are asked to evaluate a 12-year-old boy with a history of Tourette disorder and obsessive-compulsive disorder. He is brought in to the appointment with his parents, who describe the severity of his illness and how he is often teased in school. During the interview the boy intermittently makes obscene gestures.

13. Which of the following terms best describes this symptom?

(A) blepharospasm
(B) bruxism
(C) copropraxia
(D) echopraxia
(E) torticollis

14. While obtaining the history, the patient is also noted to repeat phrases you use immediately after you say them. Which of the following terms best describes this symptom?

(A) coprolalia
(B) dysarthria
(C) echolalia
(D) palilalia
(E) parapraxis

Questions 15 and 16

A wealthy, divorced 48-year-old woman presents to you after being arrested for shoplifting. The patient admits that she has been stealing for years, although she is easily able to afford the objects stolen. She states that she steals "on the spur of the moment" and that these impulses seem foreign and distressing.

15. Which of the following diagnoses is most likely?

(A) antisocial personality disorder
(B) intermittent explosive disorder
(C) kleptomania
(D) pyromania
(E) trichotillomania

16. Which of the following terms applies to the fact that these impulses are distressing to her?

(A) delusional
(B) ego-dystonic
(C) ego-syntonic
(D) mood congruent
(E) mood incongruent

17. A 49-year-old man comes to you complaining of headaches, memory loss, disorientation, and occasional paralysis that affects his arms and lasts several hours. During the MSE, you notice that the patient is giving vague answers to many questions (eg, there are six toes on the foot and 2 + 2 = 5). You also notice that the patient is talking past the point. Which of the following terms best describes this presentation?

(A) amok
(B) fugue state
(C) Ganser syndrome
(D) malingering
(E) piblokto

18. A psychiatrist discovers that she is frustrated and easily angered with one of her patients for no obvious reason. While talking to a colleague, she admits that the patient reminds her of her abusive father. Which of the following best describes the clinician's reaction?

(A) countertransference
(B) displacement
(C) projection
(D) reaction formation
(E) transference

Questions 19 and 20

A 19-year-old woman presents with complaints of fear, apprehension, and trembling without any known predisposing situations. On examination, you note brown skin, smoky brown rings on the outer cornea, and occasional rapid, jerky, purposeless swinging of the arms which appear to worsen with voluntary movement.

19. Which of the following terms best describes the patient's ocular findings?

(A) arcus senilis

(B) Brushfield spots

(C) Kayser-Fleischer rings

(D) subconjunctival hemorrhage

(E) xanthelasma

20. Which of the following terms best describes the abnormal movements seen in this patient?

(A) athetoid

(B) choreiform

(C) hemiballismus

(D) myoclonus

(E) myotonia

Questions 21 and 22

A 21-year-old woman is brought to the psychiatric emergency department after calling the police to turn herself in. She claims that she was responsible for the loss of her neighbor's pregnancy. She believes her negative thoughts toward the woman caused her miscarriage. On further questioning, she tells you that she felt threatened by her neighbor because she believed her thoughts could be heard through the walls. She feels that this is an invasion of her privacy.

21. Which of the following terms best describes the belief that the patient's thoughts toward the neighbor were responsible for the lost pregnancy?

(A) displacement

(B) ideas of reference

(C) magical thinking

(D) projection

(E) reaction formation

22. Which of the following terms best describes the patient's fear that her thoughts could be overheard?

(A) echolalia

(B) thought broadcasting

(C) thought control

(D) thought insertion

(E) transference

Questions 23 and 24

A 25-year-old man presents to the emergency room after being brought in by his girlfriend. She has been concerned as "he has not been acting right." She states he has been staying up all night over the last several days but still "very active" during the daytime. He has rearranged the furniture and attempted to remodel their bathroom, despite his lack of experience with construction. He hasn't shown up for work recently, and she is afraid he will be fired. While he admits that he hasn't slept, he claims to feel "great"! He is somewhat difficult to interview as he walks around the room, handling all the equipment. When confronted with his not going to his work, he states "Why should I... I am on the verge of discovering a cure for AIDS, which also happens to be a formula for economics, which will also get rid of poverty." He denies alcohol or drugs, but upon questioning, admits to a period in his late teens when he felt depressed, with difficulty sleeping, weight loss, low energy, guilt, and helplessness/hopelessness. He was subsequently treated with "some sort of antidepressant" for approximately 18 months, but he never followed up after that time.

23. Which of the following is the most appropriate diagnosis for this patient?

(A) bipolar disorder I

(B) bipolar disorder II

(C) cyclothymic disorder

(D) major depressive disorder with psychotic features

(E) schizophrenia

24. Which of the following medications would be the most appropriate to prescribe?

(A) amitriptyline

(B) clozapine

(C) fluoxetine

(D) haloperidol

(E) valproic acid

25. A 36-year-old woman was placed on alprazolam (Xanax) 3 years ago for panic disorder. After watching a news report on television, she became frightened about addiction. She abruptly stopped the medication and during the next 3 days experienced increased anxiety attacks, but claims that she is now doing better. She denies any tremor, sweating, increased heart rate, or uneasiness except in relation to the panic attacks. Which of the following best describes this phenomenon?

(A) akathisia

(B) dystonic reaction

(C) rebound

(D) recurrence

(E) withdrawal

Questions 26 and 27

A devout husband finds that his wife is having an affair with his best friend. One week later, he finds that he cannot walk. A thorough neurologic workup fails to reveal a cause to his sudden paraplegia. His neurologic examination is not consistent with upper or lower motor neuron findings. Despite this dramatic disability, he seems quite unaffected by it emotionally.

26. Which of the following diagnoses would be the most appropriate in this patient?

(A) conversion disorder

(B) factitious disorder

(C) hypochondriasis

(D) malingering

(E) somatization disorder

27. Which of the following terms best describes this patient's minimization of the severity of his symptoms?

(A) déjà entendu

(B) déjà vu

(C) folie à deux

(D) jamais vu

(E) la belle indifférence

28. A 67-year-old woman with pulmonary carcinoma and secondary brain metastases recently drafted a will in the presence of her family attorney. She has a history of major depressive disorder (MDD) that is now in remission. She decides that her children who are well-established in their careers do not need any inheritance and that her estate would best serve charity. To secure the validity of the will, the patient asks her psychiatrist to submit a letter to her attorney regarding her competency. Which of the following would be the most important factor in determining this woman's testamentary capacity?

(A) actus reus

(B) a history of MDD

(C) knowledge of her natural heirs

(D) the presence of a conservator of person

(E) the presence of a judge to witness the signing of the will

29. You are consulted to see a 77-year-old Hispanic male with chronic schizoaffective disorder, admitted to the hospital for chest pain. His workup has revealed a pulmonary embolism, and the medical team wishes to place a chest tube in the patient, but the patient refuses. The primary team has asked you to determine his capacity to refuse the procedure. Which of the following features is the most important in determining decision-making capacity in this patient?

(A) ability to communicate

(B) age of patient

(C) agreement with treatment team recommendations

(D) presence of psychosis

(E) Spanish speaking

30. A deputy sheriff serves you a subpoena for the records of one of your patients who is the defendant in a civil liability lawsuit. Which of the following is the most appropriate course of action?

    (A) Release the patient's records to the plaintiff because the subpoena overrides patient consent.

    (B) Hand over only the information that is relevant to the case.

    (C) Contact the patient and ask if she or he would like the information released.

    (D) Release the patient's records directly to the court.

    (E) Refuse to speak to the sheriff in order to maintain confidentiality.

31. A 23-year-old graduate student you have been seeing in long-term psychotherapy has stopped paying his bills despite being reimbursed by his insurance company. Which of the following is the next most appropriate course of action?

    (A) Notify a collection agency to obtain reimbursement.

    (B) Contact the patient's insurance company and request that they issue you another payment.

    (C) Inquire with family members whether the patient has financial problems.

    (D) Directly address this issue with the patient at the next scheduled appointment.

    (E) Send the patient a letter of termination.

Questions 32 and 33

You are asked to perform a "competency to stand trial" evaluation of an 18-year-old man who was arrested for violently assaulting his girlfriend. The patient has no past psychiatric history, and friends report that he has never demonstrated any violent tendencies. The patient reports that his relationship with his girlfriend "went downhill" shortly after they graduated from high school and his girlfriend stopped calling him. On MSE, his affect is constricted and his mood is reported as "crazy." Thought processes are goal-directed, and he denies any hallucinations or delusions. The patient is unable to correctly perform simple calculations. Each time he is asked to multiply, subtract, or add a pair of numbers, his answers are wrong by one or two digits. For example, he responds "22" when asked to multiply 7 by 3.

32. Which of the following diagnoses is the most likely in this case?

    (A) conversion disorder
    (B) dementia
    (C) factitious disorder
    (D) malingering
    (E) schizophrenia

33. Which of the following statements best describes the above patient's production of symptoms and motivation?

    (A) Conscious production of symptoms to assume the sick role.

    (B) Conscious production of symptoms to obtain secondary gain.

    (C) Unconscious production of symptoms due to unconscious conflicts.

    (D) Unconscious production of symptoms to assume the sick role.

    (E) Unconscious production of symptoms to obtain secondary gain.

34. You are asked to evaluate a 68-year-old man on the inpatient medicine service for increasing confusion. The patient was admitted 2 days earlier for pneumonia. After performing a mental status evaluation, you suspect delirium. Further history from the patient's wife indicates that the patient dropped out of school in the seventh grade. Which of the following tests would best assess his ability to maintain and focus attention?

    (A) counting by 2s to 20
    (B) random letter test
    (C) serial sevens
    (D) serial threes
    (E) simple calculations

35. A 7-year-old girl is brought to the emergency department for evaluation of a sore throat and fever. Her parents took her to the pediatrician's office about 1 week ago and he recommended

fluids and bed rest. Within the last 2 days, the patient developed dysphagia and severe abdominal pain. History from the parents indicates the patient has been anxious and impulsive over the last month. There has also been a marked decline in school performance, and she has not been interested in playing with her friends. Physical examination is remarkable for significant erythema over the posterior pharynx with gray exudate. There are abrasions in the region of the patient's labia. Complete blood count shows a white blood cell (WBC) count of 14,000/µL with a left shift. Which of the following is the next appropriate step?

(A) Detain the parents while you notify the police.

(B) Arrange for a family meeting to determine a safe disposition.

(C) Refer the patient to the family's pediatrician.

(D) Notify the probate court to have the patient legally removed from the alleged perpetrator.

(E) Contact the state's Child Protective Services while keeping the patient safe.

Questions 36 and 37

A 48-year-old male is brought into the emergency room (ER) via an ambulance. He smells of alcohol, is covered in vomit, and not responsive to questions. He is unsteady and uncooperative with the physical examination, but he is noted to have disconjugate eye movements.

36. Which of the following would be the most appropriate next step in the management of this patient?

(A) Administer thiamine orally (PO) before IV fluids and glucose.

(B) Administer thiamine intravenously (IV) before IV fluids and glucose.

(C) Administer thiamine IV after IV fluids and glucose.

(D) Administer naloxone IV before IV fluids and glucose.

(E) Administer naloxone IV after IV fluids and glucose.

37. The above patient is stabilized and admitted to the ICU. After 3 days, he begins to become confused again, with visual hallucinations, tremors, diaphoresis, and elevated blood pressure and pulse. Which of the following is the most appropriate treatment for this patient?

(A) Administer a barbiturate.

(B) Administer a benzodiazepine.

(C) Administer additional thiamine.

(D) Administer an antipsychotic.

(E) Administer hydralazine.

38. A young white male, age unknown, is brought into the emergency room unresponsive to questioning. His vitals demonstrate a normal temperature, a low pulse and blood pressure, and decreased respirations. He appears pale, with pupils that are constricted and minimally responsive. Administration of which of the following would be most likely to improve his condition?

(A) disulfiram (Antabuse)

(B) benzodiazepines

(C) flumazenil

(D) naloxone

(E) thiamine

39. A 77-year-old woman without prior psychiatric history is brought into her family physician's office with her husband. He is concerned that she is "depressed" and needs treatment. He describes her withdrawing emotionally over the past year or two, with a gradual decline in her ability to care for herself. They have been unable to take part in their usual social activities, and the patient "just wanders around the house during the day." He has also noticed that she is forgetful, often misplacing items, and mixing up names of acquaintances. When asked, the patient denies any difficulties, stating she feels "fine," and that her husband worries too much. She adamantly refutes problems with her memory, instead blaming him for "moving things around in our house." She has no significant medical problems. Upon MSE, she is pleasant and cooperative with questions, although defensive at times. Her affect is neutral but full. There is no suicidal or homicidal ideation, and she denies any psychotic symptoms. Her Mini-Mental State Examination is 20/30. Her physical is essentially unremarkable. Which of the following is the most appropriate primary treatment for this patient?

    (A) citalopram
    (B) galantamine
    (C) ginkgo biloba
    (D) memantine
    (E) ziprasidone

Questions 40 and 41

You are asked to see a 37-year-old white Catholic female with end-stage ovarian cancer because she has told her oncologist that she wants to die. When you approach the patient's bed, you see a cachectic but smiling woman surrounded by her husband and two young daughters. She has a history of depression but is not under any treatment for it now. "I am ready to go, Doctor," she says to you. Her oncologist has told you that he would like to try a new chemotherapy for which the patient is a good candidate, but the patient has refused; he is concerned about her suicidal potential.

40. Which of the following characteristics increase this particular patient's risk of committing suicide?

    (A) age
    (B) gender
    (C) marital status
    (D) race
    (E) religion

41. The patient waits until her family and primary care team leave the room. She then asks you to help her commit suicide, as her prognosis is very poor. What is the most appropriate next course of action?

    (A) Discuss her reasons for suicide in more detail.
    (B) Explain how she can obtain lethal doses of medication.
    (C) Inform the family immediately.
    (D) Place the patient in restraints.
    (E) Refer her to a physician who performs euthanasia.

DIRECTIONS (Questions 42 through 49): Match the clinical presentation with the appropriate neuropsychological test. Each lettered heading may be selected once, more than once, or not at all.

    (A) Beck Depression Inventory (BDI)
    (B) Bender Gestalt Test
    (C) Blessed Rating Scale
    (D) Boston Diagnostic Aphasia Examination
    (E) Folstein Mini-Mental State Examination (MMSE)
    (F) Minnesota Multiphasic Personality Inventory 2 (MMPI-2)
    (G) Rey-Osterrieth Test
    (H) Rorschach Test
    (I) Stroop Test
    (J) Wada Test
    (K) Wechsler Adult Intelligence Scale—Revised (WAIS-R)
    (L) Wisconsin Card Sorting Test (WCST)

42. A 40-year-old woman who scores a 26/30 on the Folstein MMSE gave many answers of, "I don't know, I'm too tired to answer." You want to assess for the possibility of depression.

43. A 65-year-old man has difficulty organizing, sequencing, and planning activities but no impairment in memory.

44. The family of an 80-year-old man with mild dementia has asked you to evaluate his ability to continue to live in his current environment. You wish to ask his family and friends their opinion of how he has been doing.

45. A 16-year-old boy with a family history of mental retardation presents with longstanding poor school performance and aggressive behavior toward peers.

46. A 37-year-old man has a history of avoiding social situations, no close friends, and a preference for being alone. He has been described by others as unemotional and detached. You would like to evaluate this patient's personality style with a projective test.

47. You would like to quickly assess for dementia in a 75-year-old woman admitted to the emergency department for failure to thrive.

48. A 45-year-old woman has a long history of unstable relationships, self-injurious behavior, and affective instability. She does not meet criteria for an Axis I disorder. You wish to employ an objective test to give further evidence for an Axis II disorder.

49. You are asked to preoperatively evaluate hemispheric dominance in an 18-year-old left-handed woman with a history of seizure disorder who is about to undergo surgery to remove a seizure focus in her left hemisphere.

DIRECTIONS (Questions 50 through 83): For each of the multiple choice questions in this section select the lettered answer that is the one best response in each case.

50. A 16-year-old girl is brought to your office by her parents to get a pregnancy test. She consents for the evaluation but requests that you keep the results confidential. Beta–human chorionic gonadotropin is positive. The patient's parents demand to know the results. Which of the following is the most appropriate course of action?

(A) Notify the parents of the results because they pay her medical bills.
(B) Encourage the patient to discuss the results with her parents.
(C) Report the results to Child Protective Services.
(D) Invoke testimonial privilege.
(E) Disclose the results in a meeting with the patient and her parents.

Questions 51 and 52

The patient is a 31-year-old, divorced male, referred by his work for evaluation. He states he has felt "down" since his separation and divorce several months ago. He has been sleeping poorly, frequently waking up during the night, then feeling "exhausted" during the day. He has had little interest in food, losing 10 lb, and he has been easily distracted at work, resulting in mistakes and a reprimand. While he feels helpless and that "I'll never feel better," he denies any suicidal ideation or homicidal ideation. He drinks 1 to 2 beers on the weekends and denies illicit drug use. He smokes 1/2 pack of cigarettes per day and has no major medical problems except for borderline hypertension. He takes a multivitamin but no other medications regularly. After further discussion, he agrees to begin a trial of a medication. The patient is begun on fluoxetine 20 mg daily. While he experiences very few side effects, he does not display significant improvement. You continue to increase the fluoxetine, finally recommending to increase to the maximum dose.

51. How long should you continue the current treatment before switching to another antidepressant?

(A) 4 days
(B) 1 week
(C) 2 weeks
(D) 3 weeks
(E) 5 weeks

52. What do you tell him is his approximate risk of developing a further episode in the future?

(A) 10%
(B) 20%
(C) 30%
(D) 40%
(E) 50%

Questions 53 and 54

A 35-year-old woman presents to your office with a referral from a psychologist for psychiatric treatment. She has been suffering "the blues" for several months, including crying spells, low energy, and insomnia. She is convinced that her fiancé is about to break up with her because she has been eating more than usual. Sometimes, however, she feels "just fine."

53. Which of the following would be the most appropriate treatment of choice for this patient?

   (A) amitriptyline (Elavil)
   (B) divalproex sodium (Depakote)
   (C) fluoxetine (Prozac)
   (D) phenelzine (Nardil)
   (E) ziprasidone (Geodon)

54. The patient responds well to treatment and after several months returns to your office for a follow-up visit. She tells you she has just been married and would like to become pregnant. She and her husband have been having unprotected sex for a month. Which of the following would be the most appropriate next course of action?

   (A) Tell her to stop her medication immediately.
   (B) Ask how important pregnancy is to her.
   (C) Refer her for electroconvulsive therapy (ECT).
   (D) Discuss the risks and benefits of continuing her treatment during pregnancy.
   (E) Add another antidepressant to prevent postpartum depression.

55. A 45-year-old man is brought to the psychiatric emergency room by police after being found screaming while cutting down a tree in the local park. He tells you that the ghost of his wife, who died 3 months ago, is living in the tree. The man has no previous psychiatric history, but he reports being "very depressed" since the death of his wife and has had suicidal ideation. He is disheveled and appears to have ignored his personal hygiene for some time. His vital signs are normal. Which of the following is the most appropriate next course of action?

   (A) Obtain a urine toxicology screen.
   (B) Prescribe an antidepressant.

   (C) Prescribe an antipsychotic.
   (D) Prescribe an antipsychotic and an antidepressant.
   (E) Prescribe a mood stabilizer.

Questions 56 and 57

You are seeing a 56-year-old man with a history of alcoholism. He complains about not being able to sleep and requests a sleeping aid. He denies pervasive depression or any change in his appetite, energy, or concentration. He claims that "everything is going well."

56. Which of the following medications would be the most appropriate to prescribe for this patient?

   (A) alprazolam (Xanax)
   (B) diazepam (Valium)
   (C) trazodone (Desyrel)
   (D) zaleplon (Sonata)
   (E) zolpidem (Ambien)

57. He agrees to begin the medication above. Which of the following side effects do you most warn him about?

   (A) anorgasmia
   (B) impotence
   (C) incontinence
   (D) priapism
   (E) retrograde ejaculation

Questions 58 and 59

58. You are seeing a 9-year-old boy with a history of depression and suicidal ideation. He has been taking fluoxetine (Prozac) for 6 months and has had a good response. His mother asks to see you after his appointment and tells you that she is concerned about news reports saying that serotonin-specific reuptake inhibitors (SSRIs) increase the risk of suicide in children. She asks you to consider stopping the medication. Which of the following is the best course of action?

   (A) Stop the fluoxetine immediately as the patient is a minor and it is his mother's wish.
   (B) Switch to paroxetine (Paxil) because it does not increase suicide risk.

(C) Ask the mother, "What's really bothering you about your son being on antidepressants?"

(D) Switch to amitriptyline (Elavil).

(E) Discuss the risks and benefits of fluoxetine and other SSRIs in the pediatric population.

59. A month later, the boy and his mother return to your office. She informs you that after her son's last appointment, she has been giving him St. John's wort because she believes he needs a "natural remedy." Which of the following would be the most appropriate course of action?

(A) Tell the mother to stop the St. John's wort immediately.

(B) Tell the mother there is no evidence that St. John's wort is an effective treatment for depression.

(C) Tell the mother to watch out for side effects including photosensitivity and dizziness.

(D) Refer the case to social services for child abuse.

(E) Increase the dose of his antidepressant as St. John's wort will lower blood concentrations of the antidepressant.

Questions 60 and 61

A 38-year-old patient with a history of bipolar disorder had his first (and only) manic episode 18 months ago. He was treated for 1 year with a mood stabilizer, and has not taken any psychotropics since that time. He has come in for an evaluation at the urging of his wife, who is concerned about his frequent crying spells. The patient admits that he has felt more depressed over the last several weeks, with associated insomnia, low energy, poor appetite and 5 lb weight loss, difficulty concentrating, and anhedonia. He denies any suicidal ideation. Fortunately, these symptoms have not interfered with his work. He has no major medical problems and is on no medications. He drinks 1 to 2 glasses of wine "on special occasions" and denies drug use.

60. Which of the following medications would be the most appropriate to prescribe this patient?

(A) bupropion
(B) fluoxetine
(C) haloperidol
(D) lamotrigine
(E) valproic acid

61. Which of the following side effects would be the most important to discuss with the patient prior to starting?

(A) ataxia
(B) nausea
(C) neutropenia
(D) rash
(E) sedation

Questions 62 and 63

A 60-year-old white female widow is brought to your clinic by her daughter, who reports that her mother said to her this afternoon that she "wanted to end it all." She reports thoughts of overdosing on her pills, which she has stockpiled. This patient has no prior history of suicide attempts but has had thoughts of suicide on multiple prior occasions over the course of her near-lifelong history of depression. She lost her husband to a sudden heart attack 1 year ago, but her daughter says that she still has many very supportive friends with whom she spends significant amounts of time. She still carries on her avid hobby of gardening, although "at a slower pace" because of her worsening arthritis. She expresses worries over a recent "big drop" in the value of retirement stocks she has.

62. Which of the following is the most significant factor mitigating her risk for suicide?

(A) gardening hobby
(B) no prior suicide attempts
(C) race
(D) slower movements secondary to arthritis
(E) social supports

63. Which of the following medical conditions would be the most important to rule out as a potential cause of depression in this patient?

    (A) basement membrane disorders
    (B) hypercholesterolemia
    (C) phospholipid metabolism disorders
    (D) thyroid illness
    (E) tryptophan deficiency

Questions 64 and 65

A 20-year-old college sophomore is brought to the emergency department after being found passed out in her bathroom. She had been vomiting, which she admits now was self-induced. Her history is notable for a breakup 4 months ago with her boyfriend of 2 years. Her weight is in the 82nd percentile for her height. She is amenorrheic. There is no history of binge eating.

64. Which of the following do you most expect to find on her physical examination?

    (A) café au lait spots
    (B) dental decay
    (C) palpable spleen
    (D) pectus excavatum
    (E) pitting fingernails

65. What is the likelihood that with treatment she will make a full recovery over the next 10 years?

    (A) 5%
    (B) 10%
    (C) 25%
    (D) 50%
    (E) 75%

66. A 14-month-old girl presents with her parents who report that she has become less responsive to them and less interactive with her 6-year-old brother. In addition, her gait has become clumsy, and, most recently, she has been noted to habitually rub her knuckles together. The parents also bring the chart from their daughter's pediatrician with a note indicating that, although her head circumference was normally sized at birth, it has now fallen into the 10th percentile for her age. Which of the following would be the most accurate diagnosis?

    (A) Asperger disorder
    (B) autistic disorder
    (C) childhood disintegrative disorder
    (D) childhood-onset schizophrenia
    (E) Rett disorder

67. A 24-year-old man with a history of schizophrenia presents to the emergency department. He had previously taken haloperidol (Haldol), but now refuses to take it. Because the patient did not take the haloperidol, you decide to try fluphenazine (Prolixin), which seems to mitigate his symptoms. One week later, he leaves the hospital. He continues the medications you prescribed and on a follow-up visit you notice he moves slowly and has a festinating gait. Blockade of which of the following receptors most likely accounts for the above side effect?

    (A) basal ganglia acetylcholine receptors
    (B) D_4 receptors
    (C) 5-hydroxytryptamine-2 (5-HT$_2$)
    (D) mesolimbic D_2 receptors
    (E) nigrostriatal D_2 receptors

68. A 16-year-old boy began having repetitive eye blinking at the age of 6. By age 12, he began blurting stereotyped phrases such as "Balls!" and "Shitty!" as well as making kissing noises. Concomitant with this, he had increasing difficulty with paying attention in school and occasionally displayed wild, disinhibited behavior. Which of the following is the most effective treatment for the primary (initial) condition in this case?

    (A) clonidine (Catapres)
    (B) fluoxetine (Prozac)
    (C) methylphenidate (Ritalin)
    (D) risperidone (Risperdal)
    (E) topiramate (Topamax)

69. A 12-year-old boy has recently been arrested for setting fire to a neighbor's barn. He has been in trouble before for playing with fireworks in the neighborhood, and when he was 10 years old he was suspended for lighting matches at his school. Which of the following diagnoses would most likely be comorbid in this patient?

(A) conduct disorder

(B) major depressive disorder

(C) mental retardation

(D) pervasive developmental disorder

(E) tic disorder

Questions 70 and 71

A 9-year-old boy with a history of normal developmental milestones has been wetting his bed for the last 6 months. His parents report that the bed-wetting initially occurred sporadically, but for the last 2 months it has been happening about every other night. This has caused him a significant amount of shame and has been limiting his social interactions as he is unable to go to sleepovers or away to camp.

70. Which of the following interventions would be the most appropriate?

   (A) behavioral therapy

   (B) cognitive therapy

   (C) dialectical behavioral therapy

   (D) psychodynamic psychotherapy

   (E) punishment

71. The child undergoes a lengthy trial of the recommended therapy as above, but his condition continues without significant improvement. Which of the following would be the most appropriate pharmacologic treatment of choice?

   (A) carbamazepine (Tegretol)

   (B) clonidine

   (C) diphenhydramine (Benadryl)

   (D) haloperidol (Haldol)

   (E) imipramine (Tofranil)

Questions 72 and 73

An 11-year-old boy is referred by his pediatrician for further evaluation. His history is notable for being adopted at age 6 months. His family history is significant for a biological mother with severe alcohol dependence. He has been in a special education school due to his global learning difficulties and his intelligence quotient (IQ) has recently been measured at 60.

72. Which of the following would be this child's most appropriate diagnosis?

   (A) borderline intellectual functioning

   (B) mild mental retardation

   (C) moderate mental retardation

   (D) severe mental retardation

   (E) profound mental retardation

73. Given the above patient's history, which of the following would most likely be expected?

   (A) cleft palate

   (B) congenital blindness

   (C) hyperextensible joints

   (D) microcephaly

   (E) prominent jaw

74. A 5-year-old girl has come under the care of state Child Protection Services. Her mother was known to be using crack cocaine and IV heroin, and supporting her habit with prostitution. The girl's temporary foster parents reported to state workers that she was indiscriminately social with adults and unusually "clingy." In her social interactions with other 5-year-old children at her preschool, she was described as being inappropriately aggressive with them. Which of the following would be the most appropriate diagnosis in this case?

   (A) attention-deficit hyperactivity disorder (ADHD)

   (B) childhood disintegrative disorder

   (C) conduct disorder

   (D) mixed receptive-expressive language disorder

   (E) reactive attachment disorder of infancy and early childhood

75. A 39-year-old man is arrested after being found in a department store, masturbating by rubbing a woman's shoe along his penis. He reluctantly admits that he has committed this act on numerous occasions although has not gotten caught or arrested. He feels a great deal of shame and guilt, but he is unable to stop the behavior. Which of the following is the most likely diagnosis?

    (A) fetishism
    (B) frotteurism
    (C) pedophilia
    (D) transvestic fetishism
    (E) voyeurism

Questions 76 and 77

A 27-year-old law student presents to you as a referral for treatment of a first episode of major depression, initially diagnosed by his primary care physician 8 weeks ago. On his mental status examination, the patient's speech is extremely rapid, difficult to interrupt, and he quickly jumps from one topic to another. He says that his mood has improved greatly since he last saw his primary care doctor: "In fact, I'm on top of the world." The patient reports 3 to 4 hours of sleep per night for the last week, "not that I need that much sleep anyway." The patient has been spending all of his money buying first edition textbooks and rearranging the furniture in the law school administration building. However, he has been skipping classes and not turning in assignments as he believes he will "automatically graduate and pass the bar because they understand my true genius."

76. Which of the following would be the most likely diagnosis for this patient?

    (A) bipolar disorder, most recent episode depressed
    (B) bipolar disorder, most recent episode manic
    (C) cyclothymic disorder
    (D) dysthymic disorder
    (E) schizoaffective disorder, bipolar type

77. Which of the following would be the most appropriate pharmacologic treatment for this patient?

    (A) citalopram (Celexa)
    (B) divalproex sodium (Depakote)
    (C) fluoxetine
    (D) imipramine
    (E) lorazepam (Ativan)

Questions 78 and 79

A 36-year-old woman presents with 7 weeks of a depressed mood most of the time (although was happy for a short period when she won $150 in the lottery), a sense of hopelessness, and thoughts of suicide for the last month. She also reports increased appetite and has been sleeping up to 16 hours a day. On mental status examination, her mood and affect are dysphoric most of the time, but she laughs in response to humorous statements.

78. Which of the following diagnoses would be the most appropriate in this patient?

    (A) bipolar I disorder, most recent episode depressed
    (B) bipolar II disorder, most recent episode depressed
    (C) dysthymic disorder
    (D) major depressive disorder, with atypical features
    (E) major depressive disorder, with melancholic features

79. Which of the following classes of medications would be the most effective in this patient?

    (A) anticonvulsants
    (B) lithium
    (C) monoamine oxidase inhibitors (MAOIs)
    (D) tricyclic antidepressants (TCAs)
    (E) typical (first-generation) antipsychotics

80. A 42-year-old accountant presents for long-term psychotherapy treatment. In the first session, you find that he has been divorced three times. The poor quality of his romantic and other relationships are the focus of his concerns. Over the course of months, you find out that he is a perfectionist and inflexible within relationships. He typically idealizes his partner, then devalues her, before ending the relationship suddenly. At times, he loses "a sense of

self" in relationships, not knowing who he is or what he wants. During this time, he relies on others to advise him on what he should do. However, if he takes this advice and his plans fail, he uses this to devalue the one who advised him. The patient makes it very clear that he sought your treatment as a psychotherapist "because I'll only accept the best in the city." The patient also reports to you that he has some unique abilities of perception that allow him to detect what or who will provide the best possible outcome for him. For example, he picked you as a therapist not only because of your reputation, but also because of your office phone number, which has digits in ascending value order. Which of the following diagnoses is the most appropriate for this patient?

(A) borderline personality disorder
(B) narcissistic personality disorder
(C) obsessive personality disorder
(D) personality disorder not otherwise specified
(E) schizotypal personality disorder

81. A 43-year-old woman is hospitalized during a psychotic episode in which she had the delusion that she is being shot with invisible laser beams from satellites in Earth orbit. According to her family, she stopped taking her regimen of haloperidol and lithium 4 weeks before this admission to the hospital, and she has been telling her family about her concerns regarding the laser beams for the last 2 weeks. The patient's past psychiatric history is significant for three prior hospitalizations over the last 20 years. At the time of her first admission, she presented with a 3-week history of manic symptoms and psychosis. During her second hospitalization, she was suicidal and noted to be depressed with psychotic symptoms. During her third admission, she was again depressed with prominent disorganized behavior. Her mental status examination upon presentation to the hospital reveals looseness of association and delusional symptoms without a prominent mood component. Which of the following is the most appropriate diagnosis for this patient?

(A) bipolar disorder, with psychotic features
(B) major depressive disorder (MDD) with psychotic features
(C) psychotic disorder not otherwise specified
(D) schizoaffective disorder
(E) schizophrenia

Questions 82 and 83

The medical team on an inpatient service calls you to help them with a 72-year-old female patient who was admitted for congestive heart failure. They report that at night she becomes confused, thinking that she is in a hotel. She makes unreasonable demands of the nursing staff and becomes disruptive on the ward, interfering in the nurses' work. She has the most difficulty from 10 PM until about 2 AM, when she usually falls asleep. In the morning, she is better oriented and much more cooperative. A review of her medications reveals that she is taking cimetidine 400 mg PO bid, furosemide 40 mg PO qd, atenolol 50 mg PO qd, digoxin 0.125 mg PO qd, and diphenhydramine 50 mg PO qhs and 25 mg PO qhs (second dose 3 hours post first dose for insomnia).

82. Which of the following medications is most likely to cause this patient's confusion?

(A) atenolol
(B) cimetidine
(C) digoxin
(D) diphenhydramine
(E) furosemide

83. Which of the following neurotransmitter systems is most directly implicated in the etiology of her confusion?

(A) acetylcholine
(B) dopamine
(C) gamma-aminobutyric acid (GABA)
(D) serotonin
(E) norepinephrine

DIRECTIONS (Questions 84 through 89): The following question is preceded by a list of lettered options. For each of the questions in this section match the clinical vignette with the most appropriate medication to prescribe.

Match the clinical vignette with the most appropriate medication to prescribe.

(A) aripiprazole
(B) bupropion
(C) chlorpromazine
(D) clozapine
(E) haloperidol
(F) lamotrigine
(G) lithium
(H) nortriptyline
(I) paroxetine
(J) risperidone
(K) risperidone Consta
(L) sertraline
(M) valproic acid
(N) venlafaxine

84. A 32-year-old man with schizoaffective disorder has good benefit with antipsychotic medications but is poorly compliant due to lack of insight and reduced cognition.

85. A 28-year-old divorced woman has a history of four manic episodes and at least one depressive episode per year, resulting in frequent hospitalizations.

86. A 41-year-old woman with chronic schizophrenia has been tried on several first- and second-generation antipsychotics at therapeutic doses, but she remains psychotic, with auditory hallucinations telling her to kill herself.

87. A 53-year-old married male with a history of major depressive disorder and poor compliance due to significant sexual dysfunction now presents with a recurrence of depressive symptoms with marked hypersomnia and low energy.

88. A 22-year-old female graduate student with bipolar disorder becomes pregnant.

89. A 37-year-old man with a history of manic episodes now has 3 weeks of depression, with insomnia, poor appetite, weight loss, low energy, and decreased concentration.

DIRECTIONS (Questions 90 through 112): For each of the multiple choice questions in this section select the lettered answer that is the one best response in each case.

90. A clinical research psychiatrist at university A has been running a double-blind placebo-controlled trial of a new antidepressant. The psychiatrist concludes after a statistical analysis of the data that there is no better effect of the drug compared to placebo. The psychiatrist's colleagues at five separate institutions (universities B, C, D, E, and F) have run identical studies and determine that there is a treatment effect of the drug compared to placebo. Given this information, one may conclude that the research trial at university A resulted in which of the following?

(A) high variance
(B) low-predictive value
(C) standard error
(D) type I error
(E) type II error

Questions 91 and 92

A 56-year-old man with a history of chronic paranoid schizophrenia has been taking his chlorpromazine regularly for 27 years. His symptoms are reasonably well-controlled, with occasional, non-command hallucinations and some paranoia. He has been able to work as a volunteer and lives in a group home. About 5 years ago, he developed writhing movements of his wrists and fingers that disappear when he goes to sleep.

91. Which of the following side effects is most consistent with this case?

(A) akathisia
(B) dystonia
(C) neuroleptic malignant syndrome (NMS)
(D) parkinsonism
(E) tardive dyskinesia

92. Which of the following anatomic structures is most likely implicated in the etiology of his movements?

(A) basal ganglia
(B) cerebellum
(C) frontal cortex
(D) midbrain
(E) motor cortex

93. You are seeing a 62-year-old Vietnam veteran at a Veteran's Administration hospital. He has been hospitalized numerous times with similar presentations. He complains of ongoing nightmares regarding fighting in Vietnam, with frequent flashbacks, intrusive thoughts, poor sleep, and increased startle. Other than coming in for his appointments, he has been unable to go out in public because he often feels that he is under attack, fearing that someone is going to jump out of the bushes and "ambush" him. He has been treated with the following medications, all with only moderate improvement in his symptoms: fluoxetine, sertraline, paroxetine, citalopram, mirtazapine, imipramine, and amitriptyline. He has been compliant with venlafaxine 375 mg daily. He has been sober from alcohol and heroin for 10 years. Which of the following medications would be the most beneficial for this patient?

(A) bupropion
(B) haloperidol
(C) lorazepam
(D) prazosin
(E) valproic acid

94. A 29-year-old married man presents to your outpatient psychiatric clinic complaining of anxiety and depression. His social history reveals that he is a junior faculty member of a local university, working about 60 hours per week. He enjoys his job but reports stress arising from his marital relationship because his wife accuses him of not spending "quality time" with her and his being "married to the job." According to Erik Erikson, in which stage of development does this patient currently have a conflict?

(A) autonomy versus shame and doubt
(B) identity versus role diffusion
(C) industry versus inferiority
(D) intimacy versus isolation
(E) trust versus mistrust

Questions 95 and 96

A 46-year-old man presents with episodes of "blacking out," where he will not remember periods lasting for several minutes. During those times, he is told by others that he has an "odd expression" on his face and doesn't respond to his name. In addition, he complains of difficulty in relationships due to decreased sex drive and irritability. He spends a great deal of time writing down his thoughts in his memoirs.

95. Which of the following additional symptoms would be most likely present in this patient?

(A) depression
(B) hyperreligiosity
(C) obsessive-compulsive behaviors
(D) sleep disorders
(E) urinary incontinence

96. A sleep-deprived electroencephalogram is performed on the patient as part of his complete workup. Which of the following lobes of the brain would most likely demonstrate abnormalities in this patient?

(A) frontal
(B) cerebellar
(C) occipital
(D) parietal
(E) temporal

97. After being called to the emergency department to evaluate a young woman who overdosed on barbiturates, you find her in bed with her eyes closed. She opens her eyes briefly in response to pain and demonstrates flexion from pain but makes no sounds. Which of the following best represents her Glasgow Coma Scale score?

(A) 7
(B) 6
(C) 5
(D) 4
(E) 3

Questions 98 and 99

You have been treating a 34-year-old man for major depression with a serotonin-specific reuptake inhibitor (SSRI) for the last 2 months. He was initially started on fluoxetine 20 mg/d for the first month, and then you raised the dose to 40 mg/d for the last month. While he has tolerated the medication without significant side effects, his depressive symptoms have remained refractory despite the increase in dosage. You have decided to switch his medication to phenelzine (Nardil), a monoamine oxidase inhibitor (MAOI), in hopes of eliciting a better antidepressant response.

98. Which of the following would be the best strategy in making the transition from the SSRI to the MAOI?

   (A) Begin tapering the dose of the SSRI while increasing the dose of the MAOI simultaneously.
   (B) Start the MAOI until therapeutic levels have been reached, then taper the SSRI.
   (C) Stop the SSRI abruptly and begin the MAOI at an equipotent dose the following day.
   (D) Stop the SSRI abruptly and immediately begin increasing the MAOI.
   (E) Taper the SSRI and 5 weeks after the last dose begin increasing the MAOI.

99. After he is switched to the phenelzine, which of the following foods/drink should the patient most avoid?

   (A) beets
   (B) lima beans
   (C) liver
   (D) peanuts
   (E) white wine

100. A 46-year-old man with a history of schizophrenia had been maintained on thioridazine (Mellaril) 700 mg qd since he was diagnosed at the age of 20. Over the last 8 months, he has been complaining of hearing derogatory voices, and his dose has been gradually increased to 1000 mg qd. He has no signs of tardive dyskinesia. Which of the following side effects would be the most concerning at this dose?

   (A) constipation
   (B) dry eyes
   (C) nephrogenic diabetes insipidus
   (D) pigmentary retinopathy
   (E) urinary retention

101. A 24-year-old man without prior psychiatric history is admitted to the psychiatric ward with disorganization, paranoia, agitation, and command suicidal auditory hallucinations. He is given two doses of haloperidol 5 mg orally. Approximately 8 hours later, he develops torticollis. Which of the following would be the most appropriate treatment?

   (A) acetaminophen
   (B) benztropine
   (C) cyclobenzaprine
   (D) ibuprofen
   (E) propranolol

102. A 28-year-old woman with a history of bipolar disorder is admitted to the medical service because of weakness, mental status changes, and a serum sodium of 154 mmol/L. According to her boyfriend, for the last 2 weeks she has been drinking "loads and loads of water" but complaining of being thirsty often, and also frequently urinating. Which of the following medications would be most likely responsible for this patient's presentation?

   (A) carbamazepine
   (B) haloperidol
   (C) lithium carbonate
   (D) quetiapine
   (E) valproic acid

Questions 103 and 104

A 58-year-old man with a long history of opiate addiction has been using intravenous heroin daily, approximately $50-60 per day. He has not been able to maintain any significant sobriety despite numerous inpatient and residential rehabilitation programs. He last used heroin 12 hours ago and has subsequently been admitted to the inpatient psychiatric ward for detoxification.

103. Which of the following medications would be the most appropriate to treat his withdrawal symptoms?

(A) amantadine (Symmetrel)
(B) clonidine
(C) haloperidol
(D) lorazepam
(E) naloxone

104. After the patient completes his detoxification on the unit, he continues to be motivated to abstain from heroin use. He is referred to an outpatient addictions program, but wishes to take a medication to decrease his heroin use after discharge. Which of the following medications would be the most appropriate to prescribe?

(A) dantrolene
(B) disulfiram
(C) flumazenil
(D) methadone
(E) sertraline

Questions 105 and 106

A 75-year-old man with Alzheimer dementia presents with his wife to your clinic for evaluation. She is concerned because he has been "down" recently, complaining of depression. His sleep has been worse, and his appetite and energy have been poor. The patient denies any suicidal ideation. His past medical history is significant for diabetes mellitus, two myocardial infarctions, atrial fibrillation, and a coronary artery bypass graft. The patient's wife wishes him to start a medication.

105. Which of the following antidepressants should be most avoided in this particular patient?

(A) bupropion
(B) imipramine
(C) mirtazapine
(D) sertraline
(E) venlafaxine

106. Which of the following antidepressants would most likely result in a cognitive decline in this patient?

(A) bupropion
(B) citalopram
(C) fluoxetine
(D) paroxetine
(E) venlafaxine

107. A 35-year-old woman with bipolar disorder and frequent hospitalizations presents to the emergency department after taking an overdose of lithium in a suicide attempt. Which of the following signs would be most likely to occur?

(A) abdominal pain
(B) acute dystonia
(C) leg pain
(D) paranoid delusions
(E) paresthesias

Questions 108 and 109

A 67-year-old woman presents to your office with a long history of major depression. She has tried a number of different antidepressant medications in the past but has not had a remission with any of them. Currently, she is on lithium, venlafaxine (Effexor), nortriptyline (Pamelor), lorazepam, risperidone, and benztropine. She is starting to believe that her next-door neighbors are out to harm her. You decide to begin a trial of electroconvulsive therapy (ECT).

108. Which of the following minimum times should the seizure last for optimal effectiveness in this patient?

(A) 10 seconds
(B) 25 seconds
(C) 60 seconds
(D) 120 seconds
(E) 180 seconds

109. Which of the following adverse effects would be the most likely during the course of ECT?

(A) brain damage
(B) catatonia
(C) fractures
(D) memory impairment
(E) vomiting

Questions 110 and 111

A 26-year-old man without prior psychiatric history presents to a psychiatric emergency department with paranoia, visual hallucinations, feelings of unreality, depersonalization, and extreme agitation. A urine toxicology screen is positive for phencyclidine (PCP).

110. Which of the following would be the best immediate treatment for the agitation in this patient?

   (A) chlorpromazine
   (B) fluoxetine
   (C) haloperidol
   (D) trazodone
   (E) trihexyphenidyl (Artane)

111. Which of the following treatments would be the most appropriate if this patient were not agitated?

   (A) cheese
   (B) haloperidol
   (C) supportive care
   (D) vitamin B_{12}
   (E) vitamin E

112. A 45-year-old woman with a prior history of depression is admitted to the psychiatric inpatient ward. She has been severely depressed, with poor sleep, decreased appetite, low energy, and suicidal ideation. She now believes that her neighbors are conspiring to murder her, and occasionally can hear a man's voice that tells her she should die. After speaking with the neighbors, you find out that they brought her to the hospital. They have been good friends for 20 years and have noticed the patient has not been leaving the house much, has taken to looking out of her windows with suspicious glances, and has not cleaned her house in the last 2 months. Which of the following medication combinations would be the most appropriate treatment for this patient?

   (A) fluoxetine and risperidone
   (B) lorazepam and clozapine
   (C) paroxetine and thyroid augmentation
   (D) sertraline and lithium
   (E) sertraline and lorazepam

Questions 113 through 116

Match the clinical vignette with the most likely substance-induced disorder. Each lettered option may be used once, multiple times, or not at all.

   (A) alcohol intoxication
   (B) alcohol withdrawal
   (C) cannabis intoxication
   (D) cocaine intoxication
   (E) cocaine withdrawal
   (F) heroin intoxication
   (G) heroin withdrawal
   (H) inhalant intoxication
   (I) methamphetamine intoxication
   (J) nicotine withdrawal
   (K) nitrous oxide intoxication
   (L) PCP intoxication
   (M) psilocybin withdrawal
   (N) 3,4-methylenedioxymethamphetamine (MDMA) (Ecstasy) intoxication

113. A 23-year-old man is brought to the emergency department by the police. He shows agitation, vertical nystagmus, and analgesia.

114. A 62-year-old homeless man admitted to a psychiatric unit begins having elevated vital signs, visual hallucinations, diaphoresis, tremor, and seizures.

115. A 43-year-old woman presents to the psychiatric emergency department complaining of depression and suicidality. She is observed to be fatigued, irritable, and with a dysphoric affect.

116. A 30-year-old musician presents in the outpatient clinic. He complains of fever and chills, runny nose, nausea, body aches, diarrhea, and abdominal cramps for the last 24 hours.

Questions 117 and 118

For the following scenarios, choose the medication most likely associated with the side effects. Each lettered option may be used once, multiple times, or not at all.

(A) benztropine

(B) clozapine

(C) desipramine (Norpramin)

(D) fluoxetine

(E) haloperidol

(F) lithium

(G) lorazepam

(H) nefazodone (Serzone)

(I) olanzapine

(J) phenelzine

(K) valproic acid

(L) venlafaxine

117. A 34-year-old man with schizophrenia presents with fever and chills. He is found to be bacteremic and has a WBC count of 900/µL.

118. A 41-year-old woman on medications for her bipolar disorder presents with fatigue, weight gain, cold intolerance, constipation, and decreased concentration.

Answers and Explanations

1. **(D)** Nefazodone is a serotonergic antidepressant, which has the advantage of not causing sexual dysfunction like most antidepressants. Unfortunately, it has a black-box warning for hepatitis and liver failure. Since this reaction is not dose-related or predictable, its use requires regular monitoring of liver function tests; therefore, nefazodone is rarely used.

2. **(G)** Venlafaxine is an antidepressant that inhibits the reuptake of both serotonin, and, in higher doses, norepinephrine. Because of this, it may cause increased blood pressure, particularly in doses above 300 mg daily.

3. **(E)** Although most antidepressants can cause a withdrawal syndrome (characterized as flu-like symptoms) if abruptly discontinued, those with shorter half-lives, especially paroxetine, are more likely to do so.

4. **(B)** Fluoxetine has a significantly longer half-life than the other listed antidepressants. This translates into fewer "withdrawal" symptoms if suddenly stopped and may also be an advantage in cases of occasional poor compliance.

5. **(E)** Most of the second-generation antipsychotics cause weight gain, including clozapine, olanzapine, quetiapine, and risperidone. However, both ziprasidone and aripiprazole are weight neutral.

6. **(B)** This patient is suffering from major depressive disorder, single episode, without psychotic features. While there are many efficacious antidepressants to choose from, serotonin-specific reuptake inhibitors (SSRIs) such as citalopram are considered first-line treatment. Aripiprazole is a second-generation (or atypical) antipsychotic. It would be appropriate if the patient had psychotic symptoms (such as hallucinations or delusions) or in the case of treatment refractory depression (which is not the case in this patient). Methylphenidate is a stimulant used for attention-deficit hyperactivity disorder, although it may be used as an adjunct in the treatment of severe depressions or in certain cases where a rapid onset is necessary (such as a dehydrated patient). Nortriptyline is a tricyclic antidepressant. While it is just as efficacious as an SSRI, it's side effects and lethality in overdose result in its not being used as a first-line medication for depression. Tranylcypromine is a monoamine oxidase inhibitor particularly useful in atypical depressive episodes (with increased appetite, weight gain, and mood reactivity), although the drug–drug interactions and dietary restrictions limit its use.

7. **(A)** This patient has described a panic attack. Panic attacks are characterized by a sudden onset of intense fear, dread, or anxiety, and accompanied by a variety of physical symptoms. Although virtually any organ system can seem to be the source of distress in panic disorder, common symptoms include diaphoresis, palpitations, shortness of breath, tremulousness, flushing, chest pain, and dizziness. Regardless of the clinical setting or psychiatric history, patients presenting with symptoms suggestive of panic disorder must be thoroughly worked up to rule-out physiologic pathology as the source of the symptoms. Reassurance may be premature until medical causes are ruled out. If the panic attacks continue, prescribing an SSRI and/or referring

her to a psychiatrist may be appropriate. Since antidepressants take several weeks to reach full benefit, benzodiazepines may be used in the interim. Untreated, panic disorder tends to run a chronic course and can cause severe disability.

8. **(D)** Neologistic speech, a positive symptom of schizophrenia, consists of words made up by the patient, having no established meaning. Clang associations are words or phrases strung together because of the sounds they make, not because of the meaning they convey. Echolalia is a symptom of catatonia, where the patient will repeat what is said by someone else, regardless of the context, and often in a repetitive manner. Flight of ideas is the rapid shifting of one idea to another and is characteristic of mania. Word salad is an illogical, incoherent collection of words or phrases.

9. **(E)** This woman suffers from dysthymic disorder, a low-grade, chronic depression. In adults, the symptoms must be present for at least 2 years. Like major depressive disorder (MDD), other than a subjective feeling of depressed mood, the key features of dysthymia are alterations in appetite and sleep, feelings of hopelessness, difficulty concentrating or making decisions, low self-esteem, and low energy or fatigue. While dysthymic disorder may not respond as robustly to medications as MDD, an adequate therapeutic trial (on a maximum dose) should last 8 weeks before deciding that it's a failure.

10. **(A)** The AIMS is a standard clinical examination and rating scale that should be administered to patients receiving neuroleptics such as haloperidol. It is useful for detecting the development of tardive dyskinesia as well as tracking changes over time. The BDI is a depression screening tool. The BPRS is a short scale developed to assess psychiatric symptomatology primarily in patients with psychosis or severe impairment. It is more often used in research settings. The PHQ is a self-administered screening tool focused on common mental problems that often present to the primary care physician (depression, panic, anxiety, alcohol abuse, binge eating, and somatoform disorders). The

PANSS is a standard test to assess treatment outcomes in studies of schizophrenia and other psychotic illnesses; it utilizes three subscales: positive symptoms, negative symptoms, and general psychopathology. Like the BPRS, it is mostly used for research rather than clinical practice.

11. **(B)** Patients with Capgras syndrome suffer from the delusion that someone familiar is an identical-appearing replacement. Cotard syndrome is a nihilistic delusion involving believing one is dead or that the body or organs are dying. Amok is a Malaysian term for a dissociative episode characterized by a period of brooding leading to a fit of violence followed by amnesia. Couvade syndrome occurs when the husband of a pregnant woman has similar symptoms of pregnancy and/or labor. Koro is a traumatic fear that the penis is shrinking into the body cavity, seen in some Asian cultures.

12. **(A)** Bereavement is the psychological reaction to a loss, often the death of a significant other. It is not considered an abnormal or pathological reaction. While symptoms may overlap with MDD (depression, appetite/sleep/energy changes), the intense symptoms of depression in bereavement do not usually last longer than 2 months, and there is little overall functional impairment. Occasional illusions or hallucinations of the deceased are not uncommon, but the individual retains insight regarding these. There is no evidence of prior or current manic episodes to justify the diagnosis of bipolar disorder. Dysthymic disorder is a chronic, low-level depression that lasts at least 2 years in adults. There is also no evidence of a primary psychotic illness consistent with schizoaffective disorder.

13. **(C)** Copropraxia is a complex motor tic occasionally seen in Tourette disorder, characterized by making obscene gestures. Bruxism is the grinding of the teeth. Blepharospasm is the spasm of the periorbital muscles causing sustained or exaggerated blinking. Echopraxia is also a complex motor tic where movements of another are repeated. It is a classic symptom of catatonia. Torticollis is a spasm of the neck

muscles such as the sternocleidomastoid on one or both sides, and can be a side effect of antipsychotic medications.

14. **(C)** Echolalia refers to repeating another's words or phrases. Coprolalia is sometimes seen in Tourette, where a patient will blurt out obscenities as part of a vocal tic. Dysarthria refers to a problem of word articulation, usually secondary to cerebellar or motor control abnormalities. Palilalia is also a repetition of words but is the repetition of one's own words as if the person "gets stuck" on the same word or phrase. Parapraxis is the term for a slip of the tongue.

15. **(C)** Kleptomania is an impulse control disorder where an individual steals objects not out of need or monetary value. Antisocial personality disorder is characterized by a lack of empathy and a chronic, maladaptive pattern of violating the rights of others; in this case, the patient is disturbed by the stealing and shows no other evidence of antisocial behavior. Intermittent explosive disorder is also an impulse control disorder where aggressive impulses result in assault or the destruction of property. Pyromania is an impulse control disorder of deliberate, recurrent fire setting that is deliberate. Trichotillomania is also an impulse control disorder where patients compulsively pull their hair resulting in appreciable hair loss.

16. **(B)** Ego-dystonic and ego-syntonic refer to whether thoughts or behaviors are distressing or not distressing to the patient, respectively. Delusions are fixed false beliefs that remain despite evidence to the contrary and are not culturally sanctioned. Mood congruent and mood incongruent refer to delusions or hallucinations in psychiatric disorders that are consistent with or not consistent with the primary mood disturbance, respectively.

17. **(C)** Ganser syndrome is considered to be a type of dissociative disorder described in prisoners. It is characterized by approximate answers and talking past the point and is associated with amnesia, disorientation, fugue, and conversion symptoms. Amok and piblokto are dissociative trance disorders that are described as disturbances in consciousness and are indigenous to particular cultures. A fugue state is where an individual takes on a new identity with amnesia for the old identity. Malingering is difficult to distinguish in these situations, but in this case a secondary gain is not identifiable.

18. **(A)** Countertransference refers to feelings the patient elicits in the therapist, versus transference, which refers to feelings the therapist elicits in the patient. Displacement is considered a neurotic defense mechanism where a feeling is directed toward another individual who is less threatening than the original object of that feeling. Projection is a primitive defense mechanism characterized by reacting to unacceptable feelings or impulses by placing them in another person. Reaction formation is another neurotic defense mechanism where an unacceptable impulse is transformed into its opposite.

19. **(C)** This patient likely has Wilson disease, an autosomal recessive error of copper metabolism. Wilson disease can present with multiple psychiatric and physical symptoms and signs. Kayser-Fleischer rings are one such sign: golden brown or gray-green rings of pigment at the corneal limbus. Arcus senilis is a light gray ring beginning superiorly and extending to the limbus. It can resemble a corneal arcus, which is associated with hypercholesterolemia, but in an elderly patient it is often a normal finding. Brushfield spots are lighter-colored areas in the outer third of the iris that can be associated with Down syndrome, but can also be a normal variant. Subconjunctival hemorrhage is the finding of blood in the areas of the eye surrounding the iris. Also associated with hypercholesterolemia is xanthelasma, raised yellow areas around the eyelids.

20. **(C)** Hemiballismus is an uncontrolled swinging of an extremity associated with Wilson disease. It is usually sudden, and once initiated it cannot be controlled. Athetoid movements, or athetosis, are slow, snake-like movements of the fingers and hands. Choreiform movements are also involuntary, irregular, and jerky but

lack the ballistic-like nature of hemiballismus. Myoclonus is a sudden muscle spasm, and myotonia is prolonged muscle contraction.

21. **(C)** Magical thinking and ideas of reference are two types of delusions that can be found in psychotic disorders, such as schizophrenia. Magical thinking is the belief that one's thoughts can control outside events. Ideas of reference are beliefs that other individuals (eg, government, entertainers, the media) are referring to or talking about the person experiencing the delusion. Displacement, projection, and reaction formation are all types of defense mechanisms. Displacement is the transferring of a feeling toward an object that is less threatening, such as the family pet or one's spouse or children. Projection is the false attribution of one's own unacceptable feelings to another. Reaction formation is the formation of thoughts that are opposite to anxiety-provoking feelings.

22. **(B)** Thought broadcasting is the delusion that one's thoughts can be heard by others. It is often seen in schizophrenia. Echolalia is the repetition of another's words or phrases, sometimes seen in catatonia. Thought control and thought insertion also can be seen in schizophrenia, and are delusions that others can control the patient's thoughts or behaviors or insert thoughts into a patient's mind, respectively. Transference, in strict terms, is the reexperiencing of past experiences with the therapist in the setting of psychotherapy. In general, this term has come to mean the transferring of emotions and feelings that one has from one's past to the physician or care provider.

23. **(A)** This patient is currently experiencing a manic episode. He had a prior major depressive episode (MDE), but regardless whether that were the case, with one manic episode he meets criteria for bipolar disorder I. Bipolar II disorder consists of a MDE and a hypomanic episode. Criteria for hypomania are the same as for mania, but the severity is less (ie, the patient is not psychotic, does not need hospitalization, or does not have significant social-occupational impairment). This patient has psychotic symptoms (grandiose delusions) and significant impairment (remodeling house, not going to work). Cyclothymic disorder consists of minor depressive episodes (ie, that do not meet criteria for MDE) alternating with hypomanic episodes. While this patient has a history of a MDE, he is currently suffering from a manic episode and not a depressive episode. While this patient is psychotic (delusional), his prior functioning and significant affective symptoms make a primary psychotic disorder such as schizophrenia unlikely.

24. **(E)** First-line pharmacotherapy for bipolar disorder, manic is either a mood stabilizer (such as valproic acid or lithium) or a second-generation ("atypical") antipsychotic (eg, risperidone, quetiapine, olanzapine). Antidepressants such as amitriptyline (a tricyclic) or fluoxetine (a serotonin-specific reuptake inhibitor) should be avoided, as they may worsen the manic episode. While clozapine is a second-generation antipsychotic, it is not a first-line medication given the risk of agranulocytosis and need for routine blood monitoring. Although first-generation ("typical") antipsychotics such as haloperidol can be used, they are not considered to be as efficacious in acute mania as mood stabilizers or the second-generation antipsychotics.

25. **(C)** Rebound is a return of symptoms that are brief and transient and is frequently associated with the abrupt discontinuation of benzodiazepines. Recurrence is the long-term return of the original symptoms. Withdrawal is characterized by a specific set of signs and symptoms specific to a particular substance. These are not necessarily similar to the original symptoms that were being treated by the medication. Akathisia is the subjective sensation of motor and mental restlessness. A dystonic reaction is an increase in muscle rigidity and spasticity that is usually associated with the use of neuroleptics.

26. **(A)** A conversion disorder is often a dramatic set of neurologic symptoms that result from unconscious conflicts. Factitious disorders involve the conscious fabrication of an illness in order to assume the sick role and be taken care of.

Hypochondriasis is the preoccupation with fears of having a serious disease based on misinterpretation of bodily sensations. Malingering is the conscious fabrication of an illness in order to obtain secondary gain (eg, avoiding military duty, work or jail, or obtaining disability). Somatization disorder is a pattern of multiple, recurring somatic complaints in different organ systems, beginning before age 30; it is seen mostly in women.

27. **(E)** La belle indifférence is the classic lack of concern shown toward a deficit or loss of function seen in a conversion disorder. Déjà entendu is the feeling that one is hearing what one has heard before. It is usually associated with anxiety states or fatigue. Déjà vu is a similar experience but refers to the sensation that something has been seen before. Jamais vu is the opposite of déjà vu in that it refers to something that should be familiar but seems quite unfamiliar. Folie à deux is a shared delusion aroused in one person by the influence of another.

28. **(C)** Testamentary capacity (the level of competence required to make a valid will) is based on the presence of all of the following: (1) an understanding of the nature of the will; (2) knowledge of one's assets; (3) knowledge of natural heirs; (4) absence of acute psychosis (ie, delusions), which might compromise rational decision making; and (5) freedom from undue influence or coercion. The validity of the will may be undermined by demonstrating that the individual failed to meet any of the above criteria. Actus reus refers to the voluntary act of committing a crime and is an element used in determining criminal responsibility. A history of mental illness is not sufficient to invalidate one's testamentary capacity. The presence of a conservator of person and history of mental illness are important only insofar as they bear upon any of the noted factors. The presence of a judge at the signing of a will is not required.

29. **(A)** Competency is a legal determination made by the court. Capacity, which is situation- and time-specific, can be made by caregivers, and is a frequent psychiatric consult question. Elements of capacity include the following abilities: to communicate one's wishes, to understand one's illness, to understand the risks and benefits of treatment and nontreatment, and to reason about one's options. The age of a patient has no bearing on the determination of capacity. Whether the patient agrees with the treatment team recommendations is not the issue; however, questions of capacity do not usually come up unless the patient disagrees with the treatment team. The presence of a psychotic illness does not, in and of itself, determine capacity. A patient being too disorganized to communicate adequately or having delusions involving the treatment proposed may indicate lack of capacity. A language barrier would not demonstrate lack of capacity, so long as the patient maintains the ability to communicate his or her preferences and reasons.

30. **(C)** Confidentiality is an integral part of the physician–patient relationship and is especially important in establishing the trust of a psychotherapeutic relationship. The physician-patient privilege should be breached only in specific instances, such as the patient's waiving of the privilege (eg, patient initiates litigation, consent to release information is obtained, there is a duty to protect, emergency situation, or in cases in which the court orders release). In this case, the information should not be released unless the patient has waived his physician–patient confidentiality privilege. Lying to or misleading the court is unethical and may subject one to prosecution. The remaining choices fail to maintain confidentiality.

31. **(D)** When a patient has stopped paying his or her bill, the physician should directly address the issue with the patient. Failure to pay one's bills may reflect underlying issues for which the patient has entered into psychotherapy or that are related to psychiatric symptoms. Contacting a collection agency before addressing the issue with the patient is inappropriate. If a patient continues to refuse payment after discussing the issue, the patient should be notified in writing of the outstanding balance and a referral to a collection agency might be made. To preserve

confidentiality, care should be taken to disclose the minimum information needed for collection (ie, date of service and charge) without referring to diagnosis or treatment rendered. Asking the insurance company to pay you after a check has been disbursed to the patient is futile because the insurance company's obligation toward the insured has been fulfilled. Disclosing the existence of a professional relationship with the patient to his family is a breach of confidentiality. Terminating the therapeutic relationship before exploring the dynamics behind the patient's payment delinquency might harm any future therapeutic alliance.

32. **(D)** Malingering is the intentional production of symptoms for secondary gain (eg, to avoid work, to evade criminal prosecution, or to gain financial rewards). A diagnosis of malingering should be suspected in medicolegal cases, in individuals with antisocial personality disorder, when symptoms are out of proportion to objective findings (as in this case), or when a patient in distress does not cooperate with evaluation/treatment. Conversion disorder describes the production of neurologic symptoms resulting from intrapsychic needs or conflicts. Dementia is unlikely in this case given the age and presenting complaints of the patient. Factitious disorder can be differentiated from malingering based on the absence of external incentives. In factitious disorder, symptoms are intentionally feigned to satisfy an intrapsychic incentive to assume the sick role. There is no evidence to suggest disorganization or psychotic symptoms consistent with schizophrenia.

33. **(B)** Individuals with malingering consciously feign symptoms for financial incentives or to avoid work/social obligations (secondary gain). The conscious production of symptoms to assume the sick role is seen in factitious disorder. Conversion disorder is the unconscious or involuntary production of symptoms resulting from intrapsychic, or unconscious, needs or conflicts. The unconscious production of symptoms to assume the sick role or to obtain secondary gain are not consistent with psychiatric illnesses.

34. **(B)** In this instance, the random letter test, which relies on concentration, cooperation, and the ability to hear, is the test of choice. It consists of telling a patient a letter and then in a monotone voice listing a random string of letters. The patient responds by raising a finger to indicate when he or she hears the key letter. The other tests rely not only on attention but also on calculation abilities, and therefore educational level.

35. **(E)** Sexual abuse is estimated to occur with an incidence of 0.25% of children per year. Known acquaintances (eg, fathers, stepfathers, and male relatives) are often the perpetrators. In this vignette, the patient likely has acquired *Neisseria gonorrhoeae* from a male perpetrator. Other physical findings may include injuries to the genitalia (ie, hymen, vagina) or the perineum. Psychiatric manifestations of sexual abuse may include anxiety, agitation, aggressive or impulsive behavior, and exhibitionism. When sexual abuse of a child is suspected, the first step is to ensure the safety of the child and immediately notify the state's Child Protective Services. Reporting is mandatory in cases of physical and sexual child abuse. The other choices fail to protect the child and do not satisfy state-mandated reporting statutes.

36. **(B)** This case represents Wernicke encephalopathy, a condition seen in chronic alcohol dependency. The etiology is acute thiamine deficiency and it presents with the classic triad of confusion, ataxia, and ophthalmoplegia. Although it is usually reversible with thiamine replacement, it is important to administer the thiamine parenterally, prior to giving fluids and glucose. Administration of glucose and fluids first may provoke a worsening of symptoms resulting in permanent damage. The administration of naloxone is used for opiate withdrawal.

37. **(B)** The patient is experiencing symptoms consistent with severe alcohol withdrawal, namely delirium tremens (DTs), characterized by delirium, confusion, combativeness, and elevated vitals signs. DTs carry a significant mortality if not treated. The treatment of choice is IM or IV benzodiazepines. Although barbiturates may

also treat withdrawal, they have a narrower therapeutic index, with a higher risk of sedation and respiratory depression. Neither thiamine nor an antipsychotic will treat the underlying alcohol withdrawal, and giving hydralazine may be dangerous as it may mask the symptoms of withdrawal.

38. **(D)** The patient is presenting with evidence of overdose with opiates, which is characterized by the triad of somnolence, respiratory depression, and pinpoint pupils. Opiate intoxication can be rapidly reversed with IV administration of an opiate antagonist, such as naloxone. Antabuse blocks acetaldehyde dehydrogenase and is given to alcoholics as an aversive stimulus to avoid alcohol consumption. Benzodiazepines would be used in cases of severe alcohol withdrawal, which would demonstrate elevated vital signs. Flumazenil is a benzodiazepine antagonist used in the emergency treatment of overdose with benzodiazepines, which does not cause pupillary constriction. Thiamine would be given in cases of Wernicke encephalopathy, caused most commonly by chronic, heavy alcohol consumption. It presents with a triad of confusion, ataxia, and ophthalmoplegia.

39. **(B)** This elderly woman is showing signs of dementia, likely Alzheimer disease, the most common cause of dementia. The primary treatment modality is to begin an anticholinesterase inhibitor, such as galantamine. Memantine, an *N*-methyl D-aspartate (NMDA) receptor antagonist, is a newer medication that may be added to the regimen additionally. Antidepressants (eg, citalopram) and antipsychotic medications (eg, ziprasidone) may be used for associated depression or agitation/psychosis, respectively, but they are not primary treatments. Ginkgo biloba has not been shown to be effective for the memory deficits in dementia.

40. **(D)** Risk factors for completed suicide include (1) age > 45, (2) male gender, (3) separated/divorced > married, (4) white race > black race, and (5) Jews/Protestants > Catholics. Women attempt suicide up to four times more frequently than men; however, men are three times more likely to complete suicide than are women.

41. **(A)** Physician-assisted suicide involves the doctor's facilitating a person's death by providing the information or equipment necessary to end his or her life. The AMA's Code of Medical Ethics strongly condemns such action as "fundamentally incompatible with the physician's role as healer." Rather, the ethical obligation of the physician is to adequately respond to a patient's end-of-life issues. Choices **(B)** and **(E)** would both be assisting the patient to commit suicide and are unethical. Informing the family would be a breach of confidentiality and not appropriate at this point, and placing the patient in restraints is not indicated.

42–49. **[42 (A), 43 (L), 44 (C), 45 (K), 46 (H), 47 (E), 48 (F), 49 (J)]** The Beck Depression Inventory **(A)** is a 21-item test with three responses per item that is an easily used screening tool to evaluate for depression. Because it would be unusual for an individual so young to have dementia and because many of the answers reflect a lack of interest, the Beck Depression Inventory, in conjunction with the Folstein MMSE, may help distinguish depression from dementia. The WCST **(L)** assesses executive functions of the brain such as organizational abilities, mental flexibility, and the ability to abstract and reason. These capacities are believed to be located in the frontal lobes. Damage to the frontal lobes can lead to abnormalities on this test. The Blessed Rating Scale **(C)** is a tool that asks friends or family of the patient to assess the ability of the patient to function in his or her usual environment. The WAIS-R **(K)** is an assessment of IQ used in ages 16 onward; it can be indicated to rule out mental retardation and help better understand the individual's intellectual level of functioning. IQ assessment will also aid the school in developing an individualized study program for students. The Rorschach Test **(H)** is a projective test that may be used to assess personality structure. The patient has characteristics of schizoid personality disorder, which may be better elucidated with a further skilled assessment in the context of his clinical history. The Folstein MMSE **(E)** is a quick, easily administered test that allows for immediate assessment of dementia. Scores of less than 24 are suggestive of a dementia. The MMPI-2 **(F)** is an objective test consisting of several hundred true/false questions used to assess an individual's personality. It is the most widely used and highly standardized test of personality. The Wada Test **(J)** is used to evaluate hemispheric language dominance prior to surgical amelioration of seizure focus. Whereas most right-handed individuals show left hemispheric dominance for language, left-handed individuals may be either right or left dominant. The test consists of injecting sodium amytal into the carotid artery and observing the transient effects on speech. Injection into the left carotid artery anesthetizes the left side of the brain, and those with left hemispheric language dominance show interrupted speech. The Bender Gestalt Test **(B)** involves copying figures, which helps to determine if organic brain disease is present. The Boston Diagnostic Aphasia Examination **(D)** is a series of tests given by an experienced clinician to evaluate and make treatment recommendations for individuals with aphasia. The Rey-Osterrieth figure **(G)** is sensitive to deficits in copying and lack of attention to detail in individuals with right-sided parietal lobe lesions. The Stroop Test **(I)** assesses executive function as the patient has to deal with distractions and has to suppress an incorrect reply before providing the correct one.

50. **(B)** Physician–patient confidentiality in the treatment of minors must be maintained unless otherwise mandated by law (eg, cases of abortion in some states) or when parental involvement is necessary in making complex and life-threatening medical decisions. In this case, the physician must respect the patient's confidentiality but should remain cognizant of the implications this will have on the family system. Therefore, it is most appropriate to encourage the minor to discuss the issue with her parents. At this point, there is no indication of child harm or neglect that would mandate reporting to Child Protective Services. Testimonial privilege refers to the privilege invoked to protect physician–patient confidentiality when medical information is subpoenaed without patient consent. The remaining two choices fail to maintain physician–patient confidentiality.

51. **(E)** This patient is experiencing major depressive disorder (MDD), single episode. Antidepressants are the treatment of choice. If the medication initially does not improve symptoms adequately, it should be increased as tolerated. An antidepressant trial should last at least 4 to 6 weeks before deciding that a medication is ineffective.

52. **(E)** MDD tends to be a chronic illness. Patients with one episode of depression have a 50% risk of having future episodes, although antidepressants help to minimize the risk.

53. **(C)** The patient is suffering from major depressive disorder (MDD). Because of their side effect profile, the treatment of choice in major depression is the serotonin-specific reuptake inhibitors (SSRIs), such as fluoxetine (Prozac). Amitriptyline and other tricyclic antidepressants include the risk of arrhythmias and can be lethal in overdose, unlike the SSRIs. While the patient reports periods during which she is "just fine," there is nothing to indicate a cycling pattern that would require a mood stabilizer such as divalproex sodium. Similarly, being convinced that her fiancé is about to leave her is not likely psychotic, but is instead a distortion that does not require an antipsychotic such as ziprasidone. Although MAOIs such as phenelzine are thought to be somewhat more effective in atypical depression—for example, eating more, rather than decreased appetite—they carry the risk of hypertensive crisis when combined with foods containing tryptophan.

54. **(D)** Fluoxetine is a class C drug, meaning that it is potentially harmful to the developing fetus, according to animal studies, although no definitive studies in humans are available. A discussion of the risks and benefits of treatment is therefore most appropriate. Fluoxetine does not have the withdrawal syndrome known to occur with paroxetine, but stopping it immediately should be avoided. Asking the patient how important pregnancy is to her would be inappropriate, since it is a personal choice, and, according to the information provided in the vignette, it is not something that puts her in danger of any kind. ECT may be an option, but not before a discussion of the risks and benefits

of her current treatment. Finally, there is no indication that she is at particular risk for post-partum depression and there is no evidence in the literature that adding a second antidepressant in pregnancy will prevent this disorder.

55. **(A)** This patient is exhibiting psychosis (cutting down a tree that his wife's ghost lives in) and depression. There are many possible etiologies, including major depressive disorder with psychotic features, bipolar disorder, and less likely, schizoaffective disorder and schizophrenia. Regardless of the eventual diagnosis, it is important to first rule out other causes of his behavior such as drug abuse. Therefore, it is premature at this point to prescribe any medications for him.

56. **(C)** Trazodone, which was developed as an antidepressant, has been shown to be an effective sleeping aid and would be useful in this patient. The benzodiazepines, such as alprazolam and diazepam, overlap with alcohol in binding to GABA receptors—hence their use in alcohol withdrawal—and should be avoided in patients with a history of alcoholism. Zaleplon is relatively contraindicated in those with severe liver dysfunction, which is a potential issue in a patient with a history of alcoholism. Zolpidem has also been shown to have similar abuse potential to the benzodiazepines.

57. **(D)** Trazodone carries a 1 in 1000 to 1 in 10,000 risk of priapism. The other sexual side effects among the choices are known to occur with the serotonin-specific reuptake inhibitors, but not particularly with trazodone. Incontinence is not a frequent side effect of any antidepressant.

58. **(E)** All of the SSRIs have been in the news because of controversy over data on increased suicidal gestures among children taking these medications. Paroxetine has been the focus of many of the reports. However, fluoxetine is the only medication indicated for treatment of childhood depression, which makes switching to paroxetine or amitriptyline inappropriate in this setting. Fluoxetine does not have the withdrawal syndrome known to occur with paroxetine, but stopping it immediately should still be avoided. Asking the child's mother what is

"really bothering her" is unlikely to be productive, as it is somewhat accusatory and not addressing her legitimate concerns.

59. **(C)** Although many individuals think of "natural remedies" such as St. John's wort as safe, these supplements can have significant side effects. In particular, St. John's wort may cause increased photosensitivity, stomach upset, rashes, fatigue, restlessness, headache, dry mouth, dizziness, and confusion. These side effects are more likely when St. John's wort is combined with SSRIs. St. John's wort has been shown to have some benefits in mild depressions and is thought to act like a monoamine oxidase inhibitor (MAOI). The precise pharmacokinetics of St. John's wort are unknown, but doses of SSRIs should be decreased while patients are taking the supplement because of possible potentiation of side effects. As with any antidepressant, it is not a good idea to stop it abruptly. There is no reason to think that child abuse is involved, as the child's mother is not putting her son in danger.

60. **(D)** This patient is presenting with bipolar disorder, most recent episode depressed. Despite the lack of data regarding bipolar depression, the impact of depressive episodes may be significantly worse than that of manic episodes. Lamotrigine, an antiepileptic medication, has demonstrated efficacy in (and has been approved for) the treatment of depressive episodes of bipolar disorder. Antidepressants such as bupropion and fluoxetine should be avoided (especially without an additional mood stabilizer) as they may precipitate a manic episode or lead to rapid cycling (>3 mood episodes per year). While second-generation antipsychotics (eg, quetiapine) are likely beneficial in the treatment of bipolar depression, first-generation neuroleptics, such as haloperidol, are not effective and may worsen depressive symptoms. Valproic acid is considered a first-line treatment of bipolar mania, but the data are far less convincing for depressed bipolar patients.

61. **(D)** Lamotrigine use has a 10% risk of a rash; unfortunately, Stevens-Johnson syndrome (a life-threatening rash) occurs in 0.1% of

patients, and because of this lamotrigine must be titrated slowly. Other significant but less concerning adverse events include ataxia, nausea, and sedation. Neutropenia is a potentially dangerous side effect of carbamazepine, not lamotrigine.

62. **(B)** Her lack of prior suicide attempts is her most significant protective factor; a lesser protective factor would be her social supports. The other factors do not play as much of a role.

63. **(D)** There are many potential medical causes of depression, including thyroid dysfunction, vitamin B_{12} deficiency, adrenal disease, and vascular disease. The other choices do not likely cause a depressive illness.

64. **(B)** This patient is most likely suffering from anorexia nervosa. Excessive dental decay is common in patients with anorexia or bulimia who purge by self-induced vomiting. Although the other choices may be present in severe starvation, excessive dental decay is the most common and appears the earliest.

65. **(C)** Anorexia nervosa has a varied course, although a poor prognosis overall. Ten-year outcome studies document that only about 25% of patients recover completely; another 50% have significantly improved symptoms and functioning. Unfortunately, the mortality rate of anorexia nervosa is approximately 7%.

66. **(E)** Rett disorder, a pervasive developmental disorder only seen in girls, presents with symptom onset between ages 5 months and 4 years with apparently normal prior development. Autistic disorder, although a pervasive developmental disorder, does not manifest with deceleration of head growth. In Asperger disorder, there is no delay in language. In childhood disintegrative disorder, as in Rett disorder, development is initially normal. However, in childhood disintegrative disorder, development is normal for at least the first 2 years after birth. Childhood schizophrenia cannot be diagnosed in children meeting criteria for a pervasive developmental disorder, and who do not have prominent delusions and hallucinations.

67. **(E)** Nigrostriatal D_2 receptors that are blocked by antipsychotic medications cause an imbalance between dopamine and acetylcholine, which accounts for the parkinsonian symptoms seen in this case. Blockade of acetylcholine receptors can help treat extrapyramidal symptoms (EPS). D_4 or 5-HT$_2$ receptor blockade does not cause EPS. Mesolimbic D_2 receptor blockade is believed to account for the antipsychotic effect of neuroleptics and does not cause extrapyramidal symptoms. Typical antipsychotics block both nigrostriatal and mesolimbic dopamine, whereas atypical antipsychotics preferentially block mesolimbic dopamine, accounting for the overall decreased extrapyramidal symptom liability.

68. **(D)** This patient is most likely suffering from Tourette syndrome. Atypical antipsychotic medications (such as risperidone) which block dopamine receptors are considered the most efficacious at decreasing vocal and motor tics. Clonidine is beneficial in treating Tourette, especially in mild cases, although it may cause excessive sedation and dizziness. Fluoxetine and topiramate may be effective for comorbid conditions found with Tourette disorder but have not been found to be specifically helpful for this primary condition. Although methylphenidate may help this patient's apparent attention-deficit hyperactivity disorder symptoms, it may also exacerbate his tic disorder.

69. **(A)** Fire setting in a repeated pattern in children often accompanies other behaviors that are defiant of rules and authority, as in conduct disorder. Although fire setting may occur in children diagnosed with mental retardation, pervasive developmental disorder, or tic disorder, it is much more unusual. Children with major depressive disorder do not engage in fire-setting as a common behavior.

70. **(A)** This child is suffering from secondary nocturnal enuresis. Utilizing a bell/buzzer and pad device (a form of behavioral therapy) is the most effective intervention, helpful in greater than 50% of children. Cognitive therapy, dialectical behavioral therapy (a form of cognitive-behavioral therapy designed for the treatment of borderline personality disorder),

and psychodynamic therapy have not been found to be effective in the treatment of enuresis. Punishment is not a type of behavioral conditioning used to treat psychiatric illnesses.

71. **(E)** More than 40 double-blind trials of imipramine have confirmed the drug's efficacy for enuresis. Carbamazepine is an anticonvulsant sometimes used as a mood stabilizer. Clonidine is an antihypertensive often used to treat opiate withdrawal. Diphenhydramine is an antihistamine with anticholinergic properties, often used for insomnia or to treat extrapyramidal symptoms. Haloperidol is a first-generation antipsychotic medication.

72. **(B)** This patient would be classified as having mild mental retardation, an IQ ranging from 50 or 55 to approximately 70. Borderline intellectual functioning refers to an IQ in the range of 71 to 84. In moderate mental retardation, the IQ is 35-40 to 50-55. In severe mental retardation, IQ ranges from 20 or 25 to 35 or 40. Profound mental retardation is diagnosed in those with IQ levels below 20 or 25.

73. **(D)** Microcephaly, short palpebral fissures, flat midface, and thin upper lip are all associated with fetal alcohol syndrome (FAS), which would be suspected in this patient with a maternal history of chronic, severe, alcohol use. Cleft palate is not specifically associated with FAS. Congenital blindness is not associated with FAS, although methyl alcohol consumption can cause blindness in adults. Hyperextensible joints and a prominent jaw are associated with fragile X syndrome.

74. **(E)** Children with reactive attachment disorder display markedly disturbed and inappropriate social relatedness associated with pathological care, such as seen in this case. Although ADHD and conduct disorder are often comorbid in those children who have histories of reactive attachment disorder, there is not enough evidence to diagnosis either at this time. Patients with childhood disintegrative disorder (a pervasive developmental disorder) show histories of decline in language and social communication that are more profound than in

reactive attachment disorder, and there is not necessarily a history of neglect or abuse. The criteria for mixed receptive-expressive language disorder do not include abnormalities in emotional communication (eg, displays of aggression toward other children) found in reactive attachment disorder.

75. **(A)** This patient would mostly likely be diagnosed with fetishism, a paraphilia characterized by the use of nonliving objects for sexual gratification. Frotteurism is also a paraphilia whereby the individual satisfies sexual urges by rubbing against nonconsenting individuals. Pedophilia involves sexual activity with a prepubescent child. The focus of transvestic fetishism involves cross-dressing, and is usually seen in heterosexual males. The paraphilia of observing unsuspecting people naked or involved in sexual activity is diagnosed as voyeurism.

76. **(B)** Despite his recent diagnosis of a major depressive disorder (MDD), this patient has symptoms consistent with a current manic episode (eg, euphoria, decreased need for sleep, impulsivity, pressured speech, impairment in functioning), and therefore would be diagnosed with bipolar disorder, most recent episode manic. Bipolar disorder, most recent episode depressed would be diagnosed in a patient with a history of mania but a current major depressive episode. Criteria for cyclothymic disorder are depressive episodes (which do not meet criterial for MDD) alternating with hypomanic episodes (symptoms of mania without impairment in functioning, psychotic symptoms, or the need for hospitalization). Dysthymic disorder is a chronic, low-level depressive illness, lasting for at least 2 years. Although the patient has manic symptoms and questionable psychosis (a grandiose delusion), there is no indication that he has had pervasive psychotic symptoms in the absence of his mood symptoms.

77. **(B)** As this patient has symptoms consistent with bipolar disorder, manic, he would most benefit from lithium or another mood stabilizer such as valproic acid. Antidepressants such as citalopram, fluoxetine, and imipramine

can exacerbate mania and should be avoided. Lorazepam, a benzodiazepine, may be used to treat psychomotor agitation and insomnia, but it does not treat the underlying disorder and has a risk of dependency if used in the long term.

78. **(D)** A major depressive episode with atypical features is characterized by mood reactivity, rejection hypersensitivity, hypersomnolence, increased appetite, and psychomotor retardation. Melancholic features include significant anhedonia, depression worse in the morning, terminal insomnia, marked psychomotor abnormalities, significant weight loss, and inappropriate guilt. To diagnose bipolar I disorder there must be at least one manic episode. Bipolar II is characterized by an episode of major depression and a hypomanic episode. Dysthymic disorder is a chronic, less-intense depression in adults, lasting 2 years and without meeting criteria for a major depressive episode.

79. **(C)** Although not commonly used because of the risk of side effects, MAOIs are considered to be the most effective class of drugs for treating atypical depression, especially compared to TCAs. SSRIs may also be effective for patients with atypical features. Some anticonvulsants and lithium are used for the treatment of bipolar disorder, but not typically for unipolar depression. First-generation antipsychotics are used to treat psychotic disorders such as schizophrenia and schizoaffective disorder.

80. **(D)** This case deliberately brings together many character traits drawn from "pure" diagnoses of personality (character) disorders, including borderline, narcissistic, dependent, obsessive-compulsive, and schizotypal personalities. In clinical practice, many patients diagnosable on Axis II do not have any specific personality disorder; such mixed cases are referred to as personality disorder not otherwise specified. Patients with pure borderline personality disorder are known for their intense personal relationships, self-destructive behaviors, anger management issues, and poor sense of self-image. Narcissistic personality disorder is marked by a grandiose sense

of self-worth, entitlement, lack of real empathy, and tendency to use others for one's own ends. Patients with obsessive-compulsive personality disorder are perfectionists, inflexible, and overly demanding of themselves and others. Schizotypal patients are known for their quirkiness and seemingly magical thinking styles.

81. **(D)** The essential features of schizoaffective disorder are prominent mood episodes (major depression, mania, or mixed episode) concurrent with symptoms consistent with schizophrenia. In addition, the diagnosis requires a period of 2 weeks of psychotic symptoms without affective symptoms which rules out bipolar disorder or major depressive disorder with psychotic features. While patients with schizophrenia may (and often do) become depressed, the mood symptoms are not present for a substantial portion of the illness. Psychotic disorder not otherwise specified is usually reserved for situations in which the clinician does not have enough historical data to know whether the patient has schizophrenia, a mood disorder with psychotic features, or a medically-caused or substance-induced psychosis.

82. **(D)** This woman is suffering from delirium, likely caused by diphenhydramine. The elderly are particularly vulnerable to medications known to have psychoactive properties or side effects. This is in part due to the decreased ability of geriatric patients to metabolize medications and the tendency of the drugs to build up to higher levels. Additionally, elderly persons are generally more vulnerable to the effects of medications that act on the central nervous system (CNS). The patient in this case is on a number of medications that may have CNS side effects at high doses. However, the significant anticholinergic properties of diphenhydramine put this patient at particular risk of memory impairment and confusion. Cimetidine and furosemide are also potential contributors to delirium, but are much less likely than diphenhydramine. Beta-blockers like atenolol have been associated with depression presumably associated with blockade of central adrenergic receptors. Additionally, in some vulnerable patients, they may reduce cardiac output enough to cause

a functional hypoperfusion of the brain causing confusion and dizziness. Digoxin may actually decrease sodium ion conduction enough in CNS neurons to produce delirium in some patients.

83. **(A)** Delirium related to blockade of cholinergic receptors is the most common cause of medication-induced delirium in the elderly. Acetylcholine is uniquely involved with memory processes in the brain, and its involvement in the pathophysiology of Alzheimer disease has been heavily researched. Drugs that alter dopamine neurotransmission are most associated with movement disorders and psychosis-related side effects. Medications affecting GABA receptors (such as benzodiazepines and barbiturates) may cause sedation and ataxia as well as memory disturbances. Drugs acting on the serotonergic system may alter sleep, appetite, and mood, although few nonpsychiatric drugs work on this system. Medications affecting central norepinephrine transmission (eg, antihypertensives) may rarely be associated with depression.

84–89. **[84 (K), 85 (M), 86 (D), 87 (B), 88 (E), 89 (F)]** Patients with mental illnesses may be noncompliant for various reasons. Long-acting antipsychotics such as risperidone Consta **(K)** are good choices in psychotic patients who benefit from and tolerate antipsychotics, but who are noncompliant due to lack of insight, confusion, or forgetfulness (not due to side effects). While lithium **(G)** is a first-line treatment for bipolar disorder, those individuals with greater than three manic or depressive episodes per year (rapid cycling) respond better to anticonvulsants such as valproic acid **(M)** or carbamazepine. Clozapine **(D)** was the first "atypical" antipsychotic developed; it is approved for treatment of patients with refractory schizophrenia and has also demonstrated efficacy in reducing suicidality in schizophrenia or schizoaffective disorder. Bupropion **(B)** is an antidepressant that is believed to block reuptake of dopamine in the brain. Although all antidepressant medications have similar efficacy, including nortriptyline **(H)** (tricyclic antidepressant), paroxetine **(I)**, and sertraline **(L)** (serotonin-specific reuptake inhibitors), and venlafaxine **(N)** (combined serotonin-norepinephrine reuptake inhibitor), only bupropion has a reduced risk of sexual

dysfunction, and in fact may be used to treat antidepressant-induced sexual dysfunction. While no psychotropic medications are proven safe in pregnancy, anti-manic agents such as carbamazepine, lithium, and valproic acid are associated with significant fetal abnormalities and should be avoided. Haloperidol **(E)** has been used safely in pregnant patients with bipolar disorder. Lamotrigine **(F)** is an antiepileptic medication indicated for the maintenance treatment of bipolar disorder (to delay the time to occurrence of mood episodes) and for the acute treatment of bipolar depression. Aripiprazole **(A)** and risperidone **(J)** are second-generation antipsychotic medications used for schizophrenia, schizoaffective disorder, and bipolar disorder. Chlorpromazine **(C)** is a typical antipsychotic with significant anticholinergic, antiadrenergic, and antidopaminergic properties.

90. **(E)** Studies that find no statistical difference between groups when there actually is a difference result in a type II error. In this case, the positive findings at the other universities make the finding at university A less likely to be correct. University A may have needed a larger number of subjects in the study to find the treatment effect. Type I errors occur more often than type II errors and cause the researcher to conclude that there is a difference between groups when in fact there is none. The variance is the sum of the differences of each data point from the mean. Positive predictive value is the proportion of abnormal test results that are true positive, while negative predictive value is the proportion of normal test results that are true negative. Standard error is the degree to which the means of several different samples would vary if they were taken repeatedly from the same population.

91. **(E)** This patient has signs most consistent with tardive dyskinesia, an extrapyramidal syndrome that usually affects perioral or limb musculature and causes choreiform movements. Its onset is usually several years after being on the medication and it is more likely to affect older patients. Akathisia is described as psychomotor restlessness that may have an onset of hours to days after beginning the neuroleptic. Dystonia is an acute reaction to

neuroleptics in which particular muscle groups (neck or ocular muscles commonly) contract involuntarily. It can be painful and should be treated immediately with anticholinergic medications. NMS is a potentially lethal but rare medical emergency in which patients may have global rigidity, mental status changes, fever, cardiovascular instability, elevated creatine phosphokinases, and risk of rhabdomyolysis. Parkinsonism may look identical to Parkinson disease (tremor, bradykinesia, masked faces) and usually has an onset within weeks to months after beginning the medication.

92. **(A)** The basal ganglia, responsible for the transmission of thought to action and for controlling the initiation and quality of motor action, is central to the pathophysiology of extrapyramidal syndromes, including dystonia, parkinsonism, akathisia, and tardive dyskinesia. The cerebellum is important in controlling the coordination of motor movements and posture. The frontal cortex is generally considered to be important for decision making, impulse control, and affect regulation. The midbrain contains nuclei that help to ensure central nervous system homeostasis by regulating neurovegetative, autonomic, and arousal functions. The motor cortex serves as the last stage of cerebral processing of motor information before it descends into the spinal cord. An intact motor cortex is required for initiation of movement.

93. **(D)** This patient is suffering from chronic post-traumatic stress disorder (PTSD) symptoms, only partially treated despite compliance with mediations and abstinence. Serotonin-specific reuptake inhibitors (SSRIs) are considered first-line treatment because of their efficacy and tolerability. Prazosin, an alpha-1 adrenergic receptor blocker has demonstrated significant efficacy in treating all three clusters of PTSD symptoms (ie, reexperiencing, hyperarousal, avoidance). Bupropion is an antidepressant used to treat major depressive disorder, but its activating properties make it not as useful for the treatment of PTSD. Antipsychotics like haloperidol should only be used in severe cases of PTSD with prominent psychotic symptoms or agitation/aggression. Lorazepam and other benzodiazepines should be avoided in patients with PTSD due to their lack of efficacy and potential for abuse and dependence. Mood stabilizers such as valproic acid may be beneficial for some patients with PTSD, but likely not as much as SSRIs or alpha-blockers like prazosin.

94. **(D)** Erik Erikson was a psychoanalyst best known for his description of eight stages of human psychological experience spanning the entire life span. He believed that successful completion of all earlier stages was necessary for successful completion of future stages. The patient in this example is able to productively work but has difficulty with intimacy in his relationship, hence the conflict between intimacy and isolation. All of Erikson's eight stages center on stage-appropriate developmental conflicts: basic trust versus mistrust (birth to 1 year); autonomy versus shame and doubt (1-3 years); initiative versus guilt (3-5 years); industry versus inferiority (6-11 years); identity versus role diffusion (11 years to end of adolescence); intimacy versus isolation (21-40 years); generativity versus stagnation (40-65 years); and integrity versus despair (65 and older).

95. **(B)** Hyperreligious thinking or preoccupation with moral behavior, altered sexual behaviors, hypergraphia or over elaborative communication styles (also referred to as viscosity), and heightened experience of emotions form a classic constellation of personality traits associated with complex partial epilepsy (or temporal lobe seizures). Depression, obsessive-compulsive symptoms, and sleep disorders may be associated with structural brain injury in frontal and subcortical areas, but they have not been described as being related specifically to complex partial epilepsy. Urinary incontinence is more often associated with normal pressure hydrocephalus or severe dementia.

96. **(E)** This patient most likely would demonstrate seizure activity in his temporal lobes, consistent with temporal lobe seizures.

97. **(B)** The Glasgow Coma Scale measures level of arousal and ranges from a scale of 3 (deep coma) to 14 (fully alert). The categories assessed are eye opening, best motor response, and best verbal response. Eye opening ranges from a

score of 4 (opening spontaneously) to 1 (not opening at all). In this case, the eyes open to pain, so a score of 2 is given. Best motor response is as follows: obeys commands, 5; localizes pain, 4; flexion, 3; extension, 2; and no response, 1. In this case, a score of 3 is given for the response. Best verbal response is also based on a scale ranging from 5 to 1. An oriented patient receives a score of 5 and no response receives a score of 1, as in this case. The scores are then added, and in this case are 2 + 3 + 1 = 6.

98. **(E)** When changing from an SSRI to an MAOI, one must allow a washout period of about five half-lives for the SSRI to be more than 90% eliminated; in the case of fluoxetine, this is approximately 5 weeks. This precaution avoids the serotonin syndrome, which may occur when significant blood levels of both drugs are present. Serotonin syndrome, which can be fatal, is marked by symptoms of tremor, diaphoresis, rigidity, myoclonus, autonomic dysregulation, hyperthermia, rhabdomyolysis, renal failure, and coma. The other choices would pose a significant risk of developing serotonin syndrome.

99. **(C)** MAOIs prevent the peripheral breakdown of tyramine, which may be ingested with certain foods such as liver, beer, red wine, aged cheeses, smoked fish, dry sausage, and fava beans. If too much tyramine builds up in the blood, it may saturate peripheral sympathetic nerve receptors and cause hypertensive crisis, a potentially fatal condition. The other choices do not contribute to hypertensive crisis.

100. **(D)** At doses of 1000 mg/d or higher, thioridazine has been associated with pigmentary retinopathy, also known as retinitis pigmentosa. Therefore, doses should not exceed 800 mg/d. Pigmentary retinopathy can cause loss of retinal response to contraction of the visual field. An early sign may be nocturnal confusion. Constipation, dry eyes, and urinary retention are all side effects from the anticholinergic properties of thioridazine, but typically are not so severe as to compromise health permanently. Nephrogenic diabetes insipidus is not associated with thioridazine.

101. **(B)** This patient is experiencing an acute dystonic reaction from the haloperidol, a high-potency first-generation (typical) antipsychotic, typically seen hours to days after initiating or increasing the antipsychotic. Acute dystonic reactions may present as muscle spasms, torticollis, oculogyric crisis, and laryngeal spasm. Benztropine 1 to 2 mg IM is useful in the treatment of acute dystonic reactions. Alternatively, diphenhydramine 50 mg IM can also be used. If the symptoms do not resolve within 20 minutes, larger doses can be given. Benzodiazepines can also be used but are not first-line treatment. For acute laryngeal dystonia, 4 mg of benztropine should be given within 10 minutes, then 2 mg of lorazepam IV if needed. None of the other choices are indicated for the treatment of acute dystonia. While analgesics such as acetaminophen and ibuprofen may help with pain, they won't resolve the underlying etiology. Cyclobenzaprine is a muscle relaxer which will not adequately treat the dystonia. Propranolol is a B-blocker, used for hypertension, but it can also be used to treat akathisia, another side effect of antipsychotics, characterized by an inner feeling of restlessness and need to move.

102. **(C)** The disorder described is nephrogenic diabetes insipidus, most likely caused by lithium. Lithium inhibits the effect of antidiuretic hormone on the kidney, causing polyuria, thirst, polydipsia, and potential hypernatremia and delirium. Although carbamazepine and valproic acid (other mood stabilizers), haloperidol (a first-generation antipsychotic), and quetiapine (a second-generation antipsychotic) are all used to treat bipolar disorder, none are associated with diabetes insipidus.

103. **(B)** Clonidine, a central alpha-2-autoreceptor agonist, has been proven useful in the treatment of the autonomic hyperactivity associated with opioid withdrawal. Amantadine is used to treat Parkinson disease and also as an anti-influenza agent. Haloperidol, an antipsychotic, and lorazepam, a benzodiazepine, may help with significant agitation occasionally seen in withdrawal, but they will not treat the underlying symptoms. Naloxone, an opiate antagonist, is used in opiate overdose and will

significantly worsen opiate withdrawal symptoms in this patient.

104. **(D)** Methadone has been proven to significantly reduce the use of heroin when used as a maintenance medication. Patients maintained on doses lower than 40 mg/d of methadone are far more likely to relapse than those on higher doses. Dantrolene is a muscle-relaxant used in the management of neuroleptic malignant syndrome, a rare side effect of antipsychotic treatment. Disulfiram is a medication used to prevent alcohol consumption by causing an aversive reaction if taken in conjunction with alcohol. Flumazenil is indicated for benzodiazepine overdose. Sertraline is a serotonin-specific reuptake inhibitor, used in the treatment of depressive and anxiety disorders, among other psychiatric illnesses. While it may be helpful for comorbid depression or anxiety, it has not been shown to decrease opiate use in dependent individuals.

105. **(B)** Imipramine is a tricyclic antidepressant (TCA). TCAs are considered class 1A antiarrhythmics because they possess quinidine-like effects that decrease conduction time through the bundle of His. They have been shown to increase mortality in cardiac patients. TCAs can also increase the heart rate anywhere from 3 to 15 beats/min, and a patient with compromised cardiac function may suffer from increased oxygen demand. Finally, TCAs are also associated with significant orthostatic hypotension, which may be further exacerbated in patients with cardiac disease. Wellbutrin, serotonin-norepinephrine reuptake inhibitors (such as mirtazapine and venlafaxine), and serotonin-specific reuptake inhibitors (SSRIs) like sertraline may all be safely used in patients with cardiac disease; however, attention should be paid to potential hypertension caused or worsened by venlafaxine and any cardiac medicines metabolized through the P-450 cytochrome system as some SSRIs (eg, fluoxetine) may alter the medication levels.

106. **(D)** Acetylcholine is the neurotransmitter most implicated in cognitive functioning. Anticholinergic effects of medications are frequently implicated in cognitive decline and drug-induced delirium. Of the medications listed, paroxetine has the most anticholinergic effect, and therefore should be avoided in this patient with dementia.

107. **(A)** Lithium toxicity is characterized early on by dysarthria, ataxia, coarse tremor, and abdominal pain. Later manifestations include seizures, neuromuscular irritability, and impaired consciousness (delirium to coma). Acute dystonias are associated with the use of typical antipsychotics. Leg pain and paresthesias are not associated with lithium. Paranoid delusions are part of the symptom profile of schizophrenia and sometimes of bipolar disorder.

108. **(B)** For ECT to be effective, the seizure should last at least 25 seconds. Prolonged seizures greater than 180 seconds should be terminated with barbiturates or intravenous diazepam.

109. **(D)** Memory impairment (mostly during the treatment) is quite common, although most patients return to their baseline by 6 months. There is no indication that ECT causes brain damage. ECT may actually be used to treat patients with catatonia. Fractures and vomiting are uncommonly seen in ECT since the use of muscle relaxants and antiemetics.

110. **(C)** For extreme agitation, the butyrophenone antipsychotic haloperidol is often useful. Benzodiazepines may also be used for this symptom. Phenothiazine antipsychotics such as chlorpromazine can cause autonomic instability when given to a patient with PCP intoxication. Trazodone, used commonly for insomnia, and fluoxetine, an SSRI, are antidepressants, and will not help with agitation. Trihexyphenidyl is used to combat extrapyramidal symptoms associated with antipsychotic use and not for agitated states.

111. **(C)** Supportive care is the best treatment for PCP intoxication that is not complicated by extreme agitation or violence. Haloperidol, a typical antipsychotic, is useful for extreme agitation. Despite urban myths, neither cheese nor vitamins have particular therapeutic benefits for PCP intoxication.

112. (A) This patient is most likely suffering from major depression with psychotic features. Neither antidepressants nor antipsychotics alone will adequately treat major depression with psychotic features; both must be initiated. The combination of lorazepam and clozapine (an atypical antipsychotic) will not treat the depression. Similarly, the combination of sertraline and lorazepam will not adequately treat the psychotic symptoms. Lithium and synthroid can both effectively augment antidepressants such as paroxetine and sertraline. Lorazepam, a benzodiazepine, may help with anxiety, but will not be effective against psychosis or depression.

113. (L) PCP (aka "angel dust") intoxication produces agitation, vertical nystagmus, and analgesia as well as hyperthermia, depersonalization, and hallucinations in auditory, tactile, and visual modalities.

114. (B) Alcohol withdrawal may begin within 24 hours after the last drink, and can progress to seizures by 24 to 48 hours and delirium tremens (DTs) after approximately 72 hours. DTs are associated with a significant risk of mortality.

115. (E) Symptoms associated with cocaine withdrawal tend to be mild and last 1 to 2 days after the last use. Occasionally, however, the depression can be severe enough to raise the risk of self-injurious behavior or suicide attempts.

116. (G) Heroin withdrawal peaks at about 72 hours after the last use in dependent users. It is experienced as many flu-like symptoms and gastrointestinal complaints, such as fever and chills, runny nose, nausea, body aches, diarrhea, and abdominal cramps. The appearance of piloerection in the syndrome gave rise to the slang term "cold turkey" to describe the action of total cessation of use of the drug. Alcohol intoxication **(A)** involves characteristic behavioral changes, as well as slurred speech, ataxia, and other neurologic findings. It can progress to coma if severe. Cannabis intoxication **(C)** heightens sensitivity to external stimuli and impairs motor skills, along with conjunctival injection and increased appetite ("the munchies"). Cocaine intoxication **(D)** is marked by elated mood, decreased sleep, hallucinations, and agitation. Heroin intoxication **(F)** is marked by an altered mood, psychomotor retardation, and drowsiness, along with pinpoint pupils and constipation. Intoxication by inhalants **(H)** (volatile substances such as gasoline fumes) is marked by euphoria, disorientation, fear, and facial rash, although the symptoms are short-lived. The syndromes of methamphetamine **(I)** and MDMA **(N)** intoxication are similar to those of cocaine intoxication. MDMA users typically report an increased "sense of closeness" with other people. Nicotine withdrawal **(J)** is characterized by depressed mood, insomnia, irritability, difficulty concentrating, decreased heart rate, and increased appetite. Nitrous oxide intoxication **(K)** produces euphoria and light-headedness and usually subsides within hours without treatment. Withdrawal from psilocybin **(M)**, a hallucinogen derived from mushrooms, is not well described.

117. (B) Clozapine (an atypical antipsychotic) causes agranulocytosis in about 1% of patients. For this reason, weekly blood counts are measured for the first 6 months of treatment, every 2 weeks for the next 6 months, then every 4 weeks thereafter (unless there is a significant drop in white blood cell counts).

118. (F) Lithium is associated with clinical hypothyroidism in about 5% of patients, most commonly women. Thyroid supplementation may be added to counter this side effect. Up to 30% of patients may show elevated thyroid-stimulating hormone levels.

Bibliography

American Medical Association. AMA's Code of Medical Ethics, Principles, Opinions and Reports. Available at: http://www. ama-assn.org/ama/pub/physician-resources/medical- ethics/code-medical-ethics.shtml. Accessed July 1,2010.

American Psychiatric Association. "The Opinions of the Ethics Committee on the Principles of Medical Ethics". 2009 Edition. 1-95. Available at: http://psych.org/ MainMenu/PsychiatricPractice/Ethics/ ResourcesStandards/ OpinionsofPrinciples.aspx. Accessed July 1,2010.

American Psychiatric Association. *The Principles of Medical Ethics with Annotations Especially Applicable to Psychiatry*; 2009, Revised. Web. 1-39. Available at: http://psych.org/MainMenu/PsychiatricPractice/ Ethics/ResourcesStandards/ PrinciplesofMedicalEthics.aspx. Accessed July 1,2010.

American Psychiatric Association. Task Force on DSM-IV. *DSM IV-TR*. Washington, DC: American Psychiatric Association; 2000. ISBN 0890420254.

Boyer EW, Shannon M. Serotonin syndrome. *N Engl J Med.* 2005;352:1112-1120.

Chambers CD, Hernandez-Diaz S, Van Marter LJ, et al. Selective serotonin-reuptake inhibitors and risk of persistent pulmonary hypertension of the newborn. *N Engl J Med.* 2006;354:579-587.

Cohen LS, Altshuler LL, Harlow BL, et al. Relapse of major depression during pregnancy in women who maintain or discontinue antidepressant treatment. *JAMA.* 2006;295:499-507.

Ghaemi SN. *Mood Disorders: A Practical Guide.* Philadelphia, PA: Lippincott Williams & Wilkins; 2003.

Janicak PG, Davis JM, Preskorn SH, Ayd FJ, Pavulur MN. *Principles and Practice of Psychopharmacotherapy.* 4th ed. Philadelphia, PA: Lippincott Williams & Wilkins; 2006.

Kaplan and Sadock's Comprehensive Textbook of Psychiatry. 9th ed. Philadelphia, PA: Lippincott Williams & Wilkins; June 8, 2009.

Kane JM, Fleischhacker WW, Hansen L, et al. Akathisia: An updated review focusing on second-generation antipsychotics. *J Clin Psychiatry.* 2009;70(5):627-643.

Lieberman JA, Stroup TS, McEvoy JP, et al. Effectiveness of antipsychotic drugs in patients with chronic schizophrenia. *N Engl J Med.* 2005; 53:1209-1223.

Miller L. Postpartum depression. *JAMA.* 2002;287:762-765.

Rosenbaum JF et al. Handbook of Psychiatric Drug Therapy, 5th Ed. Philadelphia, PA: Lippincott Williams & Wilkins, 2005.

Sadock B, Sadock V. Forensic psychiatry. *Synopsis of Psychiatry.* 9th ed. Philadelphia, PA:Lippincott Williams and Wilkins; 2003:1351-1364.

Sadock B, Sadock V. Ethics in psychiatry. *Synopsis of Psychiatry.* 9th ed. Philadelphia, PA: Lippincott Williams and Wilkins; 2003:1365-1373.

Sadock BJ, Sadock VA. *Kaplan and Sadock's Comprehensive Textbook of Psychiatry.* 7th ed. Philadelphia, PA: Lippincott Williams & Wilkins; 2000. ISBN 0781723884.

Stoffers J, Völlm BA, Rücker G, et al. Pharmacological interventions for borderline personality disorder. *Cochrane Database Syst Rev.* 2010; 6:CD005653.

Sadock BJ, Sadock VA. Kaplan & Sadock's Synopsis of Psychiatry, 10th ed. Philadelphia, PA: Lippincott Williams & Wilkins, 2007.

Strawn JR, Keck PE Jr, Caroff SN. Neuroleptic malignant syndrome. *Am J Psychiatry.* 2007;164(6):870-876.

Schiffer RB, Rao SM, Fogel BS. *Neuropsychiatry.* 2nd ed. Philadelphia, PA: Lippincott Williams & Wilkins; 2003.

Trivedi MH, Rush AJ, Wisniewski SR, et al. Evaluation of outcomes with Citalopram for depression using measurement-based care in STAR*D: Implications for clinical practice. *Am J Psychiatry.* 2006; 163:28-40.

Wijkstra J, Lijmer J, Balk F, Geddes J, Nolen WA. Pharmacological treatment for psychotic depression. *Cochrane Database Syst Rev.* 2005 Oct 19;(4):CD004044.

Yonkers KA, Wisner KL, Stowe Z, et al. Management of bipolar disorder during pregnancy and the postpartum period. *Am J Psychiatry.* 2004;161:608-620.

Wiener D. *Textbook of Child and Adolescent Psychiatry.* 3rd ed. Arlington, VA: American Psychiatric Publishing; 2004.

Index